T0202171

The Cancer Problem

The Cancer Problem offers the first medical, cultural, and social history of cancer in nineteenth-century Britain. It begins by looking at a community of doctors and patients who lived and worked in the streets surrounding the Middlesex Hospital in London. It follows in their footsteps as they walked the labyrinthine lanes and passages that branched off Tottenham Court Road; then, through seven chapters, its focus expands to successively include the rivers, lakes, and forests of England, the mountains, poverty, and hunger of the four nations of the British Isles, the reluctant and resistant inhabitants of the British Empire, and the networks of scientists and doctors spread across Europe and North America.

The Cancer Problem: Malignancy in Nineteenth-Century Britain argues that it was in the nineteenth century that cancer acquired the unique emotional, symbolic, and politicized status it maintains today. Through an interrogation of the construction, deployment, and emotional consequences of the disease's incurability, this book reframes our conceptualization of the relationship between medicine and modern life and reshapes our understanding of chronic and incurable maladies, both past and present.

The Cancer Problem

Malignancy in Nineteenth-Century Britain

AGNES ARNOLD-FORSTER

Chancellor's Fellow,
University of Edinburgh

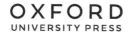

OXFORD
UNIVERSITY PRESS

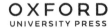

OXFORD
UNIVERSITY PRESS

Great Clarendon Street, Oxford, OX2 6DP,
United Kingdom

Oxford University Press is a department of the University of Oxford.
It furthers the University's objective of excellence in research, scholarship,
and education by publishing worldwide. Oxford is a registered trade mark of
Oxford University Press in the UK and in certain other countries

First published 2021
First published in paperback 2023

Published in the United States of America by Oxford University Press
198 Madison Avenue, New York, NY 10016, United States of America

British Library Cataloguing in Publication Data
Data available

Library of Congress Cataloging in Publication Data
Data available

ISBN 978–0–19–886614–5 (Hbk.)
ISBN 978–0–19–888509–2 (Pbk.)

DOI: 10.1093/oso/9780198866145.001.0001

Acknowledgements

Despite the many hours I have spent alone researching in archives and writing in libraries, this book—as is true for all historical scholarship—has been a collaborative endeavour. There are, therefore, many people I would like to thank. Without them, the commencement and completion of this book, and the PhD thesis before it, would have been impossible. I would not have been able to start my postgraduate studies without funding and I am indebted to the Arts and Humanities Research Council for funding both my MSc and PhD. I would also like to thank the Society for the Social History of Medicine, the American Association for the History of Medicine, the British Society for the History of Science, and King's College London for providing financial support for research trips and conference attendance.

I have been extraordinarily lucky and have managed to acquire a highly supportive network of scholars—both junior and senior—who have read too many of my words and listened to me talk for far too long. My PhD supervisors were consistently supportive, diligent, and critical. With her endless patience and attention to detail, Professor Abigail Woods transformed my intellectual approach and writing style. She provided consistent, incisive commentary. Dr Caitjan Gainty was, and continues to be, a source of advice, enthusiasm, and creative insight. Her analytical eye pushed my work in new directions and I thank her for her unwavering kindness. I am also very grateful to my two examiners, Professor Keir Waddington and Dr Carsten Timmerman, and to the anonymous readers of this manuscript. Together, they made the book immeasurably better and any errors or omissions that remain are, of course, very much my own.

The community of fellow PhD students at King's was a major source of support and scholarly insight. I am particularly grateful to Professor Paul Readman for convening the Modern British History Reading Group. Its members read and reflected on my work more times than I can count and continue to provide crucial intellectual and emotional support in these uneasy early career times. I would also like to thank Dr Will Tullett for patiently reading chapters and lending a sympathetic ear.

Since completing my PhD, I have expanded the community of scholars in which I work and with whom I collaborate. Without them, I could not have navigated the transition from thesis to book. I am particularly grateful to Dr Michael Brown and Professor Thomas Dixon who are responsible not only for my gainful employment post-PhD—an essential condition for writing a book it turns out—but for my intellectual development. Without Dr Alison Moulds, moving from fixed-term contract to fixed-term contract could have been a lonely and isolating experience.

This book could not have been written without my friends and family. My friends, Isabel Asquith, Phoebe Arnold, Isabelle Fraser, and Bronya Arciszewska have listened to me talk about cancer with almost unwavering stoicism and for that I am truly grateful. My parents and siblings, Jake Arnold-Forster, Dr Rebecca Jewell, Theo Arnold-Forster, and Dora Arnold-Forster, have also suffered the brunt of my myopia, and only responded by taking me on holiday, cooking me delicious meals, and providing endless emotional support. Most importantly, for his pragmatism and love, I would like to thank my partner Ben. Finally, this book is dedicated to my grandmother, Dr Juliet Clutton-Brock, an academic who died from cancer while I was writing my thesis. Her advice and gentle criticism would have been so welcome.

Contents

List of Figures

Introduction

Malignancy in Nineteenth-Century Britain

In 1899, the English doctor and writer Woods Hutchinson turned his pen to the 'Cancer Problem' and, in a metaphorically rich essay articulated a series of anxieties about medical failure, professional identity, and biological fragility. Hutchinson was born in Yorkshire in 1862. As a child, he moved with his parents to the American Midwest and received his medical degree from the University of Michigan in 1884. Not unusually for the era, he pursued a transatlantic literary and academic career, lecturing at both the University of Buffalo and in London. A vivid writer, he had a taste for the fashionable and melodramatic. His theatrical titles included *The Gospel According to Darwin* (1898), *Conquest of Consumption* (1910), and *The Doctor in War* (1918). He died in 1930, his life a brief footnote in the history of turn-of-the-century medicine, yet his experiences were representative of contemporaneous medical life, and he had an uncanny ability to capture the anxieties peculiar to his age.

In 'The Cancer Problem', Hutchinson argued that while nineteenth-century state, society, and science had reined-in the powers of epidemic disease, cancer remained 'a riddle of the sphinx'.[1] Despite multiple medical successes—anaesthesia, asepsis, sewage systems, and bacteriology—nineteenth-century doctors and scientists had failed in one of their key aims: to understand and effectively treat malignancy. In 1899, cancer remained the 'dread disease' and the 'emperor of all maladies'—equal parts incurable and unknown. Its deadly and mysterious status increasingly set it apart from other diseases that medicine now thought it understood, and, in some cases, could manage. Cancer was, therefore, particularly troubling for a profession newly fashioning itself as socially useful and scientifically competent. Hutchinson's essay was replete with frantic commentary on modern medicine's inability to even *comprehend* cancer, let alone treat it; he even made the troubling suggestion that this mysterious disease seemed to be taking advantage of medical practitioners' ignorance, increasing in incidence and capacity to kill. Cancer, therefore, undermined the increasingly prevalent belief in the teleology of medical progress and the cumulative nature of scientific knowledge. In 1884, the *Pall Mall Gazette* reported, 'Cancer . . . stands almost alone as a

---

[1] Woods Hutchinson, 'The Cancer Problem: Or, Treason in the Republic of the Body', *The Contemporary Review* (July 1899), 105–17, at 105.

The Cancer Problem: Malignancy in Nineteenth-Century Britain. Agnes Arnold-Forster, Oxford University Press (2021).
© Agnes Arnold-Forster. DOI: 10.1093/oso/9780198866145.003.0001

disease which increases with our prosperity, and while our health laws are raising the standard of public health, the mortality from cancer stands forth as a blot upon the results, detracting in part at least from the measure of the success which has thus far been obtained.'[2]

Some nineteenth-century medical men argued, therefore, that cancer—despite all the rationalization by modern and innovative technologies—was resistant to improvement. The Sisyphean nature of their efforts rendered practitioners and social commentators miserable—fatalistic about what this failure said about the nature of body and society and their parallel tendencies towards decline, and pessimistic about the ineptitude of medical science. The intensity of these abstract emotions was matched or superseded by those felt by the men and women who, across the nineteenth century, inhabited and encountered cancerous bodies. Disgust, abjection, sorrow, pity, fear, dread, pain, frustration, hope, love, and sympathy all marked the 'cancer experience' and structured both doctor and patient decision-making.

This is the first book about the history of cancer in nineteenth-century Britain. It narrates the disease's pre-twentieth-century story and, in doing so, demonstrates that it was then that cancer acquired the unique symbolic, emotional, and politicized status it maintains today. As I will show, there was no 'conspiracy of silence' surrounding cancer in the nineteenth century.[3] Not only did it maintain a not-insignificant incidence, cancer also played a symbolically laden role in nineteenth-century life. British vital statistics from the 1850s identify cancer as the cause of death for about 2 per cent of the population—a figure which increased as the century progressed and likely under-represented the actual burden of the disease.[4] Then as now, observers tied cancer to environment, diet, and morality; and malignancy was a prominent feature of the social, political, and cultural landscape. Cancer appeared in hospital casebooks, the diaries and letters of the elite, medical textbooks, the pages of periodicals, on the maps, charts, and urban plans of the British Isles, and in parliamentary debates. Using this array of source material, this book focuses on two interrelated concerns: one, the lasting formation of cancer's identity as an uncommonly incurable—and therefore uncommonly dreadful—disease; and two, how cancer was made into a malady of modern life, a pathology of progress, and a product of civilization.

After c.1792 cancer was defined as not just incurable, but as unusually so. However, the story I am telling here is not just a tale of death, despondency, and

---

[2] Hugh P. Dunn, 'The Increase of Cancer', *Pall Mall Gazette*, 12 May 1884.

[3] Susan Sontag argues that, 'conventions of treating cancer as no mere disease but a demonic enemy make [it] not just a lethal disease but a shameful one'. Susan Sontag, *Illness as Metaphor and AIDs and its Metaphors* (London, 2013), 6.

[4] George Graham, 'Causes of Death in England, and in Each Division and County in 1851', in George Graham, *Fourteenth Annual Report of the Registrar-General* (London, 1855), 126. This figure corresponds approximately with the incidence of scarlatina, whooping cough, and dysentery.

disease—it is one of creativity, pragmatism, and productivity. I will show how cancer can make us think critically about what nineteenth-century practitioners and patients understood by the very notion of incurability. What, if any, was their distinction between incurable people and incurable diseases? Did they differentiate between those maladies that were resolved by 'nature' and those cured by 'art' (or, in other words, medical intervention)? Could you have a temporary or periodic cure? Was a cure an action or an outcome? Did 'to cure' mean to eradicate the disease from the body or simply to apply a treatment or palliate suffering? In this book, I take a more expansive understanding of incurability to allow us to see the concept, perhaps paradoxically, as productive. Cancer's incurability was not just an obstacle to overthrow, but a galvanizing and intellectually provocative idea that shifted the concepts and practices of medicine, health care, and professional identity in profound and lasting ways. Indeed, this book shows how cancer's incurability enabled the construction of professional credentials and community values; made hospitals into places for treating 'terminal' illness; made possible the invention of palliative surgery as a means of relieving suffering without performing a 'complete' cure; and brought into being certain modes of investigating cancer, such as mapping, the microscope, and discourses of progress and decline.

This book also argues that this incurability was implicated in cancer's complex relationship with 'modern medicine'. 'Modern medicine' was a phrase frequently used in the nineteenth century and its prevalence then reveals the past preoccupation with the connections among health, progress, and modern life. 'Modern medicine' was something that doctors and allied practitioners were seeking to achieve—a set of ideologies, practices, and participants that were optimistic, preoccupied with progress, institutionalized, and professionalized. It was self-conscious and self-aggrandizing—seeking to elevate the social and intellectual status of medicine, surgery, and the life sciences. These processes of self-definition, professionalization, and institutionalization have been well studied. Here, I argue that nineteenth-century versions of 'modern medicine' were inextricably linked to cancer and its unusual characteristics, that cancer was perceived as a product and pathology of progress, and that the disease was made emblematic of medicine and its many and various promises for the future. This book seeks, therefore, to explain what was understood as 'modern' about cancer then, and elucidate the connections between the disease and the era's new institutions.

It also explores what elements of nineteenth-century medicine and society were made 'modern' *by* cancer. How did Britain and its people adapt to the disease and the unique, or at least unusual, pressures it applied to communities, health-care institutions, and the healing professions? In following these two lines of enquiry, this book not only offers an innovative history of cancer, but a new and synthetic account of the social, emotional, and medical world of nineteenth-century Britain. It enables us to think differently about the purposes of medicine and health care;

prompts us to reconsider the identities and attitudes of practitioners (heterodox and orthodox alike); and pushes us to interrogate the creative and productive potential of death and disease.

Cancer's relationship to modernity has often been asserted, yet only rarely scrutinized. We tend to locate the emergence of cancer as the 'dread disease' in the middle of the twentieth century, when cancer charities portrayed the malady as 'an insidious, dreadful, relentless invader' and presidents of the United States of America waged war on malignancy.[5] Indeed, it is a well-known and often rehashed trope that cancer today constitutes an unintended consequence of progress. Or, as Charles E. Rosenberg puts it, 'the notion that the incidence of much late-twentieth-century chronic disease reflects a poor fit between modern styles of life and humankind's genetic heritage'.[6] Roy Porter called cancer 'the modern disease *par excellence*' and Siddhartha Mukherjee described it as 'the quintessential product of modernity'; however, both locate that 'modernity' in the decades after the Second World War.[7] As Joanna Bourke observes, in 1957 the physician and cancer educationalist George W. Crile blamed those cancer charities for having 'fashioned a devil out of cancer'. Crile lamented, 'They have created a new disease, cancerphobia, a contagious disease that spread from mouth to ear.'[8] Key to this 'cancerphobia', Crile argued, was the belief that the disease was incurable. Crile was making an astute observation about the fear that surrounded malignancy in the 1950s, but he misidentified the origin and chronology of that fear. 'Cancerphobia' existed in nineteenth-, not just twentieth-century, Britain.

Indeed, this observation has been made by several scholars of medieval and early modern medicine. Historians such as Alanna Skuse, Luke Demaitre, Marjo Kaartinen, and Michael Stolberg have all examined cancer before the twentieth century and all dealt with a disease that had much in common with the malady we encounter today.[9] However, while these few scholars have made inroads into medieval and early modern Britain, far more have traversed the disease's twentieth-century terrain.[10] This asymmetry can be partly explained by the ways

---

[5] Quoted in Joanna Bourke, *Fear: A Cultural History* (London, 2015), 234.

[6] Charles E. Rosenberg, 'Pathologies of Progress: The Idea of Civilization as Risk', *Bulletin of the History of Medicine*, 72 (1998), 714–30, at 714.

[7] Roy Porter, *The Greatest Benefi1t to Mankind: A Medical History of Humanity from Antiquity to the Present* (London, 1999), 574; Siddhartha Mukherjee, *The Emperor of All Maladies: A Biography of Cancer* (New York, 2011), 241.

[8] Quoted in Bourke, *Fear*, 234.

[9] For medieval and early modern accounts of cancer see Luke Demaitre, 'Medieval Notions of Cancer: Malignancy and Metaphor', *Bulletin of the History of Medicine*, 72 (1994), 609–37; Marjo Kaartinen, *Breast Cancer in the Eighteenth Century* (London, 2013); Alanna Skuse, 'Wombs, Worms and Wolves: Constructing Cancer in Early Modern England', *Social History of Medicine*, 27 (2014), 632–48; Alanna Skuse, *Constructions of Cancer in Early Modern England: Ravenous Natures* (Basingstoke, 2015); and Michael Stolberg, 'Metaphors and Images of Cancer in Early Modern Europe', *Bulletin of the History of Medicine*, 88 (2014), 48–74.

[10] Unlike for the nineteenth century, cancer in the twentieth century is a well-studied field. See, for example, Emm Barnes Johnstone and Joanna Baines, *The Changing Faces of Childhood Cancer: Clinical*

in which cancer and chronic disease have been constrained by a version of periodization that serves to tie certain maladies—or malady types—to specific epochs. Medical historians, epidemiologists, and demographers have conceptualized the nineteenth century as the 'epidemic century', with infectious diseases and their control occupying the forefront of historical investigation. This periodization is most clearly articulated by Abdel Omran's 'citation classic', published in 1971, on the theory of epidemiological transition.[11] He posited three phases: 'the age of pestilence and famine'—roughly corresponding to medieval and early modern Europe; 'the age of receding pandemics'—the long nineteenth century; and 'the age of degenerative and man-made diseases'—intimately associated with 'civilisation' and the development of 'modern' health care and medicine.[12] Omran's model has been nuanced, expanded, and countered by public and global health professionals who have critiqued its determinism, international homogeneity, and its limited explanatory power with respect to the quintessential late modern pandemic: AIDS.[13]

However, this periodization persists and it is unhelpful for the medical historian, not least because it has obscured cancer from our vision of the nineteenth century. Instead, scholars of nineteenth-century medicine have tended to focus on epidemic diseases—cholera, relapsing fever, tuberculosis—whereas those of the twentieth turn instead towards chronic maladies like cancer, framing them as problems of modern life.[14] Medical historians frequently betray a subtle, even

---

and Cultural Visions since 1940 (Basingstoke, 2015); David Cantor, *Cancer in the Twentieth Century* (Baltimore, MD, 2008); K. E. Gardner, *Early Detection: Women, Cancer, and Awareness Campaigns in the Twentieth-Century United States* (Chapel Hill, NC, 2006); Ilana Löwy, *Preventive Strike: Women, Precancer, and Prophylactic Surgery* (Baltimore, MD, 2010); Barron H. Lerner, *The Breast Cancer Wars: Hope, Fear, and the Pursuit of a Cure in Twentieth-Century America* (Oxford, 2001); John V. Pickstone, 'Contested Cumulations: Configurations of Cancer Treatments through the Twentieth Century', *Bulletin of the History of Medicine*, 81 (2007), 164–96; Carsten Timmermann and Elizabeth Toon (eds.), *Cancer Patients, Cancer Pathways: Historical and Sociological Perspectives* (Basingstoke, 2012).

[11] George Weisz and Jesse Olszynko-Gryn, 'The Theory of Epidemiologic Transition: The Origins of a Citation Classic', *Journal of the History of Medicine and Allied Sciences*, 65 (2010), 287–326.

[12] A. Omran, 'The Epidemiological Transition: A Theory of the Epidemiology of Population Change', *Milbank Quarterly*, 83 (1971), 731–57.

[13] Aliana Santosa, Stig Wall, Edward Fottrell, Ulf Högberg, and Peter Byass, 'The Development and Experience of Epidemiological Transition Theory over Four Decades: A Systematic Review', *Global Health Action*, 23567 (2014). For a reassessment of Omran's model of the medical past by historians see Flurin Condrau and Michael Worboys, 'Second Opinions: Epidemics and Infections in Nineteenth-Century Britain', *Social History of Medicine*, 20 (2007), 147–58; and Graham Mooney, 'Response: Infectious Disease and Epidemiological Transition in Victorian Britain? Definitely', *Social History of Medicine*, 20 (2007), 595–606.

[14] The classic nineteenth-century text on the troubled relationship between civilization and social and individual pathology is Benjamin Ward Richardson's *Diseases of Modern Life* (London, 1876). Historical analysis of this phenomenon can be found in Daniel Pick, *Faces of Degeneration: A European Disorder, c.1848–1918* (Cambridge, UK, 1989); F. Edwards Chamberlin and Sander L. Gilman (eds.), *Degeneration: The Dark Side of Progress* (New York, 1985); and the European Research Council-funded project 'Disease of Modern Life: Nineteenth-Century Perspectives' at the University of Oxford, https://diseasesofmodernlife.org/, accessed 16 April 2020. For a late twentieth-century perspective on so-called 'pathologies of progress' see S. Boyd Eaton, Melvin Konner, and Marjorie Shostak, 'Stone Agers in the

unconscious, commitment to the epidemiological transition model and its underpinning intellectual assumptions. In 1962, Rosenberg wrote, 'Cholera was the classic epidemic disease of the nineteenth century, as plague had been of the fourteenth.'[15] Similarly, in his 2009 book, *Cholera: The Biography*, Christopher Hamlin writes, 'It is in the magnitude of the *reaction* to it that cholera stands out as the signal disease of the nineteenth century. It was (apparently) new as an epidemic entity and grew up in conjunction with Enlightenment liberalism, nationalism, imperialism, and the rise of global biomedical science.'[16] This book shows that cancer, like cholera, developed in line with 'nationalism, imperialism, and the rise of global biomedical science'. Crucially, however, I will not excavate the epidemiological burden of cancer in the nineteenth century or contribute to a debate over quantitative shifts in causes of death. I will, instead, historicize and problematize the notion that certain diseases 'belong' to, or are representative of, certain time periods and demonstrate that simplistic models of epidemiological transitions cannot be sustained.

Incurability

While cancer existed in the eighteenth century and before, from *c.*1792 onwards, and within the context of a newly established hospital setting, cancer was constructed, configured, and conceptualized differently to how it had been so before and increasingly in line with how we see it today. Moreover, key to this new or altered definition was its identity as an unusually incurable malady. Over the ensuing century, this identity was subject to constant renegotiation by doctor, patient, and the public. However, throughout this period, elite, 'regular', or 'learned' surgeons and physicians were ambivalent about the efficacy of *any* form of medical or surgical intervention in cases of cancer, and the only semblance of a consensus was over the *inability* of both art and nature to 'remove and banish' the disease from the body.

This history of cancer shows that there were many different, coexisting versions of 'incurability' and 'cured' in the nineteenth century. Historians such as Roy Porter and Pat Jalland have pointed out that 'Therapeutic medicine had very limited power to cure disease before the advent of sulphonamide drugs in the 1930s.'[17] However, while many diseases were people's last, I argue that nineteenth-century practitioners set cancer apart. Then, many maladies killed and

Fast Lane: Chronic Degenerative Diseases in Evolutionary Perspective', *American Journal of Medicine*, 84 (1988), 739–49.
[15] Charles E. Rosenberg, *The Cholera Years: The United States in 1832, 1849, and 1866* (Chicago, 1962), 1.
[16] Christopher Hamlin, *Cholera: The Biography* (Oxford, 2009), 4.
[17] Pat Jalland, *Death in the Victorian Family* (Oxford, 1996), 77.

yet cancer was still conceptualized as unusual, even unique. Fevers might prove deadly, but they might also resolve themselves. Even consumption had its own patterns of relapse and remission that could be invoked by both doctor and patient as evidence for the curative powers of various treatments. In contrast, cancer set its sufferers on an irreversible and inevitable period of decline. Diagnosis became prognosis and from the moment of identification, their fate was decided. In 1816, surgeon and man-midwife Thomas Denman, insisted, 'Of all diseases deemed incurable, that which is denominated Cancer has been most generally allowed to be so.'[18]

There have been many histories of disease and death. Hannah Newton argues that historians have a 'general penchant for sad topics' and suggests that the field of the history of emotions is preoccupied with the tragic, the fearful, and the despondent.[19] Historians of science, technology, and medicine tend instead to focus on innovation and success—albeit contingent, caveated, and contextualized.[20] Carsten Timmermann posits that progressive accounts provide scholars with a practicable narrative framework, suggesting that stories of incurability are more difficult to write. Cancer in particular has an uneasy relationship with the key 'moments' of medical history—the 'bacteriological revolution', the professionalization of health care, and the development of modern biomedicine. The disease frustrates any easy narrative of Victorian social, political, and medical progress. Cancer offers us, therefore, an unusual opportunity to write a history of what Timmermann calls therapeutic and theoretical 'failure and disappointment'.[21] Failure and disappointment did not, however, cause cancer investigation and management to stagnate. Instead, the early nineteenth-century codification of cancer as an incurable disease was the origin of a period of intense creativity, intellectual debate, and therapeutic innovation. Cancer offered a challenge to the medical and scientific community—a challenge that prompted a range of productive, pragmatic, and potential solutions to the 'cancer problem'.

Some of what I say about cancer also applies to all chronic and incurable diseases in the nineteenth century. These maladies were symbolically laden and approaches to death, dying, and cancer altered across the period. Moreover, and following the work of historian Jason Szabo on nineteenth-century France, I suggest that the experience of having an incurable disease is best understood 'as the product of an intricate series of negotiations and interactions among various social actors—patients, families, physicians, alternative healers, religious and political authorities—each with his or her own agenda and challenges'.[22]

[18] Thomas Denman, *Observations on the Cure of Cancer, with Some Remarks upon Mr Young's Treatment of that Disease* (London, 1816), 3.

[19] Hannah Newton, *Misery to Mirth: Recovery from Illness in Early Modern England* (Oxford, 2018), 1.

[20] Carsten Timmermann, *A History of Lung Cancer* (Basingstoke, 2013), 8.   [21] Ibid.

[22] Jason Szabo, *Incurable and Intolerable: Chronic Disease and Slow Death in Nineteenth-Century France* (New Brunswick, NJ, 2009), 6.

Cancer acquired and developed a social role and function that was both unique and telling about the nature and purpose of illness and medical intervention alike. Having, treating, and investigating an incurable disease all had their own complex matrices of motivations and experiences, and understanding this complexity allows us to move beyond the predictable if conflicting narratives of suffering, despondency, and disappointment on the one hand, and heroism and success on the other.

Modern Medicine

In the nineteenth century, cancer was subject to an anxious and active public commentary in newspapers, periodicals, and political debate. It was treated in dedicated hospitals and wards with innovative, adversarial treatments and patients were cared for by practitioners who wielded palliative tools. A variety of different practitioners and professionals believed that diet, housing, environment, age, habits, gender, accidents, and behaviour were causes of cancer. It was studied in specialized clinics and investigated by scientists working in a network of laboratories that spread across the globe. Philanthropic individuals, charitable organizations, and governments invested money and time into countering the 'cancer problem'. And desperate dying people sought untested remedies and found solace in alternative medical means. These various features of cancer were formed by nineteenth-century ideas and institutions, and cancer exerted its own influence on a range of organizations and projects, from hospitals, to the General Register Office, laboratories, governments, and public health practices. These various structures and systems were also a key component of an industrializing, civilizing, nation state. Crucially, too, cancer's influence on these organizations and projects was made possible by the disease's incurability. The construction of cancer as an intractable malady was key to the processes by which it was made 'modern'.

Disease—and particularly cancer—was increasingly a marker of industrial and technological modernity, an unintended consequence of progress, and a potent if paradoxical component of national identity. As I have suggested, cancer is widely perceived today as a product of progress in the late twentieth century, and this book shows that similar patterns of thought were present in nineteenth-century meditations on malignancy. Indeed, our recent anxieties about cancer's relationship to our current lifestyles can be backdated to the 1800s and were formed in response to specific nineteenth-century concerns. Cancer was, therefore, deployed to rationalize national and racial hierarchies in the context of modernity and modernization, and its perceived prevalence used to affirm the superior status of British social, economic, and medical institutions.

Incurability had, therefore, an intriguing relationship with notions of nineteenth-century progress and 'modern medicine'. There is a paradox in the fact that our twenty-first-century version of modern medicine is so marked by a malady that we neither fully understand nor can effectively treat. Indeed, nineteenth-century medical men were engaged in a project of professionalization and 'self-improvement' that increasingly attempted to make medicine out as progressive, socially useful, and, in their own terms, 'modern'. At the same time, the same medical men were repeatedly re-inscribing cancer's incurability and insisting on their identification of its intractability as a marker of their professional skill and insight. That tension—that modern medical professionals must identify their own limitations—continues today and makes cancer peculiarly problematic and particularly productive.

This book is, after all, not just a medical history, but a social and cultural account of cancer, the institutions it inhabited, and the bodies it infiltrated. To that end, it explores what elements of nineteenth-century Britain were made 'modern' *by* cancer. Other scholars have demonstrated that medicine and ideas about health were key to the development and definition of modernity in the nineteenth century. Roger Cooter identified neurasthenia alongside degeneration in his study of 'medicine and modernity' as one of those 'new-fangled theories' that 'were themselves signs of modernity in medicine', as they 'cut new social paths in medical thinking at the same time as they established new medicalised ways of thinking about society and identity'.[23] In redirecting attention towards chronic and incurable disease; towards accommodation rather than cure; and towards aging and the elderly; cancer restructured medicine, society, and politics along the lines of nineteenth-century notions of 'modern life'. Thus, medical theories and treatments of the so-called 'modern maladies' were not only deeply embedded in social and cultural operations, but modernity itself was actively constructed and deployed from within nineteenth-century cancer discourses.

Definitions and Parameters

But what was cancer in nineteenth-century Britain? Throughout the period covered in this book, c.1792 to 1914, cancer was a capacious disease category and there was plenty of room for variation and disagreement. However, almost all diseases designated cancer shared a selection of essential characteristics which were determined by the clinical environment of the hospital and its capacity to provide practitioners with extended observation of a large number of patients. Cancer was a chronic disease with a long duration; it had an irreversible capacity

---

[23] Roger Cooter, 'Medicine and Modernity', in Mark Jackson (ed.), *The Oxford Handbook of the History of Medicine* (Oxford, 2015), 103.

for growth and spread; it manifested as a physical lesion or tumour; and it was incurable. While all of these aspects had existed in the eighteenth century and before as incidental observations, with the hospitalization of cancer they were converted into defining and identifying features. Chapter 1, 'From Home to Hospital', devotes space to a further anatomization of the disease and a more comprehensive account of its perceived causes and characteristics. However, it is worth setting out here what cancer was not—or rather, how I have chosen to approach cancer in two ways that differ from those of other historians of the disease. First, I do not conceptualize cancer as a peculiarly female disease; and, second, I approach cancer as an integrated disease category.

The prominence of breast cancer in contemporary culture and society has made the disease a fertile ground for historians of medicine. Frances Burney's account of her 1811 mastectomy has proven particularly alluring for feminist critiques of the male and medical gaze, and investigations into her words and experience form a substantial part of our knowledge and understanding of nineteenth-century cancer. Burney was an English gentlewoman who lived in France at the turn of the eighteenth century. She recorded a vivid account of her own pre-anaesthesia mastectomy. S. Mediratta and J. E. Epstein have both looked at Burney's narrative, exploring issues of gender and maternity. As Mediratta observes, Burney's account reveals her breasts' essential association with motherhood and suggests that the mastectomy cut to the very heart of her 'feminine identity as defined by late eighteenth and early nineteenth-century culture'.[24] Gender historians have also argued that cancer, irrespective of site, was constructed as a peculiarly 'female' disease with supposedly 'female' characteristics. For example, its capacity for growth and extension was conceptualized as reproductive and generative.[25] While I do not deny the role of gender in the comprehension and experience of cancer—and this book acknowledges the prevailing historical idea that the nineteenth century was a time of particular change with respect to women and their bodies—it is not the only way to think through the disease in this period.[26] Not only are there other useful categories—class, race, region—but attending to

---

[24] S. Mediratta, 'Beauty and the Breast: The Poetics of Physical Absence and Narrative Presence in Frances Burney's Mastectomy Letter (1811)', *Women: A Cultural Review*, 19 (2008), 188–207, at 188; J. E. Epstein, 'Writing the Unspeakable: Fanny Burney's Mastectomy and the Fictive Body', *Representations*, 16 (1986), 131–66.

[25] Tammy Duerden Comeau, 'Gender Ideology and Disease Theory: Classifying Cancer in Nineteenth Century Britain', *Journal of Historical Sociology*, 20 (2007), 158–81.

[26] Feminist critiques of the Victorian doctor, first put forward in the 1970s, suggest that the nineteenth century was a 'new Fall' for the medical management of female bodies; and that professionals were uncaring, even sadistic, in their approach to their women patients. See C. M. Scholten, '"On the Importance of the Obstetrick Art": Changing Customs of Childbirth in America 1760–1825', *William and Mary Quarterly*, 3rd ser., 34 (1977), 426–45; M. S. Hartman and L. Banner (eds.), *Clio's Consciousness Raised: New Perspectives on the History of Women* (New York, 1974); and Ornella Moscucci, *The Science of Woman: Gynaecology and Gender in England, 1800–1929* (Cambridge, UK, 1993).

gender alone also risks reifying a pervasive stereotype of the nineteenth-century medical professional as unfeeling or even quasi-sadistic.

The few historians of malignancy in nineteenth-century Britain have tended to focus on site-specific cancers—books on the history of breast, uterine, and lung cancers are more common than texts on the disease as a whole.[27] In contrast, I address cancer as an integrative, rather than site-specific, disease category. This is partly because historians' differentiation between cancers located in different organs is more appropriate for the twentieth than the nineteenth century. That is not to suggest that histories of site-specific cancers in the nineteenth century are not useful or relevant. After all, and as I argue in Chapters 1 and 6, most of the cancers diagnosed in the nineteenth century were located close to the surface of the body or in accessible places (e.g. the female reproductive organs). In other cases, cancerous growths may have been suspected, but could only be conclusively identified in post-mortem examinations. The prognoses of various cancer types also improved unevenly and there were increasingly detailed investigations into the cellular structures and natures of a range of site-specific and stage-specific malignancies.

However, while medical men did distinguish between cancers of different type, site, and stage; they also conceived of cancer as a useful, emotive, and politically generative 'umbrella term' that could be deployed in case notes, medical journal articles, and the popular press to communicate a shared understanding of a single—albeit complex and multifaceted—disease. After all, even today any evidence in support of disaggregating the singular category 'cancer' has not transformed the collective imaginary of the disease. While cancer experiences and expectations differ widely, for most, cancer is still cancer, whether it is in the breast, lung, or pancreas. In the nineteenth, twentieth, and twenty-first centuries alike, it is just as reasonable to speak of a broad 'cancer experience', shared by people living with a range of different site-specific cancers, because the disease had and continues to have an undifferentiated social and cultural significance. While practitioners might distinguish between different types, the disease moved and moves through medicine and society as an integrated unit.

Sources and Structure

This book begins by looking at a community of doctors and patients who lived and worked in the streets surrounding The Middlesex Hospital on Mortimer

[27] See Ilana Löwy, ' "Because of their Praiseworthy Modesty, They Consult Too Late": Regime of Hope and Cancer of the Womb, 1800–1910', *Bulletin of the History of Medicine*, 85 (2011), 356–83; Ornella Moscucci, *Gender and Cancer in England, 1860–1948* (London, 2016); Ornella Moscucci, 'Gender and Cancer in Britain, 1860–1910', *American Journal of Public Health*, 95 (2005), 1312–21; Timmermann, *A History of Lung Cancer*

Street in London. It follows in their footsteps as they walked the labyrinthine lanes
and passages that branched off Tottenham Court Road; then, through seven
chapters, its focus expands to successively include the rivers, lakes, and forests
of England; the mountains, poverty, and hunger of the four nations of the British
Isles; the reluctant and resistant inhabitants of the British Empire; and the
networks of scientists and doctors spread across Europe and North America,
while always keeping Britain at its centre.

The book is divided into two parts—'Characteristics and Cures' and 'Causes'—
with the thread of incurability running throughout. In this book, I show how the
medical and scientific community responded creatively and optimistically to
cancer's intractability. I trace these responses through a variety of spaces and
settings and argue that incurability was productive of new medical categories and
knowledge. In doing so, this book intersects with a body of historical literature
that suggests that different places and projects produced variant medical theory
and practice. Following, albeit unintentionally, the classic trifecta of nineteenth-
century medicine—bedside, hospital, laboratory—this book begins with the establishment of Britain's first cancer-specific institution in 1792, at The Middlesex
Hospital in London, and ends on the eve of the First World War.[28] The intervening period of just over a century saw a proliferation of cancer hospitals, with
surgical approaches to the disease increasingly situated within the hospital walls.
In early modern Britain, hospitals were primarily seen as philanthropic institutions that provided for the poor. Social rather than medical criteria determined
admission and most doctor–patient interactions took place in the home, at the
'bedside'. Over the course of the nineteenth century, hospitals lost their charitable
associations and became sites of scientific research and the primary loci of medical
education and care. Finally, in the fin de siècle, with the advent of an experimental
paradigm, medical investigation took up residence in the laboratory. This book
tracks cancer through these three locations—home, hospital, and laboratory—and
shows how each produced distinctive medical cosmologies and patterns of social
interaction.[29]

Part I, 'Characteristics and Cures', explores diagnosis, treatment, and prognosis, drawing on The Middlesex Hospital's extensive archive, published surgical
tracts and treatises, medical journals, narrative and autobiographical accounts,
general-interest periodicals, and the popular press. I look at cancer from the
viewpoint of practitioners and try to read against the grain to access the patient

[28] The classic trifecta is drawn from both Nicholas D. Jewson and John V. Pickstone. Nicholas
D. Jewson, 'The Disappearance of the Sick-Man from Medical Cosmology, 1770–1870', *Sociology*, 10
(1976), 225–44; John V. Pickstone, 'Commentary: From History of Medicine to a General History of
"Working Knowledges"', *International Journal of Epidemiology*, 38 (2009), 646–9.
[29] Foremost in the construction of this narrative was Michel Foucault. He posited the 'birth of the
clinic' and coined the term 'medical gaze' to indicate the medical separation of body and identity that
supposedly took place within the nineteenth-century hospital context. M. Foucault, *The Birth of the
Clinic: An Archaeology of Medical Perception* (London, 1973).

perspective. Founded as the Middlesex Infirmary in 1745 on Windmill Street, the renamed hospital moved to its later location in 1757. Since 1792, it had housed two cancer wards, one for women and one for men, making it the first institution in the world with space and staff dedicated to the care of cancer. In contrast to most eighteenth-century hospitals that did not tolerate long stays by chronic and incurable inhabitants, The Middlesex Hospital's cancer ward insisted that, 'such [cancer] Patients be not hurried out of the Hospital under an idea that they are incurable, for these of all cases call aloud for time and patience'.[30]

The first chapter, 'From Home to Hospital', pivots around this shift from exclusion to inclusion and explores the senses and emotions that attended living with and dying from cancer in the early nineteenth century. The archives of The Middlesex Hospital consist of registers of cancer patients from 1792 through to the twentieth century, and a potted selection of casebooks. This chapter, therefore, tells the stories of sixty patients from 1805 to 1836. From these case notes we can add flesh and blood to the lived experience of cancer and go some way towards recovering the patient voice. We can follow in their footsteps from home to hospital, and in multiple literal and metaphorical ways appreciate the distances they travelled in their 'cancer journeys'.

Cancer's incurability was an emotional and sensory experience as much as it was an intellectual construction. An emphasis on incurability allows us to explore the mechanisms used by sufferers and the medical community to cope with and manage this persistent and profoundly troubling problem. Cancer sufferers felt pain and discomfort, saw their own disfigurements, were touched by practitioners seeking to diagnose and treat; and were seen and smelt by others and marked out as representative of decline and death. I trace these sensory engagements— between two different bodies and between a person and their own body—and in doing so 'flesh out' the people who suffered in the past. Appreciating this character of cancer then allows us to cut across the words and impositions of practitioners— who were almost always male and part of the social elite—to access the experiences of women and the disempowered. But even in cases of cancer in the Victorian aristocracy, an attention to embodiment and the senses equips us with empathy. It humanizes individuals who might otherwise be homogenized as a nameless collection of 'cancer patients'.

Power is laced through these encounters between doctor and patient. The establishment of The Middlesex Hospital's cancer ward subjected the disease to 'hospital medicine' and the distinctive medical cosmologies and patterns of social interaction that accompanied this. For Erwin H. Ackerknecht and others, the decades following the French Revolution saw a 'political and technological revolution'.[31] This 'revolution' led directly to a 'new medicine': one that was closely

---

[30] UCLH Archive, London, 'Weekly Board Meeting', Middlesex Hospital Minutes, 10 January 1792.
[31] Erwin H. Ackerknecht, *Medicine at the Paris Hospital, 1794–1848* (Baltimore, MD, 1967), xi.

tied to the hospital context and 'based on physical examination by hand and eye, on pathological anatomy, on statistics, and on the concept of the lesion'.[32] Following Ackerknecht, and expanding upon many of Foucault's ideas, the historical sociologist Nicholas Jewson suggested his own tripartite history—of private patronage, of state hospitals, and of laboratories—linking the late eighteenth century to the present day.[33] He argued that the end of the eighteenth century saw a transition from 'bedside' to 'hospital' medicine. In 'bedside medicine', symptoms and the patient's voice were prominent in the diagnostic process because both were explicit manifestations of the individual disease.

In the 'clinic' (i.e. the Paris hospital), the symptom and its signification became detached: the symptom was no longer synonymous with the disease. The new paradigm of 'hospital medicine' sought the underlying anatomical correlate—the physical lesion was now the sign of the illness, which rendered the patient's symptoms and feelings irrelevant to the diagnosis. The doctor found truth through an objective gaze that was directed at those new disembodied signs. Jewson claims that because of this reconceptualization, the 'sickman [sic] disappeared' in the early nineteenth century along with 'his [sic] narrative'.[34] These patterns of power and disempowerment are apparent in the early nineteenth-century cancer ward's case notes. While men and women travelled from all over the country seeking medical advice from the surgeons at the Middlesex, the hospital primarily served the surrounding areas of intense urban poverty and most of those treated in the institution were members of the metropolitan poor. They slipped in and out of employment, shifted occupations across their lifespan, and were likely unable to afford private medical treatment for their cancers. In addition, most cancer patients in the nineteenth century were women—a fact observed and problematized by contemporaries—and their over-representation was likely because their tumours more often appeared in accessible and visible organs: breasts and genitals. Thus, while I do not think of cancer as an exclusively, or inherently, 'female' disease, women and their bodies are nonetheless prominent in this book, and most of the clinical encounters I interrogate took place between a male surgeon or physician and their female patients. The people treated in the Middlesex were often doubly, if not triply, disempowered by their social status, gender, and sometimes age.

However, my research suggests that the materiality of cancer—with its widely recognized external lesions, long life history that necessitated an extensive patient narrative, and chronic and incurable nature—posed a specific set of problems to the hospital doctor and, later, the laboratory scientist, and their methods of diagnosis. As a result, cancer patients being treated in hospitals retained perhaps unusual agency—at least in directing the meaning and implications of their

[32] Ibid.   [33] Jewson, 'The Disappearance of the Sick-Man'.   [34] Ibid.

disease—in the nineteenth century. Long, descriptive case notes remained a prominent part of The Middlesex Hospital's archive throughout the period in question. Moreover, this book provides an alternative portrayal to that of the crude and dispassionate nineteenth-century surgeon or physician. Linda Payne argues that the development of a culture of emotional detachment was—by the end of the eighteenth century—an essential component of operative surgery.[35] In analyses of the nineteenth century, such detachment has often been reframed as insensitivity. The surgeon, impervious to the pain and suffering of his patient, is a familiar caricature. As this book shows, however, this conceptualization is unsatisfying and leaves out the many and various ways that nineteenth-century practitioners made use of 'compassion and intersubjectivity' in the formation of their culture and identity.[36] Doctors were not immune to the emotional intensity associated with living with and dying from cancer.

This attendance to emotions, the senses, and discourse marks this book out as a cultural history; and indeed, it owes much to the 'linguistic turn' and its attendant focus on textual representation.[37] Cancer has a vibrant rhetorical history. Today, the disease is a potent metaphor for anything evil, malevolent, or menacing. It has become almost a platitude of political discourse and equips moralizers of many stripes with a culturally resonant high ground. This was also true in the nineteenth century. Cancer was synonymous with 'malignancy'—an evocative term that meant both the ability to metastasize and something with malevolent intention. Medical writers described it as the 'dread and excruciating disease', synonymous with death and decline, and feared by doctor and patient.[38] It was, 'of all the ills to which the human frame is liable', the most 'poignant'.[39] This book explores the utility and deployment of these metaphors and argues that their persistence depended on their mutability and continued applicability to the peculiar social and political context of nineteenth-century Britain. Cancer lay, therefore, at the intersection between the material and the metaphorical. While I contend that historians must take seriously the lived experience of cancer—and consider carefully the pain and suffering it inflicted—cancer was not just a biological or experiential phenomenon but, as anthropologist S. Lochlann Jain argues, 'a

---

[35] Lynda Payne, *With Words and Knives: Learning Medical Dispassion in Early Modern England* (London, 2007).

[36] See the work of Michael Brown, whose recent project, 'A Theatre of Emotions: The Affective Landscape of Nineteenth-Century British Surgery', explores the place of emotion in the practice, politics, and representation of nineteenth-century surgery. Michael Brown, 'Surgery and Emotion: The Era before Anaesthesia', in Thomas Schlich (ed.), *The Palgrave Handbook of the History of Surgery* (Basingstoke, 2017).

[37] James Vernon, 'Who's Afraid of the Linguistic Turn? The Politics of Social History and its Discontents', *Social History*, 19 (1994), 81–97.

[38] 'The Increasing Fatality of Cancer', *BMJ*, 1 (1883), 969–71, at 970.

[39] Thomas Pope, 'On Cancer', *Association Medical Journal*, 3 (1855), 859–60, at 859.

politics' or a cultural product that cannot be fully comprehended without its rhetorical trappings.[40]

In Chapter 2, 'Incurability and the Clinic', I show how the hospitalization of cancer gave the care of the disease new legitimacy, tied it closely to the investigative and charitable projects of the metropolitan medical elite, and provided cancer with a presence in London's built environment. It was in this early nineteenth-century moment that the disease moved out of the confines of the sickbed and entered the culture, politics, and social world of the early Victorian metropolis. The chapter reveals how, because of their new, concentrated, and hospital-based study of the disease, the capital's medical elite defined cancer as an incurable malady and as a problem that they, as a collective, needed to overcome. It argues that the hospitalization of the disease codified cancer and transformed characteristics—such as incurability—that had long been observed by practitioners into essential, identifying features. Now that practitioners could see sufferers in aggregate, they could extract shared symptoms and experiences, and observe the patient and their illness from beginning to end.

Cancer's new incurable status was, therefore, not just a biological observation, but had great rhetorical power. Practitioners used this identity to establish certain professional credentials, such as humanity, restraint, and intellectual nuance; they also articulated a professional chronology and progressive teleology. For while surgeons and physicians derived social and intellectual capital from lamentations and doubt, they also professed profound optimism and contrasted current incurability with future, inevitable medical mastery over cancer. Incurability was repeatedly deployed by a range of practitioners in the construction of their professional selves. Indeed, it was in the nineteenth century that various health-care practitioners— apothecaries, physicians, surgeons, and general practitioners—pursued professionalizing agendas in the form of structural and institutional reform. The Apothecaries' Act (1815), the Anatomy Act (1832), and the Medical Act (1858) all attempted to differentiate various professionals from each other and distinguish them from unorthodox practitioners or 'quacks'.[41] Moreover, medical men used a variety of rhetorical techniques to express shared goals and articulate the differences between practitioners of different types.

Over the course of the nineteenth century, surgeons progressively claimed priority in the management, treatment, and control of cancer. As a result, in Chapter 3, 'Cancer Therapeutics', I pay particular attention to these practitioners.

---

[40] S. Lochlann Jain, *Malignant: How Cancer Becomes Us* (Berkeley, CA, 2013), 14.

[41] Historians such as Roger French, A. Wear, Ivan Waddington, and Susan C. Lawrence have explored these structural aspects of professionalization in detail. R. French and A. Wear (eds.), *British Medicine in an Age of Reform* (London, 1991); Susan C. Lawrence, 'Private Enterprise and Public Interests: Medical Education and the Apothecaries' Act, 1780–1825', in French and Wear (eds.), *British Medicine in an Age of Reform*; Ivan Waddington, *The Medical Profession in the Industrial Revolution* (London, 1984).

The professionalization of surgery was accomplished by a rhetorical and semantic arsenal that elevated their craft to the 'scientific' level and gentility of internal medicine. Christopher Lawrence has delineated a phenomenon whereby surgeons habitually boosted their own era by denigrating former regimes as barbaric or inadequate.[42] To combat such accusations from contemporaries, they frequently emphasized restraint, insisted on the unity of medicine and surgery, and made claims about the perfectibility of surgery as a curative practice. Historians such as Michael Brown have focused on this 'cultural history' of professionalization and looked towards surgeons' and physicians' use of language in constructing an external image and coherent identity. He argues that, 'The medical profession of the early nineteenth century was less a structural category than an imaginative concept, a point of individual and collective self-identification which was conditioned by such factors as political ideology and social/spatial location.'[43] This rhetoric comes through in writings on cancer surgery, with the apparent incurability of the disease posing a particular set of challenges to various professionals attempting to establish their authority. And yet this incurability was also an opportunity. Cancer's intractability allowed elite surgeons to set themselves apart from rivals and competitors and identify themselves as humanitarian and benevolent actors.

However, this same characteristic—its incurability—also made cancer particularly appealing to unconventional healers. Boundaries between different types of medical men were often arbitrary, those labelled alternative practitioners also pursued a professionalizing agenda. They too established hospitals, societies, and journals. Thus, the importance of rhetoric and language in framing identity, forming collective values, and differentiating between 'regular' and 'irregular' practitioners was paramount.[44] Historians have argued that nineteenth-century 'quacks' marked themselves out through bombast and self-aggrandizement, whereas elite surgeons and physicians performed their identity through the rhetoric of caution and intellectual complexity.[45] However, cancer complicates this distinction. Unorthodox practitioners also made use of incurability in their self-fashioning and, as a result, the disease frustrates any easy differentiation between the rhetorical styles of regular and irregular medical men.

[42] Christopher Lawrence, 'Democratic, Divine and Heroic: The History and Historiography of Surgery', in Christopher Lawrence (ed.), *Medical Theory, Surgical Practice: Essays in the History of Surgery* (London, 1992).

[43] Michael Brown, *Performing Medicine: Medical Culture and Identity in Provincial England, c. 1760–1850* (Manchester, 2011), 6; see also Michael Brown, 'Medicine, Reform and the "End" of Charity in Early Nineteenth-Century England', *English Historical Review*, 124 (2009), 1353–88.

[44] P. S. Brown, 'Social Context and Medical Theory in the Demarcation of Nineteenth-Century Boundaries', in W. F. Bynum and Roy Porter, *Medical Fringe and Medical Orthodoxy 1750–1850* (London, 1987), 230.

[45] Roy Porter, *Health for Sale: Quackery in England, 1660–1850* (Manchester, 1989). See also Mark S. R. Jenner and Patrick Wallis (eds.), *Medicine and the Market in England and its Colonies* (Basingstoke, 2007); Bynum and Porter, *Medical Fringe*.

Chapter 4, 'Cancer Quackery', serves to nuance the stories of nineteenth-century cancer therapeutics as set out in the first three chapters by bringing in patients and practitioners whose views on cancer diverged from those of the London and Edinburgh elites. Analysis of their perspectives demonstrates that the climate of pessimism surrounding cancer's intractability was not hegemonic, and that various voices of dissent existed both within and without the 'regular' profession. This chapter reconsiders the medical marketplace and places the concept of incurability at the centre of patient choice and professional self-fashioning. The suffering that cancer patients were willing to undergo suggests that, for many, the diagnosis of an incurable disease and subsequent offers of palliative care alone were unsatisfying. Incurability made space for a crowded medical marketplace that catered for desperately ill people and provided treatments of last resort.

In Part II, 'Causes', I continue the argument that the incurability of cancer was productive. It focuses on the medical and scientific community and their creative responses to cancer's intractability. I show how it prompted a range of new 'ways of seeing' cancer. Frustrated with therapeutic limitations, concerned by its persistent incurability, and anxious over its increasing incidence, various medical men turned their attention from treatment to cause. A range of medical 'interventions' proliferated that aimed to make sense of the nature, emergence, potential spread, and prevention of cancer. The creative and constructive nature of incurability is confirmed by these men's pursuit of these 'interventions'. Diverse practitioners used new technologies and techniques—statistics, mapping, the microscope, and discourses of progress and decline—to comprehend cancer. They required these techniques because their efforts to produce a cure had proven futile. It is a paradox, therefore, that incurability was productive rather than just tragic or restrictive. Like Part I, 'Causes' examines a wide variety of source material, including periodicals and the medical and lay press, and published tracts and treatises. It also uses maps, drawings and diagrams, letters, and the archives of institutions. 'Causes' tracks the disease's journey through a range of medical and scientific disciplines—public health, histology, bacteriology, colonial medicine—and explores its reverberations through nineteenth-century society, culture, and politics.

The quantification of the British populous from the 1840s onwards, in the form of census gathering, suggested to anxious observers that the disease's incidence was increasing. The new 'epidemic' coalesced with long-standing conceptualizations of the disease as unusually 'malignant' (with all its attendant meanings) and cemented cancer as the 'dread disease'. Chapter 5, 'Counting and Mapping Cancer', explores the practice of collecting cancer statistics and elucidates the meanings and implications of the nascent idea of the 'cancer epidemic' in the mid-nineteenth-century. This sets the scene for Part II of the book and its shift in focus from treatment to cause. In response to the supposed increasing incidence of cancer, some medical men sought strategies beyond the clinic to elucidate the evasive malady. The continued therapeutic futility with respect to cancer provoked a diversification of investigative efforts, and elements of the medical community refocused on the disease's causes, prevention, transmission, and potential communication.

Chapter 5 explores the ways in which practitioners interested in cancer—little-known characters like Alfred Haviland, Charles H. Moore, and Charles E. Green—mapped cancer incidence, understood the disease to be produced by certain environments, and conceptualized the disease spatially and according to scale. Urban space was, for many, the underbelly of modernity—the dark side of progress. Cancer, however, forced nineteenth-century observers to question this correlation between disease and urban modernity. Instead, cancer map-makers were preoccupied with the countryside and connected the disease to bucolic locales rather than areas of urban squalor. In this alternative geography of Britain, unexpected places could have therapeutic or pathological potential. Not only does this chapter add the countryside to our map of the diseases of modern life, it also interrogates an early step along the road towards a later conceptualization of cancer as a disease of health and affluence.

Chapter 6, 'Cancer under the Microscope', reveals how mapping was but one tool deployed in the decoding of the 'cancer problem' in the latter half of the nineteenth century. Running parallel to the activities of Haviland, Moore, and Green, biologists, pathologists, and histologists took up the microscope with gusto and spawned a vibrant debate between cell theorists, bacteriologists, and parasitologists. This chapter thus traces the introduction of the microscope into the landscape of cancer theory and practice, explores the development of cell theories of malignancy, and interrogates the many and various 'germ theories' of the disease. I argue that despite their close relationship with the microscope and its scientific and progressive associations, all three theories appealed in part because they recapitulated and reframed very old ideas about cancer's causes and characteristics.

The final chapter, 'Making Cancer Modern', analyses and assesses the medical practitioners and social commentators—like Woods Hutchinson—who searched for an explanation for the new 'cancer epidemic' in late Victorian modernity. While Chapters 5 and 6 looked at medical men who, using a range of techniques and technologies, attempted to decode the aetiology of cancer and explain and arrest its expansion, the limited success of these efforts prompted some observers to suggest that perhaps the origin of malignancy could be found in the very fabric of late nineteenth-century society. If it was not latent in the landscape, nor a waxing and waning infectious disease, then maybe cancer's increasing incidence was a sign of some change in the bodies and lifestyles of the nation and its inhabitants. Finally, this chapter will reconsider the fin-de-siècle moment, and situate cancer within broader debates over the simultaneous promise and peril posed by the coming century. It will track the troubled relationship among professional optimism, pessimism, and realism; it will also argue that cancer's incurability and its unusual relationship with longevity provided the medical community with ample opportunity to articulate a coherent identity and exposed fundamental limits to what they could offer both to the individuals they treated and to British society writ large.

PART I
CHARACTERISTICS AND CURES

1

From Home to Hospital

In the early summer of 1805, forty-two-year-old Dorothy Bullock walked the short distance from her home in St Giles to The Middlesex Hospital on Mortimer Street, London.[1] Dorothy was a married woman and a mother and she came seeking advice about her cancerous left breast. Dorothy's home, St Giles, was one of the poorest parts of London. Appearing in Hogarth and later in Dickens, it was the iconic Victorian slum. Known as the 'rookery', it was notorious for its drunkenness, licentiousness, and Irish immigrant population. According to nineteenth-century surveyors, some of its four-roomed houses were home to up to ninety people at a time.[2] But Dorothy only had to walk ten minutes to reach the relative calm of The Middlesex Hospital, just a stone's throw from what is now Euston Road, which in 1805 marked London's northern boundary with nothing but fields and villages beyond.

Dorothy had fair skin and flushed cheeks. She claimed that no one in her family had ever suffered from cancer before—everyone on entry to the hospital was asked whether they had any hereditary predisposition to the disease—but her left breast was 'hardened' and 'fibrous' and there were tumours evident in her armpit and in her right breast.[3] She told the surgeon that she had first noticed the growths several months ago and that she could not think of any reason or explanation for their appearance. Her left arm was swollen and heavy to lift. Dorothy was admitted and spent nine months in and out of the ward, until her death in March 1806. From the post-mortem, investigators determined that her cancer had spread to her lungs and it was this that had caused her death. Her surgeon remarked in her notes that she had declined, breathless, more quickly than they had expected.

Dorothy had received the very best treatment available. She was operated on and provided with palliative care in the form of pain relief (opium) and home comforts (nourishing food and the occasional stiff drink). Dorothy would have paid nothing for her treatment and was entitled to remain under the care of hospital staff, 'until relieved by Art, or released by Death'.[4] Dorothy's experience was not unusual. In 1805, thirty-three-year-old Hannah Cressford was also

---

[1] UCLH Archive, London, 'Dorothy Bullock', 1805, Case Notes from the Cancer Ward at the Middlesex Hospital (1805–1838).
[2] Edward Walford, *Old and New London*, vol. 4 (London, 1878).
[3] UCLH Archive, 'Dorothy Bullock'.
[4] UCLH Archive, London, 'Weekly Board Meeting', Middlesex Hospital Minutes, 10 January 1792.

The Cancer Problem: Malignancy in Nineteenth-Century Britain. Agnes Arnold-Forster, Oxford University Press (2021).
© Agnes Arnold-Forster. DOI: 10.1093/oso/9780198866145.003.0002

admitted to the same ward. She was also married, a mother, and suffering from breast cancer.[5] For three months, she had watched her tumours grow and multiply before she, too, walked the short distance from her home in Somers Town (near King's Cross) to The Middlesex Hospital. In September, she underwent a mastectomy without anaesthetic. Within weeks her tumours had returned and as 'no prospect of cure was held out', she returned home to die with her friends.[6]

Between 1805 and 1838, the surgeon to The Middlesex Hospital's cancer ward kept detailed case notes of all the female patients he treated (the male equivalent was either never made or does not survive). Bound in leather folios, these meticulous, handwritten records fill whole pages and narrate the lives and deaths of women whose stories are rarely told. Poor and female, these case notes add flesh and blood to the lived experiences of cancer in early nineteenth-century London. With help from the casebooks, we can follow in their footsteps from home to hospital, and in multiple literal and metaphorical ways appreciate the distances they travelled in their 'cancer journeys'.

These experiences are important. Not only were they new but they mark the moment when cancer entered the hospital walls. Eighteenth-century hospitals did not tolerate long stays by chronic and incurable inhabitants. As a result, before the establishment of the cancer wards in 1792, poor men and women were left to die, their suffering often unalleviated, at home or in the workhouse. In contrast, The Middlesex Hospital's cancer ward allowed such patients to remain in the hospital until they either died or their condition improved.[7] The foundation of the Middlesex did not, however, just alter the experience of cancer sufferers—it transformed how cancer was understood and investigated. Prior to 1792, medical men's interactions with the disease would have been limited to the occasional visit from a private patient or a letter from a concerned sufferer.

The impetus behind this institutionalization of cancer patients was not predicated on new ideas about the disease; however, hospitals did provide new contexts for pre-existing understandings to be collated, elaborated, and confirmed. Surgeons and physicians could now see sufferers in aggregate, extract shared symptoms and experiences, and observe the patient and their disease from diagnosis through to death. Through the study of large numbers of patients over long periods of times, cancer was codified. Medical men transformed incidental observations into defining features of the disease and published their findings as texts referred to as 'Classifications'.[8] The year 1792, therefore, marked a transformative moment in the history of the cancer. First, it ushered in a new and very

---

[5] UCLH Archive, London, 'Hannah Cressford', 1805, Case Notes from the Cancer Ward at the Middlesex Hospital (1805–1838).

[6] Ibid.   [7] UCLH Archive, 'Weekly Board Meeting', 10 January 1792.

[8] John Abernethy, *Surgical Observations on Tumours* (London, 1811), x.

'modern' experience—dying on the hospital wards. Second, it remade cancer into an identifiable and diagnosable disease with a set of standard characteristics.

In what follows, I will narrate a brief history of The Middlesex Hospital and contextualize the foundations of its cancer wards, before moving on to describing the lives and circumstances of the patients who sought medical care from the institution. Then I will use the surviving case notes to map out the characteristics of early nineteenth-century cancer, and particularly its identity as a disease with a physical, tangible manifestation—the tumour. Touch was crucial to this identification process. While Roy Porter argues that the nineteenth century was the period in which 'the physical examination became the *pièce de résistance* of the bedside encounter',[9] touch plays only a minimal role in the historiography of nineteenth-century medicine. Mark Jenner has analysed the ways in which the early modern physician Sir John Floyer made use of his senses (including, and sometimes especially, touch) in his diagnosis and experimentation, and Olivia Weisser has made a similar case for practitioners in the eighteenth century. However, histories of nineteenth-century medicine have tended to focus on touch in anatomical pedagogy and surgical treatment. For example, Carin Berkowitz has examined the philosophical and practical defence of touch in Charles Bell's *Bridgewater Thesis*, and Thomas Schlich has written about the uneven adoption of surgical gloves in late nineteenth-century surgery and the changing value of haptic sensitivity.[10] There is, therefore, still much to be written about the sensory experiences of care and treatment.

Finally, this chapter also explores the 'life course' of cancer and seeks to understand the various stages people's bodies experienced. As I will show, the disease was also defined by its long duration, its irreversible capacity for growth and spread, and ultimately its incurability. While dependent on the words of the elite and the educated, in this chapter I attempt to read against the grain of case histories and other written materials to partially represent the experiences of poor people who lived in London and died from cancer in the first few decades of the nineteenth century.

This is important because much of what we know about cancer in nineteenth-century Britain relies on analysis of the words and experiences of wealthy people. Frances Burney and Ada Lovelace were both diagnosed with cancer and the latter

[9] Roy Porter, 'The Rise of Physical Examination', in W. F. Bynum and Roy Porter (eds.), *Medicine and the Five Senses* (Cambridge, 2005), 183.

[10] See Mark Jenner, 'Tasting Lichfield, Touching China: Sir John Floyer's Senses', *Historical Journal*, 53 (2010), 650–1; Roy Porter, 'The Rise of Physical Examination', in W. F. Bynum and Roy Porter (eds.), *Medicine and the Five Senses* (Cambridge, 2005); Carin Berkowitz, 'Charles Bell's Seeing Hand: Teaching Anatomy to the Senses in Britain, 1750–1840', *History of Science*, 52 (2014), 377–400; Thomas Schlich, 'Why Were Surgical Gloves Not Used Earlier? History of Medicine and Alternative Paths of Innovation', *The Lancet*, 386 (2015), 1234–5; Susan C. Lawrence, 'Educating the Senses: Students, Teachers and Medical Rhetoric in Eighteenth-Century London', in Bynum and Porter, *Medicine and the Five Senses*; and Olivia Weisser, 'Boils, Pushes, and Wheals: Reading Bumps on the Body in Early Modern England', *Social History of Medicine*, 22 (2009), 321–39.

died a slow and painful death meticulously recorded by her relatives. While their narratives are valuable—not least for what they can tell us about the gendered nature of illness experiences and medical care—they represent the lives of an elite few. Neither received treatment in hospitals and both had access to the most expensive surgeons and physicians around. Unlike for Burney and Lovelace, we do not have access to words written by the poor women who died on The Middlesex Hospital cancer ward. We must make do with accounts mediated by their doctors and with descriptions those men made of their patients' bodies. Writing a history of nineteenth-century cancer that takes the experiences of poor people as its starting point requires, therefore, some imagination.

The Middlesex Hospital

In November 1792, The Middlesex Hospital established the first cancer-specific institution or ward in Britain, and only the second in the world.[11] It received 'a contribution of three Thousand Pounds for establishing a Fund for the endowment of a Ward for the reception of Persons afflicted with that disorder [cancer], and four Hundred Pounds to fit up the Ward'.[12] The surgeon, Mr Howard of Argyll Street, outlined a detailed plan for how the ward would be set up and managed. To relieve 'persons afflicted with Cancer', he suggested

> That an airy Ward of the Middlesex Hospital might be appropriated to this specific Disease and to this Disease only, that the diseased might there find such alleviation of their sufferings as their respective situations should require, and that for an unlimited time.[13]

He proposed that the ward be divided into two, one side for men and the other for women, 'containing ten or twelve Beds ... [and] the usual function of ... bowls, candles, board'. They predicted that there would be about forty inpatients per year.[14]

In this period, medical men shared humanitarian values with the local elites who subscribed to the charitable hospitals, asylums, and dispensaries that were established across the British Isles. The Middlesex cancer ward's unnamed financial backer and chief supporter in parliament, Samuel Whitbread (1764–1815), had broad altruistic obligations and was interested in reforming the system of poverty relief at the end of the eighteenth century. He was a Whig MP from Bedford and supported Poor Law legislation and other measures intended for the

---

[11] The first was likely in Reims, France, in the 1740s: Victor Richards, *Cancer: The Wayward Cell, Its Origins, Nature and Treatment* (Berkeley, CA, 1978), 85.
[12] UCLH Archive, 'Weekly Board Meeting', 10 January 1792.   [13] Ibid.   [14] Ibid.

relief of the dispossessed and disenfranchised. He took an active interest in the affairs of The Middlesex Hospital and shortly before his death, on the eve of Waterloo, he arranged the appointment of Charles Bell (1774–1842) as its surgeon.[15] Whitbread also had a personal connection to the disease. His sister had died from cancer and his commitment to the amelioration of malignancy stretched beyond his initial financial support of the two wards.[16]

This institutionalization and concentrated study of cancer was at once new and predicated on a pre-existing hospital system that was already incorporating a greater number of sufferers and a greater diversity of diseases than had been admitted one hundred years earlier. While the two royal hospitals— St Bartholomew's in West Smithfield and St Thomas' in Southwark—had existed in some form or another since the twelfth and thirteenth centuries; from the mid-eighteenth century onwards, various voluntary hospitals were founded in London by philanthropic men who wished to improve the lives of the poor, contribute to the increasing population and prosperity of the nation, and enhance their own social position.[17] Voluntary hospitals relied on philanthropy and other private sources of funding. They were administered by committees of volunteer lay (non-medical) governors and were staffed by surgeons and physicians working in unpaid posts. Institutional provision for the sick and infirm grew in eighteenth-century London, and by 1800 there were almost twenty hospitals in the capital.[18]

Admission to the voluntary hospitals was never automatic. Instead, it depended on the patient meeting certain diagnostic and financial criteria. Sufferers typically required some combination of a payment of fees, nomination by a governor or subscriber, and the provision of a surety who guaranteed to pay the burial expenses if the patient died. In many cases, fees were paid by friends and family, or by the parish, though in some cases of extreme need hospitals waived the fees. It was usually expected that patients who lived in London should be paid for by their parish, although they could also be supported by a military or naval officer in the case of wounded soldiers or sailors, or by employers or commercial bondsmen. Most hospital patients were from the lower orders as wealthier Londoners preferred to pay doctors to attend to them in the comfort of their own homes.[19]

However, even from these institutions tailored to the care of the poor, most cancer patients found little relief because hospitals in the eighteenth century

[15] D. R. Fisher, 'Whitbread, Samuel (1764–1815)', in *Oxford Dictionary of National Biography* (Oxford, 2004).

[16] Samuel Whitbread, 'Address: To the Governors of the Middlesex Hospital', in Samuel Young, *Minutes of Cases of Cancer and Cancerous Tendencies Successfully Treated by Mr Samuel Young* (London, 1815).

[17] Lindsay Granshaw and Roy Porter (eds.), *The Hospital in History* (London, 1991).

[18] See https://www.londonlives.org/static/Hospitals.jsp, accessed 17 April 2017.

[19] However, Keir Waddington has observed that London's hospitals 'could never be only for the working classes'; Keir Waddington, 'Unsuitable Cases: The Debate over Outpatient Admission, the Medical Profession and Late-Victorian London Hospitals', *Medical History*, 42 (1998), 26–46, at 32.

tended not to admit people with fatal maladies. Acceptance onto their wards was dictated by the patient's diagnosis and prognosis and various institutions had their conditions of entry written into their foundational documents. For example, Leeds General Infirmary's 'Rules and Orders', written in 1771, recorded that, 'no Persons apprehended to be in a dying condition or incurable, be admitted as In-Patients'.[20] This meant that prior to the establishment of The Middlesex Hospital's cancer wards—tailored to the care and treatment of malignancy—surgeons' and phys-icians' interactions with the disease would have been limited to their private practice or to the occasional appearance in hospital by people who had somehow managed to circumvent the rules.[21] Thus, while cancer patients do appear in the case notes of other hospitals in the eighteenth and the early nineteenth century, the Middlesex was the only institution that mandated their acceptance onto its wards.

Indeed, in contrast to most eighteenth-century hospitals that did not tolerate long stays by chronic and incurable inhabitants, The Middlesex Hospital's cancer ward insisted that

> Patients labouring under cases of Cancer requiring Operation, spreading ulcer-ated Cancers, and Cancers returning after Operation, shall remain an unlimited time, until either relieved by Art, or released by Death.[22]

Thus, people could be housed for months or even years, and frequently made repeat visits to the hospital for increasingly lengthy stretches of time. Martha Tatham, for example, was treated by the Middlesex for six years before she died in January 1845.[23] Amelia Foley's first stay for cancer of the uterus lasted from March until May 1843, but she returned for another six months later that year.[24] Hannah Russell was discharged after a month-long stay in 1843 for a cancerous breast, before being readmitted two years later and dying in September 1845.[25]

The Patients

These women were free to come and go as they pleased; however, their institu-tionalization was likely structured as much by their socio-economic status as by

---

[20] *Rules and Order of the General Infirmary at Leeds* (Leeds, 1771), 13.

[21] Later in the century, other hospitals increasingly treated cancer and new institutions were founded that tended specifically to the disease. For example, the Free Cancer Hospital, now the Royal Marsden Hospital, was founded in 1851. See Eve Wiltshaw, *A History of the Royal Marsden Hospital* (Edgware, 1998).

[22] UCLH Archive, 'Weekly Board Meeting', 10 January 1792.

[23] UCLH Archive, London, 'Martha Tatham', Cancerous Patients Register (1829–1846).

[24] UCLH Archive, London, 'Amelia Foley', Cancerous Patients Register (1829–1846).

[25] UCLH Archive, London, 'Hannah Russell', Cancerous Patients Register (1829–1846).

their ill-health. Both published and unpublished histories refer to patients 'returning to the country' when the hospital no longer met their needs; but it is likely that the men and women who sought care at the Middlesex were more or less representative of 'plebeian London'.[26] They were frequently unemployed, regularly changed jobs, and probably could not afford to be treated in their own homes.[27] The Middlesex served the surrounding area of intense urban poverty, and the only institutional alternative to the voluntary hospital was the workhouse, which loomed large on the eighteenth- and nineteenth-century London landscape. While initially intended to provide housing and occupation for an able adult male population, the workhouse soon provided for almost anyone in need of food and lodging. The metropolis' plebeian population was likely partially or periodically reliant on what Joanna Innes calls a 'mixed economy of welfare'.[28]

However, the workhouse was not designed to provide its inhabitants with the kind of specialized care that cancer patients required.[29] Moreover, most of the people treated for cancer in the Middlesex were post-menopausal women who were not only beset by the double disempowerment of gender and social status, but also their age.[30] The necessity of institutionalization is partly reflected in the Middlesex patients' movement from one establishment to another. Barbara Daves, who was admitted to the cancer ward in September 1824, spent several months in the hospital, before moving to the workhouse due to her supposed insanity (not the asylum, as one might expect).[31] As a fifty-four-year-old widow, her care was left to the responsibility of various metropolitan institutions. While in practice these men and women could enter and exit the hospital as they wished, as their suffering and abjection increased they were likely unable to return home, and the alternative institutional options for an incurable pauper were limited.

The Middlesex cancer ward was not just a charitable enterprise, but a medical endeavour. Bringing cancer within the hospital walls in a new, systematic, way altered how the disease was conceptualized because practitioners could now see sufferers in aggregate and extract shared symptoms and experiences, and because the surgeons and physicians could observe the patient and their disease from beginning through to the end. To enable the practitioner to derive generalities and make sense of the presented symptoms the founder of The Middlesex Hospital

---

[26] The phrase is borrowed from Tim Hitchcock and Robert Shoemaker, *London Lives: Poverty, Crime and the Making of a Modern City, 1690–1800* (Cambridge, UK, 2015), 4.

[27] Ibid.

[28] Joanna Innes, 'The "Mixed Economy of Welfare" in Early Modern England: Assessments of the Options from Hale to Malthus (c.1683–1803)', in Martin J. Daunton (ed.), *Charity, Self-Interest and Welfare in the English Past* (New York, 1996).

[29] Jonathan Reinartz and Leonard Schwarz, *Medicine and the Workhouse* (Rochester, NY, 2013).

[30] This can be understood as part of the increasing medicalization and institutionalization of the elderly across the eighteenth and nineteenth centuries. Susannah Ottoway, 'The Elderly in the Eighteenth-Century Workhouse', in Reinartz and Schwarz, *Medicine and the Workhouse*.

[31] UCLH Archive, London, 'Barbara Daves', Case Notes from the Cancer Ward at the Middlesex Hospital (1805–1838), 1824.

cancer ward advocated for the keeping of a detailed case history for each patient admitted:

> In order to improve a subject... I propose, that a faithful account of the history and circumstances of every case be kept, its antecedents and consequences should be marked, the effects of medicines and of Operations, when necessary, noted, together with all the collateral details.[32]

The cancer wards, therefore, aligned with the so-called 'Paris medicine' that had its origins in the decades following the French Revolution.[33] This context allowed for new regimes of care that enabled the comparative study of cancer's material manifestations and privileged the physical examination of the patient's body.

Case Notes, Clinical Touch, and Observation

These new regimes of care included frequent ward rounds by surgeons, long durations of stay, and systematic post-mortem examinations. Together, these means confirmed cancer as a disease indicated by the presence of a tumour—one that could be seen and touched by an external observer as well as felt by the patients themselves. Thus, while in early modern cosmologies, cancer was broadly understood as a 'systemic', 'general', or 'constitutional' disease, in the first few decades of the nineteenth century it was reconstructed as a 'local' disease—a physical and tangible entity that originated in a single bodily location. A small lump was no longer an indication of a systemic problem, but rather a diseased object that had only *the potential* for extension into the constitution. While some medical men at the turn of the nineteenth century, such as John Abernethy, argued that cancer arose from 'a disordered state of the health in general', by the 1840s, Irish surgeon Walter Hayle Walshe spoke for the majority when he argued that cancer began its 'life' as a physical mass, locally confined, before spreading around the body and appearing in distant organs and far-off tissue.[34] This transition had implications for who treated and investigated cancer. The shift from constitutional to local meant that surgeons were increasingly involved in the care of malignancy. Cancer transformed from a 'medical' to a 'surgical' disease.

---

[32] UCLH Archive, 'Weekly Board Meeting', 10 January 1792.

[33] See Erwin H. Ackerknecht, *Medicine at the Paris Hospital, 1794–1848* (Baltimore, MD, 1967); Mary E. Fissell, 'The Disappearance of the Patient's Narrative and the Invention of Hospital Medicine', in R. French and A. Wear (eds.), *British Medicine in an Age of Reform* (London, 1991); Michel Foucault, *The Birth of the Clinic: An Archaeology of Medical Perception* (London, 1973); Nicholas D. Jewson, 'The Disappearance of the Sick-Man from Medical Cosmology, 1770–1870', *Sociology*, 10 (1976), 225–44.

[34] Abernethy, *Surgical Observations on Tumours*, 88–9; Walter Hayle Walshe, *The Nature and Treatment of Cancer* (London, 1846), 92.

This transformation—while neither easy nor complete—resulted from a complex combination of scientific and social factors.

The prevailing historical narrative charts a linear transition across the nineteenth century, from constitutional understandings of cancer at the beginning of the period to local imaginings at the end. For example, Ornella Moscucci writes that 'the belief that cancer was a "local" disease' developed in the late nineteenth century, and Barron H. Lerner suggests that William Halsted's radical mastectomy was justified by late-century evidence that proved a local origin of breast cancer.[35] However, not only do we see evidence of localism much earlier than either of these historians suggest, but the transition was not as radical as we might suppose. Even in the seventeenth century, language that zoomorphized the disease implied that it was in some way distinct from the body—not an integral part of its constitution— and we know that mastectomies and other operations to remove cancerous masses were practised throughout the early modern period.[36] If early modern practitioners believed cancer to be constitutional then surely surgery would offer little hope of success. Moreover, there continued to be dissenting voices well into the late nineteenth century, and debates over cancer's causes and characteristics flourished rather than withered. Nonetheless, my evidence demonstrates that the early nineteenth century was a time of intense theoretical and professional flux within the medical community and that it witnessed a new insistence on cancer's localism. There was, therefore, an uneven shift from medical to surgical understandings of the disease, which was due to a range of transformations in the institutionalization and conceptualization of cancer after c.1800, and related to broader changes in medical knowledge and practice, including the decline in humoral theories, an increase in hospitalization, and the rising status of surgeons as compared to physicians and apothecaries.

The practitioners in this chapter were all operating at the end of humoral theory's predominance. In the eighteenth century, cancer was understood in terms of physiology and pathology that reflected a reworking of Galenic theory. In this schema, all diseases were explained by an imbalance in 'humours' that consisted of black bile, yellow bile, blood, and phlegm. Cancer was an overfilling of black bile or 'cancerous humour'—caused by some systemic blockage or the

[35] Ornella Moscucci, *Gender and Cancer in England, 1860–1948* (London, 2016), 47. Barron H. Lerner, *The Breast Cancer Wars: Fear, Hope, and the Pursuit of a Cure in Twentieth-Century America* (Oxford, 2011), 17. Alanna Skuse and Ilana Löwy have both nuanced this narrative. Skuse suggests that some practitioners saw cancer as a local malady in early modern England. Alanna Skuse, *Constructions of Cancer in Early Modern England: Ravenous Natures* (Basingstoke, 2015), 80. Löwy 'seeks to nuance a view of the history of cancer focused on late- nineteenth- and early-twentieth-century cognitive and practical ruptures'. Ilana Löwy, ' "Because of their Praiseworthy Modesty, They Consult Too Late": Regime of Hope and Cancer of the Womb, 1800–1910', *Bulletin of the History of Medicine*, 85 (2011), 356–83, at 358.

[36] Skuse, *Constructions of Cancer in Early Modern England*, 80.

degeneration of a local accumulation of a more benign substance.[37] This system rendered women particularly vulnerable to cancer, and helped to explain the increase in incidence once they had experienced menopause. Breast and uterine cancers became more common after the cessation of the menses because the women had ceased to self-regulate bodily flows.

Humoral theory also helped explain why eighteenth- and nineteenth-century patients and practitioners believed that physical trauma could provoke the formation of a cancerous deposit by rupturing normal passages of fluid. In 1807, Susan Squires was admitted to the Middlesex with a tumour in her breast that had 'commenced three years ago from a blow'.[38] However, it is important to note that there was no one dogmatic schema, and practitioners and theorists were frequently flexible in their interpretations of humoralism. Moreover, the abandonment of humoral theory was not immediate and elements persisted in medical, biological, and cultural thinking throughout the nineteenth century. Indeed, right up to 1900 The Middlesex Hospital's cancer ward recorded the 'predisposing' and 'exciting' causes of their patients' diseases in the case notes. In the Cancer Registers for 1887–91, 'exciting causes' included 'tooth?', 'blow probably', 'suckling baby for 18 months', 'attributes it to lifting a bundle of clothes'.[39] The explanatory system that identified physical trauma as an exciting cause of cancer was pervasive and resilient.[40]

In 1804, surgeon James Nooth congratulated his 'fair countrywomen' on their 'easy and elegant mode of dress, free from the unnatural and dangerous pressure of stays ... I have extirpated a great number of scirrhous tumours which originated from that absurdity.'[41] A domestic medicine manual from 1847 warned against the cancer-causing 'modern barbarisms of fashionable dress'.[42] Similarly, in 1874, *Berrow's Worcester Journal* reported on a case at the County Court. Major Baker sued his brother, David Baker, for £50 for damages for injuries sustained by his wife. David was accused of striking Mrs Baker on the breast, and, 'from the effects of the blow on the breast a cancer formed, and the woman had to undergo an operation'. Mr George Ashmead was 'called to give scientific evidence' and he agreed that 'cancers were generally produced by some external injury'.[43]

---

[37] Michael Stolberg, 'Metaphors and Images of Cancer in Early Modern Europe', *Bulletin of the History of Medicine*, 88 (2014), 48–74, at 57.

[38] UCLH Archive, 'Susan Squires', Case Notes from the Cancer Ward at the Middlesex Hospital (1805–1838), 1807.

[39] UCLH Archive, London, Cancer Registers (1887–1891).

[40] It is remarkable how enduring ideas about cancer causation have been, even into the twentieth century. See Elizabeth Toon, ' "Cancer as the General Population Knows It": Knowledge, Fear, and Lay Education in 1950s Britain', *Bulletin of the History of Medicine*, 81:1 (2007), 116–38.

[41] James Nooth, *Observations on the Treatment of Scirrhous Tumours, and Cancers of the Breast* (London, 1804), 82.

[42] *Woman and Her Diseases, from the Cradle to the Grave: Adapted Exclusively to Her Instruction in the Physiology of her System and all the Diseases of her Critical Periods* (New York, 1847), 215.

[43] *Berrow's Worcester Journal*, 2 May 1874, 3.

Historian Mary E. Fissell calls this emphasis on long-term causation of disease, 'the central interpretative structure in early modern medical thought, popular and professional'.[44] Galenic influences have persisted into the twenty-first century too. People might be described as 'hot-headed', or they might 'catch' a 'cold' from the temperature of the air or the changing season.

Thus, cancer's reframing as a surgical entity with a tangible manifestation was as much dependent on the shifting balance of power between surgeons and physicians as it was on the decline of humoral theories. The conventional hierarchy situated physicians above surgeons—with apothecaries and alternative practitioners somewhere below the two. Physicians traditionally trained at either Oxford or Cambridge, and received broad, humanistic educations replete with classical literature, ethics, and physiology. Surgeons were trained by apprenticeships, and had only recently divested themselves from their butcher brothers. However, at the end of the eighteenth century, surgeons were increasingly articulating themselves as equal—intellectually and socially—to physicians. The specialist hospital in particular was a way for peripheral practitioners—often surgeons—to climb the professional ladder and gain personal prestige.[45] This was not the case for the Middlesex—as those involved were not, by and large, men who were at the outset of their careers, or in need of a niche in which to make their names, or to 'step to fame and fortune by means of bricks and mortar'.[46] However, not only did the Middlesex make cancer into a local, 'surgical' disease, it also allowed surgeons an increasing proportion of clinical space and prestige. Most of those in prominent positions on The Middlesex Hospital's cancer ward were surgeons rather than physicians.

Bringing cancer into the hospital ward provided those surgeons with regular encounters with the disease and foregrounded the post-mortem as a primary mechanism for knowledge acquisition. In almost every case cancer was diagnosed by surgical touch, and texts privileged the haptic skill of the practitioner in identifying the disease and its prognosis. Such skills were specific to the surgeon, who was increasingly articulating his profession in terms of the craft-like status of his practice. John Pearson wrote, 'Chirurgical writers have generally enumerated *tumour* as an essential symptom of the Scirrhus [cancer]; and it is very true.'[47] Whereas in the eighteenth century this element of the surgical identity—a close association with manual labour, the butcher, and the barber—had been a 'vice' that relegated the surgeon below the intellectual and moral elitism of physician,

---

[44] Fissell, 'The Disappearance of the Patient's Narrative', 99.

[45] George Weisz, *Divide and Conquer: A Comparative History of Medical Specialization* (Oxford, 2005).

[46] Lindsay Granshaw, '"Fame and Fortune by Means of Bricks and Mortar": The Medical Profession and Specialist Hospitals in Britain', in Granshaw and Porter, *The Hospital in History*.

[47] John Pearson, *Practical Observations on Cancerous Complaints: With an Account of Some Diseases Which Have been Confounded with the Cancer* (London, 1792), 9.

in the nineteenth it was reframed as a virtue that endowed him with a special, almost artistic ability to touch and therefore to know. Indeed, throughout the nineteenth century, cancer was almost exclusively the preserve of the surgeon: they encountered the patients, treated the disease, and produced the relevant and prominent texts.

This emphasis on the tumour, and the perceived clinical value of hospital-based physical examination, is clear from The Middlesex Hospital's case notes. They described women brushing their hands over their bodies during bathing, noticing something that had not been there before. The surgeon who wrote up Barbara Daves' case of breast cancer in 1824 recorded, 'she surely discovered it by shaping her hand over it and feeling the irregularity'.[48] The women identified hard knots in soft flesh, uneven lumps in previously smooth skin, and subtle shifts in the equilibrium of the body—changes in menstruation, for example.[49] Indeed, menstruation, motherhood, and menopause were periods of intense risk. Most of the practitioners surveyed in this chapter agreed that women were more vulnerable to cancer than men, but all also acknowledged that male cancers were by no means uncommon, and even noted that men could suffer from cancers of the breast. Thomas Denman wrote, 'women who menstruate irregularly or with pain, or who have profuse discharges at each period, are suspected to be more liable to Cancer than those who are regular, or who do not suffer at those times'.[50] However, the tumour was the primary site of investigation in the clinic. Cancer was, first and foremost, an 'object' that could be identified by a trained observer (with hand or eye). Touch was, therefore, crucial in the diagnosis of cancer, and surgeons depended on haptic skill and a rich textural vocabulary in their identification and definition of the disease.

When a patient arrived at hospital they were subjected to physical examination. Case notes recorded what tumours had in common with each other, and how they differed in physical appearance and texture. Tumours were often described as either 'moveable' or 'fixed', suggesting surgeons manipulated their patient's bodies with their fingers. Abernethy wrote of one class of cancers that they could endure 'even a rough examination by the hand'.[51] His choice of words here gives a possible insight into the way he treated and handled the patients who sought his care and advice. If a growth was 'fixed' then it was likely cancerous. This diagnostic technique continues to be used today, with twenty-first-century doctors palpating tumours to identify 'site', 'size', and 'shape'.[52] The notes for Charlotte Skinnor

[48] UCLH Archive, 'Barbara Daves'.

[49] Thomas Denman, Observations on the Cure of Cancer, with Some Remarks upon Mr Young's Treatment of that Disease (London, 1816), 43.

[50] Ibid.   [51] Abernethy, Surgical Observations on Tumours, 22.

[52] As Charles E. Rosenberg has noted, there is 'social power' in the naming and diagnosis of disease. This is a power that early nineteenth-century practitioners had to fall back on in absence of therapeutic success. Charles E. Rosenberg, 'The Tyranny of Diagnosis: Specific Entities and Individual Experience', The Milbank Quarterly, 80 (2002), 237–60.

described how 'the breast is drawn in and adherent to the sternum'.[53] Tumours could be 'compact' and 'imbedded in fat'.[54] Or, 'attached' to the ribs.[55] Sarah McMurdy's breast cancer was described as 'very tender to the touch'.[56] Sarah Hill's breast cancer 'had the appearance of a cauliflower', and, 'on being opened or twisted...let out a...wheyish greenish or brownish fluid'.[57] Again, the descriptions of the surgeon's examination suggests rough handling of the patient's body—Sarah Hill's growth was 'twisted' and Sarah McMurdy likely expressed pain when her breast was examined.

In many cases, physical intervention disrupted the tumour's integrity. The investigation of cancer in the clinic was carried out by a combination of sensory interrogations—tumours were looked at, prodded, smelt, and sometimes tasted. Then, these various physical details were turned into identifying characteristics:

> The puckering of the skin, the dull leaden colour of the integuments, the knotted and uneven feel of the disease, the occasional darting pains in the part, its fixed attachment to the skin above, and muscles beneath, form so striking an assemblage of symptoms, that, when they are all present, there cannot be the smallest doubt that the tumour is a scirrhus.[58]

This 'assemblage of symptoms' guided the practitioner towards his diagnosis and privileged the surgical senses.

Case notes often used comparisons to fruit, nuts, and eggs to make clear the size, shape, and characteristics of the cancer tumour. Early stage growths were frequently described in case notes as nuts—hard objects that retained their form and were solid to the touch. Lydia Dettmer had a 'tumour of the size of a hazelnut' taken out of her left breast.[59] Cancer transformed the body into something unrecognizable—it converted previously soft, yielding skin and muscle into a new and troubling substance: the hardness of the malignant tumour.

However, as tumours grew, they invariably started to collapse at the centre. Cancer was not just a 'lump'—a rounded or smooth protuberance—but a fragile

---

[53] UCLH Archive, London, 'Charlotte Skinnor', Case Notes from the Cancer Ward at the Middlesex Hospital (1805–1838), 1814.

[54] UCLH Archive, 'Barbara Daves'.

[55] UCLH Archive, London, 'Sophia Othen', Case Notes from the Cancer Ward at the Middlesex Hospital (1805–1838), 1811.

[56] UCLH Archive, London, 'Sarah McMurdy', Case Notes from the Cancer Ward at the Middlesex Hospital (1805–1838), 1811.

[57] UCLH Archive, London, 'Sarah Hill', Case Notes from the Cancer Ward at the Middlesex Hospital (1805–1838), 1816.

[58] Samuel Cooper, *The First Lines of the Practice of Surgery: Designed as an Introduction for Students, and a Concise Book of Reference for Practitioners*, vol. 1, 4th edn (London, 1819), 257.

[59] UCLH Archive, London, 'Lydia Dettmer', 1811, Case Notes from the Cancer Ward at the Middlesex Hospital (1805–1838).

object that could and would disintegrate. This ulceration disrupted the body's boundaries.[60] One surgeon wrote:

> A softening or decaying of the cancerous matter takes place in the interior of the mass. This mass of a soft and yellowish colour, when thrown out, leaves a deep hole or cavity in the tumour...the walls of these hollows or pits gradually become decomposed, and so enlarging the cavities, while the cancer itself rapidly increases in the adjoining parts.[61]

This process described the experience of most of the Middlesex patients. Admitted to the ward in 1805, Jane Barnes' growth 'supported discharge plentifully from three small openings'; Ann Darney's breast cancer had been 'an open sore a year'; Charlotte Skinnor's nipple was 'entirely destroyed' by an 'ulcer on the right breast of about 12 months [sic] continuance'; and Ann Dawson's 'cancerous ulceration' was 'a deep cavity'.[62] These evocative descriptions call to mind the image of cancer 'eating away' at the healthy flesh and consuming the body from the inside out. They also give possible insight into the suffering—physical, emotional, and social—experienced by people living with cancer. These women had open and sometimes deep sores on their bodies for months, even years.

Fruit and eggs provided meaningful and not just practical analogies. They described cancer's capacity for putridity because they—like tumours—had the potential for decay. Both were natural objects with a tendency towards decomposition, and both could occupy that anxious territory between living and dead, growth and decline. In 1825 Ann Sharp came to the ward with a tumour in her left breast 'about the size of an orange'.[63] At around the same time, Scottish surgeon James Young Simpson wrote about finding a tumour 'the size of a small pear' attached to a woman's cervix.[64] Abernethy recorded the case of a lady 'about twenty-seven years of age', who 'had a tumour between the breast and the axilla, which had gradually increased during a year and a half to the size of a goose egg'.[65] Eggs had obvious parallels with the natural structure of a cancer tumour. They contained within them growth potential and were, quite literally, reproductive.[66]

---

[60] Barbara Duden refers to the 'strategic importance of the body and the symbolic value of its integrity'. Cancer's disruption of that integrity was, therefore, not only unpleasant but profoundly distressing. *The Woman beneath the Skin: A Doctor's Patients in Eighteenth-Century Germany*, trans. Thomas Dunlap (London, 1991), 10.

[61] J. Weldon Fell, *A Treatise on Cancer, and its Treatment* (London, 1857), 10.

[62] UCLH Archive, London, 'Jane Barnes', 1805; 'Anne Darney', 1810; 'Charlotte Skinnor', 1814; 'Anne Dawson', 1826; Case Notes from the Cancer Ward at the Middlesex Hospital (1805–1838).

[63] UCLH Archive, London, 'Ann Sharp', Case Notes from the Cancer Ward at the Middlesex Hospital (1805–1838), 1825.

[64] James Young Simpson, *Cases of Excision of the Cervix Uteri for Carcinomatous Disease* (Dublin, 1846), 4.

[65] Abernethy, *Surgical Observations on Tumours*, 41.

[66] There is a long-standing conceptualization of cancer as both 'of' the body, and separate from it. This finds expression in the ancient metaphoric connections—as identified by Susan Sontag—between cancer and a pregnancy. *Illness as Metaphor and AIDs and Its Metaphors* (London, 2013), 45.

Bringing cancer onto the ward also foregrounded the post-mortem as a primary mechanism for knowledge acquisition. While post-mortems were problematic and contested in early nineteenth-century society, the Middlesex had its own dead house, where examinations were conducted and most of the patients who died on the ward were dissected. Investigations after the patient had died assisted practitioners in the categorization of different types of tumour. Indeed, when cancer was categorized and catalogued—such as by John Abernethy in his *Surgical Observations on Tumours*—it was done so according to the tumour's materiality and appearance (the pathological anatomical approach privileged by Paris medicine), rather than site or symptoms.[67] Abernethy described one category of cancer—'pulpy or medullary sarcoma'—as resembling the brain in look and texture. He sketched (with words) its 'structure and feel' and referenced its 'pulpy consistence'.[68] Another class of tumour—pancreatic sarcoma—was

> Made up of irregularly shaped masses; in colour, texture and size resembling the larger masses which compose the pancreas. They appear also to be connected with each other, like the portions of that gland, by a fibrous substance of looser texture.[69]

This tumour was designated 'pancreatic', not because of the site in which it was most commonly found—rather, it 'more frequently occurs in the female breast'—but because of the texture it shared with that organ.[70]

The language of cancer case notes was, therefore, metaphorically rich, alluding to the reification of the disease's problematic identity. Cancers were frequently described as 'degenerating', a word that encased a litany of meanings ranging from a decline in character or qualities, an alteration from a normal type, to reduce to a lower or worse condition, and revolt. All implied something meaningful about cancer—that it had a 'natural' trajectory that involved various 'evolutionary' stages, that it manifested something corrupt in the corporeal, and that the body was rebelling against itself. The language of these notes reveals a way of conceptualizing cancer through analogy to irreversible natural processes and speedy expansions: 'decomposing', 'enlarging', 'rapidly increases', and 'destroyed'. In practical terms, those suffering from cancer, and living in the area surrounding the Middlesex, were often unable to remain at home for the duration of their illness. At some point, the ulcerating cancer tumour became too much to bear. Not only would these men and women have been excluded from full social participation, power and privilege, and be seen in some way as different and deviant, they would have suffered severe physical limitations and restrictions. Cancer could be both disfiguring and disgusting. In 1801, *The Times* ran an obituary for the Countess of Holderness, who had died 'at the advanced age of seventy-six'. Her 'complaint' was a cancerous tumour in her mouth, which had

---

[67] Abernethy, *Surgical Observations on Tumours.*   [68] Ibid., 57.   [69] Ibid.   [70] Ibid.

'destroyed the upper jaw, and part of the tongue'.[71] One woman treated on The Middlesex Hospital's cancer wards a few decades later had a breast tumour that emitted such a foul smell that even Burnett's Solution, 'employed plentifully about the bed and outside the dressing', could not counteract it.[72]

The size and stench of a tumour meant patients required constant care and attendance as they were unable to use their own bodies in accustomed ways. As their bodies became noxious, they might no longer be able to contribute to the household economy or be welcome within the home. They could have been marked out as possessing pathological bodies, which for women was a status layered on top of their already 'flawed' and 'dependent' female bodies.[73] Surgeon Samuel Cooper wrote that cancer 'in a chronic state' was 'both a deformity and an oppression; and, in an inflamed or ulcerated state, is a source of severe pain and even of fatal mischief'.[74]

Understanding the materiality of cancer allows us to appreciate why men and women might have sought cancer care in hospital. A cancer's size shaped the experience of the disease for the patient, adding to their suffering and exclusion from the world, and making the choice to enter hospital walls rational. This was particularly true for the metropolitan poor, living at close quarters and dependent on a degree of physical health for their subsistence. Moreover, the cancer hospital allowed the study of physical manifestations of cancer. In almost every case cancer was diagnosed by touch, and texts privileged the haptic and observational skills of the practitioner in identifying the disease and its prognosis. Diagnosis was made during life, and then post-mortem examination decided the category of cancer from which the patient had suffered. Such examination skills were specific to the surgeon, who was increasingly articulating his profession in terms of the craft-like status of his practice.

The Cancer 'Life Course'

Despite its tangible, tactile nature, cancer was not just a tumour. Contemporaries observed that growths, then as now, could be malignant or benign, and could only be differentiated by their behaviour over long periods of time. This is what set the hospital apart as a mechanism for redefining cancer. For while private practice and the occasional hospital visitor might allow the practitioner temporary access

---

[71] 'Obituaries', *The Times*, 16 October 1801, 3.
[72] Burnett's Solution was a popular disinfectant. Alexander Shaw, Charles H. Moore, Campbell de Morgan, and Mitchell Henry, *Report of the Surgical Staff of the Middlesex Hospital, to the Weekly Board and Governors, Upon the Treatment of Cancerous Diseases in the Hospital, on the Plan Introduced by Dr Fell* (London, 1857), 67.
[73] See Susan Wendell, 'Toward a Feminist Theory of Disability', *Hypatia*, 4 (1989), 104–24, at 104.
[74] Cooper, *The First Lines of the Practice of Surgery*, 242.

to the diseased body and its attendant tumour, the Middlesex created a 'captive' cohort of cancer sufferers who could be observed (at least periodically) over the entire 'life course' of the disease, from diagnosis through to death and beyond.

Thus, cancer was not diagnosed by the senses alone. Instead, the disease was also defined by its long duration, its irreversible capacity for growth and spread, and ultimately its incurability. Practitioners accessed these characteristics using two methods: their own observation and their patients' narratives. These 'captive' patients were not just bodies to study—they spoke too. Extensive accounts of the cancer 'life cycle' frequently appeared in the case notes. Practitioners included descriptive detail and often reproduced the patient's 'own words' in full to sketch in the story from before they arrived at the hospital. In 1825, Hannah Thirlow was admitted to the Middlesex with a tumour in her left breast and her illness narrative was recorded, 'She states that about two years ago she discovered a lump about the size of a small nut. She says that about six months previously to her having discovered this lump she fell while dusting some shelves and struck her Breast.'[75]

As a result, while the construction of cancer as a surgical disease speaks to the well-documented transition from 'bedside' to 'hospital' medicine, the disease's other characteristics problematize this shift. Historians have characterized 'bedside medicine' as an informal system of medical theory and practice in which the patient narrative was prominent in the diagnostic process; where patients exerted considerable agency in both diagnosis and treatment; and where treatment was highly individualized according to the sufferer's physiology and pathology. They posit a transition from bedside to hospital medicine that occurred at the turn of the eighteenth century. This involved a proliferation of hospital-based care and a shift from a 'patient-centred' mode of diagnosis to an 'object-centred diagnosis' in which the clinician disregarded the patient's experience and narrative.[76] In 'bedside medicine', the patient and her voice were key to the diagnostic process because doctors could not understand the individual disease without them. In the 'hospital', the symptom was no longer synonymous with the disease—denigrating the value of the patient narrative

This new 'hospital medicine' paradigm sought instead the underlying anatomical correlate. Rather than attending to the subjective words of the patient, the doctor now found truth through an objective gaze directed at the body. N. D. Jewson claims that because of this reconceptualization, the 'sickman [sic]' disappeared in the early nineteenth century along with 'his [sic] narrative'.[77] However, while the physical lesion was crucial in the diagnosis of cancer—and the hospital offered practitioners new, systematic ways to analyse the tumour

---

[75] UCLH Archive, London, 'Hannah Thirlow', Case Notes from the Cancer Ward at the Middlesex Hospital (1805–1838), 1825.
[76] Fissell, 'The Disappearance of the Patient's Narrative'; Foucault, *The Birth of the Clinic*; Jewson, 'The Disappearance of the Sick-Man'.
[77] Jewson, 'The Disappearance of the Sick-Man'.

and its various forms—because of the disease's long duration the practitioner's 'objective gaze' had to work in tandem with the patient's illness narrative. In other words, it was not enough to simply observe and touch the tumour—surgeons had to speak to their patients as well.

Only rarely did men and women seek hospital help as soon as they identified their tumours. Instead, there was often a significant time lapse between someone feeling something awry in their own bodies and being admitted to the Middlesex. Thus, illness narratives served to fill in the life cycle of the disease before the patient arrived at the hospital doors. Ann Darney waited four years after first discovering the lump in her right breast, Eliza Willis and Ann Beazley each waited a year, and Ann Bradley waited five months.[78] Hayle Walshe estimated that cancer patients suffered for an average of twenty-seven months—just over two years— but that in some cases the disease could last for decades.[79]

As we have seen, while cancer started small, and at first would have been almost imperceptible—described as a small lump, pimple, or blemish—most people who sought care and attention at the hospital did so when suffering from tumours of considerable size. Towards the end of the eighteenth century, surgeon John Pearson held a consultation with a woman whose breast was 'more than twice its natural size'.[80] Another patient treated by Pearson had a 'cancer in her right breast the bulk of a man's head'.[81] A patient cared for by John Abernethy had a tumour growing beneath the skin of her perineum, which 'descended as low as the middle of the thigh'.[82] Hayle Walshe quoted Professor P. H. Bérard, who had observed a tumour in the thigh of a woman 'as large as the body of a full-grown man', with 'veins larger than the index finger' supplying it with blood and nutrition.[83] Here, the cancer tumour was a parasite—almost humanoid in form. These extreme scales confirmed cancer as a disease with a monstrous capacity for growth and expansion—so much so that Walter Hayle Walshe wrote in 1846, 'One of the most essential attributes of cancerous substance is an unswerving tendency to grow.'[84]

This growth potential was not just about a tumour's ability to expand in size, but also cancer's tendency to metastasize. Those surgeons who felt surface cancer with their hands were well aware that these masses could be later-stage manifest-ations of an internal disease; or that breast cancer, for example, could spread to the liver or lungs. They knew that cancer could and would affect the internal organs, even if its presence there could only be verified after the person had died. The

---

[78] UCLH Archive, London, 'Anne Darney', 1810; 'Eliza Willis', 1813; 'Ann Beazley', 1814; 'Ann Bradley', 1814, Case Notes from the Cancer Ward at the Middlesex Hospital (1805–1838).

[79] Walter Hayle Walshe, *The Anatomy, Physiology, Pathology, and Treatment of Cancer* (Boston, MA, 1844), 127.

[80] Pearson, *Practical Observations on Cancerous Complaints*, 17.   [81] Ibid., 38.

[82] Abernethy, *Surgical Observations on Tumours*, 50.

[83] Hayle Walshe, *The Nature and Treatment of Cancer*, 15.   [84] Ibid., 134.

precise mechanism of spread was subject to intense debate, and ideas shifted over the course of the century. John Abernethy thought cancer might be spread through the lymphatic system and be 'communicated from one gland to another'.[85] He believed that the disease 'begins in a small spot and extends in its progress from thence in all directions, like rays from a centre'.[86]

Thomas Denman had a slightly different, more material model, 'The disease is making its progress into the constitution or the neighbouring parts, by means of the firm whitish bands.'[87] Cancer would extend its physical tendrils through the body, amassing at certain points like nodes on a web woven through the body's textures. In the 1840s, Hayle Walshe wrote about the movement of 'cancerous cells' through the bloodstream.[88] This new phase of spread was signalled by symptoms that affected the entire body, not just the site of the initial tumour. Italian surgeon Antonio Scarpa described how one patient began 'to complain of general weakness, faintness of stomach and wandering pains over the whole body'.[89] Patients might also complain of localized aches distant from the original tumour, or external signs—such as jaundice in cases of metastases in the liver— might alert the surgeon to internal extension.[90]

Thus, while the repeated study of cancerous bodies and tumours helped to construct cancer as a surgical disease and a material entity known primarily through touch and skilled observation during the patient's life and after their death, the clinic also allowed medical men to trace cancer through its life course, making possible extended observations of its duration and its tendency to grow and metastasize. Starting small, the initially innocuous cancer tumour grew to monstrous proportions, inflicting acute emotional, social, and physical suffering. Then, practitioners watched their subjects die with depressing regularity, and the intimacy of the early nineteenth-century clinical interaction likely structured a wretched experience for both doctor and patient.

These ideas about cancer's capacity for growth and metastasis also had purchase in broader cultural and political discourse. In 1791, *The Times* referred to the Grand Gallic Charter in terms that would have been familiar to Middlesex medical men:

> It may not inaptly, be compared to a cancerous excrescence, the greater part of which, in hopes of saving the patient, it is necessary to cut off; and which, after

---

[85] Abernethy, *Surgical Observations on Tumours*, 70.   [86] Ibid.

[87] Denman, *Observations on the Cure of Cancer*, 17–18.

[88] See Chapter 5 for more on cell theories of cancer. Hayle Walshe, *The Nature and Treatment of Cancer*, 62.

[89] Antonio Scarpa, *Remarks and Practical Results of Observation on Scirrhus and Cancer*, trans. James Briggs (London, 1822), 33.

[90] Such as with the case of Sarah Moore, who died at the Middlesex in 1813; UCLH Archive, London, 'Sarah Moore', 1813, Case Notes from the Cancer Ward at the Middlesex Hospital (1805–1838).

being separated from the body, will, notwithstanding, leave the germ of another excrescence.[91]

Fifty years later, an English MP described the 'unjust and miserable system of paying wages out of rates' as 'the cancer which has got such a powerful hold of the southern provinces', and which 'was gradually eating its way to the heart of England'.[92] Both quotations make recourse to the language of living creatures—'germ' and 'eating'—and in doing so reflect the mutability and applicability of cancer metaphors to the climate of Britain in the long nineteenth century. Cancer was both material and a powerful metaphorical force—one that could be deployed in various ways and to various ends.[93]

Conclusion

The Middlesex Hospital confirmed the view of cancer as a disease with a physical manifestation (the tumour) and made clear its irreversible and distressing trajectory from small to all-consuming. Of course, these characteristics were known before the hospitalization of cancer, and the disease's profile helped to justify the establishment of The Middlesex Hospital's cancer wards in the first place. Nonetheless, the institution transformed occasional or periodic observations of cancer's trajectory into essential characteristics that defined the disease and directed diagnosis and treatment. The hospital context allowed for new regimes of care that enabled the comparative study of cancer's material manifestations and privileged the physical examination of the patient's body. While in the eighteenth century and before, cancer was generally thought of as a 'constitutional' malady, by the early nineteenth century, cancer was reconfigured as a 'local' disease—something that started 'life' somewhere discrete in the body before spreading to distant parts. The hospital and the surgeons who worked there identified the tumour as the primary sign of malignancy and by bringing cancer into the institution, the Middlesex provided practitioners with frequent opportunities to observe the disease.

The value of case notes as an historical source is clear, particularly when they capture illnesses of long duration. They demonstrate that cancer was more than just an object, more than just a tumour. Instead, these growths could only be understood when watched for an extended period of time. Only then could contemporaries determine whether the tumours were malignant or benign. This requirement made the hospital—with its captive cohort of patients—the ideal place to define and identify cancer. While private practice and the odd person who

---

[91] 'France', *The Times*, 9 August 1791, 2.   [92] HC Deb., vol. 56, cc375–451, 8 February 1841.
[93] S. Lochlann Jain, *Malignant: How Cancer Becomes Us* (Berkeley, CA, 2013), 14.

managed to circumvent hospital admissions regulations allowed some practitioners brief and occasional access to people living with and dying from cancer, the institutionalization of cancer offered surgeons and physicians the opportunity to study people through the entire 'life course' of their disease.

Finally, cancer case notes and the language used to describe patients' bodies attests to the problematic identity of cancer in this period and the reification of its associated metaphors. The hospital captured and concentrated deeply felt anxieties about cancer's characteristics; such as its materiality, capacity for growth, and potential to metastasize. Moreover, the hospital also allowed practitioners to witness—on a new scale—the relentless incurability of cancer. In Chapter 2, 'Incurability and the Clinic', I delve deeper in the rationales and justifications of those who founded and first worked in The Middlesex Hospital's cancer ward and other contemporaneous institutions. I argue that such institutions were vehicles for self-fashioning and professional identity formation, and that they reified cancer's key characteristic: its incurability.

2

Incurability and the Clinic

On 28 May 1802, the philanthropist Sir Thomas Bernard (1750–1818) wrote:

> In the long train of diseases to which human nature is subject, no one is attended
> with more hopeless misery than that which is denominated cancer, whatever part
> of the body may be the seat of it. This occurs far more frequently than is generally
> supposed; and a calamity so pitiable as that of persons afflicted with cancer, in
> any rank or situation in life (all being alike subject to them) it is hardly possible to
> imagine; their suffering being aggravated by the present insufficiency of medi-
> cine, to afford any proportionate relief...In fact, little is at present known of
> cancer, but as an incurable disease; and after a great number of trials and
> attempts to discover a method of cure, the faculty seems to have been reduced
> to a state of despondency; as if both science and art were exhausted, or were
> unequal to the difficulties they have to encounter.[1]

In this passage, Bernard interlaced various threads of early nineteenth-century
cancer discourse and articulated a common set of concerns. He confirmed cancer
as an incurable disease, and elevated it above rival maladies as a superlative threat
to the human body. None of the other diseases 'to which human nature is subject'
provoked more 'hopeless misery'. He layered his lamentations with affective
pronouncements on the special suffering of cancer patients and emphasized the
harmful influence of medical 'insufficiency' on their emotional states. Bernard
wove a tapestry of repeated failure, wasted efforts, and 'despondency'; of art and
science 'exhausted' and 'unequal' to the dreaded foe. This was an adversarial
image of a losing battle with real, human costs, and cancer—the incurable
disease—as implacable foe.

Bernard was born in Lincoln and spent some of his early life in British North
America, where his father was Governor of Massachusetts. He began a course at
Harvard University but the uneven political climate of the colony forced him to
abandon his studies and return to England, where he amassed his fortune through
the dual success of his legal work and his marriage. From the late eighteenth
century, he devoted much of his time to ameliorating the living and working

---

[1] Thomas Bernard, 'Extract from an Account of the Institution for Investigating the Nature and
Cure of Cancer', in *Reports of the Society for Bettering the Condition and Increasing the Comforts of the
Poor*, vol. 3 (London, 1802), 355.

The Cancer Problem: Malignancy in Nineteenth-Century Britain. Agnes Arnold-Forster, Oxford University Press (2021).
© Agnes Arnold-Forster. DOI: 10.1093/oso/9780198866145.003.0003

conditions of the poor, and in 1796 helped to establish the Society for Bettering the Condition and Increasing the Comforts of the Poor. He continued to invest in a diverse range of interests and projects, including a school for the indigent blind, a fever hospital, and in 1802, the Society and Institution for Investigating the Nature and Cure of Cancer.

The extract at the start of this chapter comes from the preface Bernard wrote to an account of this new organization. In the account, he described how a collection of elite surgeons and physicians acquired a house near Tottenham Court Road in London and converted it into a hospital for the care of cancer patients. This institution followed in the footsteps of Middlesex Hospital's cancer ward, established in November 1792 just down the road; the latter, as we have seen in Chapter 1, received 'a contribution of three Thousand Pounds for establishing a Fund for the endowment of a Ward for the reception of Persons afflicted with that disorder [cancer], and four Hundred Pounds to fit up the Ward'.[2] Its new neighbour, however, had more ambitious national and international plans. While both were preoccupied by the observation and retention of cancer patients, the Society and Institution also wanted to develop a new network of cancer knowledge exchange, personal association, and belonging for elite medical and surgical practitioners in London and abroad.

In 1802, and in pursuit of this lofty goal, the Society and Institution issued a set of thirteen queries, designed to collate existing knowledge and to extend the community of medical men interested in cancer beyond the confines of the metropolis.[3] These were a set of basic questions to be circulated to all members of the medical community, regardless of membership in the Society and Institution.[4] The queries covered a range of subjects, and they shaped cancer investigation throughout the nineteenth century and beyond. They explored questions of causation and diagnosis and interrogated the relationship between cancer, inheritance, and contagion. They also covered climate, temperament, cancer in animals, and period of life. These questions provoked multiple responses from all over the British Isles, and various practitioners were motivated to write tracts and treatises in pursuit of some of the answers.

It was the thirteenth and final query, however, that provoked the most communication and consternation. It asked, 'Is cancer under any circumstances susceptible of a natural cure?' As shown in Chapter 1, the clinic allowed medical men to trace cancer through its life course, making possible extended observations of its duration and its tendency to grow and metastasize. Starting small, the initially innocuous cancer tumour grew to monstrous proportions, inflicting

---

[2] UCLH Archive, London, 'Weekly Board Meeting', Middlesex Hospital Minutes, 29 November 1791.
[3] Bruce Schoenberg, 'A Program for the Conquest of Cancer: 1802', *Journal of the History of Medicine and Allied Sciences*, 30 (1975), 3–22, esp. 3.
[4] Ibid., 10.

acute emotional, social, and physical suffering. Then, practitioners watched their subjects decline and die with depressing regularity. These observations, coupled with new knowledge gathered from across the medical community, transformed not only the social and cultuGral status of cancer, but codified aspects of the disease's identity that had long been suspected: namely, its incurability.

In what follows, I will show how the hospitalization and concerted study of cancer gave the care of the disease new legitimacy, tied it closely to the investigative and charitable projects of the metropolitan medical elite, and provided cancer with a presence in London's built environment. It was in this moment that the disease moved out of the confines of the sickbed and entered the culture, politics, and social world of the early nineteenth-century metropolis. This chapter reveals how the capital's medical elite defined cancer as an incurable malady and as a problem that they, as a collective needed to overcome. Cancer's new incurable status was, therefore, not just a biological observation, but had great rhetorical power. Medical men—and primarily surgeons—used the diseases' incurability to establish certain communal credentials, such as humanity, restraint and intellectual nuance; they also articulated a professional chronology and progressive teleology.

Indeed, while surgeons, physicians, and philanthropists—like Sir Thomas Bernard—derived social and intellectual capital from lamentations and doubt, they also professed profound optimism, and contrasted current incurability with future and, as they saw it, inevitable medical mastery over malignancy. This chapter will begin by establishing the boundaries and biographies of the early nineteenth-century 'cancer community' and particularly of those men who participated in the Society and Institution from its inception. Then it will examine the clinical evidence for cancer's incurability and interrogate the meaning and implications of 'cured', 'incurable', and 'to cure' in early nineteenth-century parlance and medical thought. I will end this chapter with an exploration of the different ways that incurability was deployed as a discursive tool and suggest that this disease characteristic reflected and contributed to the culture of metropolitan medicine and to the 'imagined community' of practitioners.[5]

The Cancer Community

Both the Society and Institution for Investigating the Nature and Cure of Cancer and Middlesex Hospital attracted the medical and surgical elite of turn-of-the-century London—men who participated in a pre-existing network of intellectual

---

[5] Michael Brown, 'Medicine, Reform and the "End" of Charity in Early Nineteenth-Century England', *English Historical Review*, 124 (2009), 1353–88; Michael Brown, *Performing Medicine: Medical Culture and Identity in Provincial England, c. 1760–1850* (Manchester, 2011).

communication and personal connections. In what follows, I will briefly recount the biographies of some of the men most intimately involved in the 'cancer community' and outline their criss-crossing network of relationships, both personal and professional. Thomas Denman (1733–1815) was a man-midwife and surgeon. Born in Derbyshire, at age twenty he moved to London to study medicine at St George's Hospital.[6] He was, by all accounts, cheerful and amiable. A 'well-cultivated and entertaining man', he took an active interest in public charities.[7] He had a modest background—his father was an apothecary—and soon after starting his studies he ran out of cash. In 1753, he joined the navy as a surgeons' mate and spent the next nine years abroad and aboard ship. In 1764, he gained an MD from Aberdeen University before returning to London and renting a small house off the Haymarket. In 1769, he was appointed physician-accoucheur to Middlesex Hospital but by the 1780s his professional visibility, publications, and patient numbers had increased to such an extent that he had to resign the post, although he continued to sit on the hospital's board. He was instrumental in the establishment of the cancer ward and was secretary to the Society and Institution.[8]

In 1777, Denman married Elizabeth Brodie (1747–1833), younger daughter of an army linen draper; they had one son, Thomas Denman (1779–1854), and twin daughters, one of whom married the anatomist and physician Matthew Baillie (1762–1828).[9] Baillie was John and William Hunter's nephew and, after finishing his degrees at Oxford, attended dissections and lectures at the anatomy school and museum in Great Windmill Street, just off Tottenham Court Road, in London. Baillie soon became an established anatomy lecturer himself. He was appointed physician at St George's Hospital in 1787. He was Croonian Lecturer of the Royal Society in 1791 and Goulstonian Lecturer for the Royal College of Physicians of London in 1794. He gave the Harveian Oration in 1798, and in 1805 he was a founder member of the Medical and Chirurgical Society of London, forerunner of the Royal Society of Medicine.[10] Following these various accolades, he was appointed to the Medical Committee of the Society and Institution for Investigating the Nature and Cure of Cancer in 1802.[11] Just eight years later, he was appointed Physician-Extraordinary to King George III.[12]

Everard Home (1756–1832) was a surgeon and chief curator of the Hunterian Museum. The son of a former army surgeon, he was born in Hull and educated at Westminster School.[13] Despite gaining a scholarship to Cambridge in 1773, he chose instead to become a surgical pupil of his brother-in-law, John Hunter

---

[6] Ornella Moscucci, 'Denman, Thomas (1733–1815)', in *Oxford Dictionary of National Biography* (Oxford, 2004).

[7] Ibid.   [8] Schoenberg, 'Program for the Conquest of Cancer', 10.

[9] John Jones, 'Baillie, Matthew (1761–1823)', in *Oxford Dictionary of National Biography*.

[10] Ibid.   [11] Schoenberg, 'Program for the Conquest of Cancer', 10.

[12] Jones, 'Baillie, Matthew (1761–1823)'.

[13] N. G. Coley, 'Home, Sir Everard, First Baronet (1756–1832)', in *Oxford Dictionary of National Biography*.

(1728–1793). Hunter had married Home's sister Anne in 1771 after a seven-year courtship. Home lived in Leicester Square, built up a large surgical practice, and had a glittering professional career of lectures, papers, and other successes. However, his reputation was dogged by accusations of plagiarism. Home drew heavily on Hunter's work in the papers and books which he published after his brother-in-law's death. He had most of Hunter's papers destroyed in 1823, only after he had stripped his work for his own publications.[14] In 1802, Home was appointed surgeon to the Society and Institution.[15]

John Abernethy (1764–1831) was born in London and was one of five children of John Abernethy, a merchant, and his wife, Elizabeth Weir from Ireland. At the age of fifteen he was apprenticed to Charles Blicke, surgeon to St Bartholomew's Hospital in London.[16] In 1787, he was appointed Assistant Surgeon at St Bart's, a post he held for twenty-eight years before promotion to full surgeon. He was elected a Fellow of the Royal Society in 1796 and served as Professor of Anatomy and Surgery at the Royal College of Surgeons of England from 1814 to 1817.[17] Abernethy was best known as a medical practitioner and enjoyed a large private practice in London. He was notoriously brusque and abrupt with patients, regardless of their wealth and social standing. While he was by no means everybody's idea of a good doctor, his plain speaking attracted a fierce following. Like Home, Abernethy was appointed surgeon to the Society and Institution in 1802.[18]

The illustrious list of medical men appointed to work at the institution also included: Thomas Young (1773–1829), Fellow of the Royal College of Physicians; Pelham Warren (1778–1835), Physician to St George's; Robert Willan (1757–1812), a dermatologist and successful private practitioner; James Sims (1741–1820), President of the Medical Society of London for twenty-two years; and John Pearson, Fellow of both the Royal Society and the Linnaean Society.[19] These men represented the medical orthodoxy of the time. Several of the committee members were associated with the famed anatomist John Hunter. While Hunter died in 1793, Abernethy, Home, Pearson, Baillie, and Denman had, at one time or another, studied under him.[20] The surgeons and physicians involved in the Society and Institution for Investigating the Nature and Cure of Cancer were all connected through the medical institutions and societies of London. This pre-existing network was both professional and personal; for example, Denman's daughter married Matthew Baillie and Home was Hunter's

[14] Ibid.   [15] Schoenberg, 'Program for the Conquest of Cancer', 10.
[16] L. S. Jacyna, 'Abernethy, John (1764–1831)', Oxford Dictionary of National Biography.
[17] Ibid.   [18] Schoenberg, 'Program for the Conquest of Cancer', 10.
[19] Geoffrey Cantor, 'Young, Thomas (1773–1829)', in Oxford Dictionary of National Biography; Victor A. Triolo, 'The Institution for Investigating the Nature and Cure of Cancer: A Study of Four Excerpts', Medical History, 13 (1969), 11–28, esp. 20; W. W. Webb, 'Warren, Pelham (1778–1835)', rev. Patrick Wallis, in Oxford Dictionary of National Biography.
[20] Schoenberg, 'Program for the Conquest of Cancer', 5.

brother-in-law.[21] As individuals and a collective they have been subjected to considerable historical attention. However, their interest in cancer—marked by a considerable written output—has not been explored.[22]

These individuals produced most of the tracts on cancer published in Britain in this period. Denman completed his *Observations on the Cure of Cancer* in 1810, and Home wrote two tracts on cancer, *Observations on Cancer: Connected with Histories of the Disease* in 1805 and *A Short Tract on the Formation of Tumours* in 1830.[23] Abernethy published a full text on cancer, *Surgical Observations on Tumours* (1811), but made extensive reference to the disease in four of his other published works.[24] These four texts, along with Pearson's *Practical Observations on Cancerous Complaints* (1792), provide much of the theoretical material for this chapter.

Everard Home and friends were part of an established culture of medical charity and both societies had explicit philanthropic functions. This culture reached its zenith in the late eighteenth century.[25] Much has been written about the process of hospitalization at the end of the eighteenth century, and about the move towards specialization in the nineteenth. However, the two cancer institutions pre-dated the specialist hospitals of the mid-nineteenth century by fifty years and were, perhaps, the first of their kind.[26] The Society and Institution for Investigating the Nature and Cure of Cancer also had benevolent foundations. It had 'very liberal' support, and was financed by an endowment from the Society for Bettering the Condition and Increasing the Comforts of the Poor, founded in 1796 by Bernard.[27] In 1802, as mentioned, the Society and Institution issued a set of thirteen queries.[28] In a reprint of the queries, the Society and Institution's committee wrote:

In order to form a basis of inquiry, in which the nature and cure of cancer, it is presumed, may be pursued with all the advantages of reason and experience, the

---

[21] Jones, 'Baillie, Matthew (1761–1823)'.

[22] There are two essays on the history of the Society and Institution for Investigating the Nature and Cure of Cancer, but neither situates it within the broader context of early nineteenth-century medicine. See Schoenberg, 'Program for the Conquest of Cancer' and Triolo, 'Institution for Investigating the Nature and Cure of Cancer'.

[23] Everard Home, *Observations on Cancer: Connected with Histories of the Disease* (London, 1805); Everard Home, *A Short Tract on the Formation of Tumours: And the Peculiarities that are Met with in the Structure of Those that Have become Cancerous; with their Mode of Treatment* (London, 1830).

[24] John Abernethy, *Surgical Observations on Tumours* (London, 1811).

[25] Some scholars have seen this as an attempt to rationalize the labour market, others as a form of social and moral control. Brown, 'Medicine, Reform and the "End" of Charity', 1362.

[26] See Lindsay Granshaw, '"Fame and Fortune by Means of Brick and Mortar": The Medical Profession and Specialist Hospitals in Britain, 1800–1948', in Lindsay Granshaw and Roy Porter (eds.), *The Hospital in History* (London, 1991); George Weisz, 'The Emergence of Medical Specialization in the Nineteenth Century', *Bulletin for the History of Medicine*, 77 (2003), 536–75; George Weisz, *Divide and Conquer: A Comparative History of Medical Specialization* (Oxford, 2006).

[27] Bernard, 'Extract from an Account'.   [28] Ibid., 3.

Medical Committee very early drew out and distributed the following queries, for the consideration not only of the corresponding members, but of all medical men, to whom opportunities of answering them might, by study or by accident, occur.[29]

According to its own claims, in its first year there were already over fifty international corresponding members.[30]

The thirteen queries evidently inspired other physicians and surgeons from further afield to respond. Richard Carmichael, a surgeon from Dublin, wrote *An Essay on the Effects of Carbonate, and Other Preparations of Iron, Upon Cancer* in 1809 and called it, 'An attempt to answer the queries of the Medical Society, established in London, for investigating the nature and cure of cancer.'[31] John Rodman, a physician from Paisley, wrote in the introduction to his *Practical Explanation of Cancer in the Female Breast* (1818), 'This Treatise is ... in obedience to the *London Society*, which was instituted for investigating the nature and cure of *Cancer*. The liberal basis of so laudable an Institution, requires no apology for my humble endeavours.'[32]

Cancer and Incurability

The key contribution of the Society and Institution for Investigating the Nature and Cure of Cancer was to confirm cancer as an incurable disease. They made it into a malady that was distinct from others in that, regardless of bodily constitution and medical interventions, nature was never able to provide relief or reverse its trajectory. The clinic converted incurability from an incidental characteristic into an identifying one. With depressing regularity, the patients on the ward died. Unlike other hospitals, and even unlike the workhouse, most patients admitted to the cancer institutions never left.[33] Of the sixty female patients admitted between 1805 and 1838 for whom we have case records, approximately 70 per cent died. Those who did not, left of their own accord and sought palliation elsewhere. Hannah Cressford's case notes end with a heart-wrenching line, 'No prospect of cure was held out and she returned to her friends.'[34] In the early nineteenth

[29] Bernard, 'Extract from an Account', 382.

[30] Schoenberg, 'Program for the Conquest of Cancer', 3.

[31] Richard Carmichael, *An Essay on the Effects of Carbonate, and other Preparations of Iron, upon Cancer: With an Inquiry into the Nature of that and other Diseases to which it Bears a Relation* (Dublin, 1809), 4.

[32] John Rodman, *Practical Explanation of Cancer in the Female Breast* (London, 1818), vii.

[33] Across the nineteenth century, hospital death rates were usually under 10 per cent. See https://www.londonlives.org/static/Hospitals.jsp, accessed 2 August 2017.

[34] UCLH Archive, London, 'Hannah Cressford', 1805, Case Notes from the Cancer Ward at the Middlesex Hospital (1805–1838).

century cures could be effected in one of two ways—Hayle Walshe wrote, 'A disease is capable of cure either by a natural process or by art.'[35] Cancer was subjected to a double incurability. Not only was it insusceptible to a 'natural cure', it was also resilient in the face of treatment and could be neither reversed nor removed by medical interventions.

Early modern medicine placed great faith in the healing powers of nature, which could apply to all manner of ailments from injuries and accidents, repair after surgical operations, and internal diseases. This medical model blurred the boundary between curative interventions and the periodic management of ill-health. In 1772, William Cadogan, Fellow of the College of Physicians, began a treatise on chronic disease with an unsettling rhetorical device:

> The art of physic has now been practised, more or less regularly, above two thousand years; and most assuredly there is not yet discovered any one certain remedy for any disease. Ought not this to make us suspect that there is no such thing?[36]

He was not, however, suggesting that his chosen craft was futile and that all maladies were incurable, but was instead gesturing towards a subtle truism of medicine in that period—that medicine alone could never secure health for the body and could only be effective in deferent collaboration with nature. He wrote, 'The skilful in medicine, and learned in nature, know well that health is not to be established by medicine; for its effects are but momentary, and the frequent repetition of it destructive to the strongest frames.'[37] Medicine's role was, there-fore, to 'gently call...forth the powers of the body to act for themselves, intro-ducing gradually a little more and more activity, chosen diet, and, above all, peace of mind, changing intirely [sic] that course of life which first brought on the disease, medicine co-operating a little'.[38]

The relationship between health and ill-health was thus governed by nature—and she had long been endowed by the medical community and the laity alike with impressive curative powers. In the eighteenth century, sicknesses were commonly seen as the body's way of coping with imbalances or poisons in the system; hence, a malady was self-limiting and possessed its own internal logic. The humours would go awry, the body would display troubling symptoms, and then order would return. Thus, the mantra of the medical man at the turn of the eighteenth century was that he must—in most cases—allow nature to take its course.

---

[35] Walter Hayle Walshe, *The Anatomy, Physiology, Pathology, and Treatment of Cancer* (Boston, MA, 1844), 146.

[36] William Cadogan, *A Dissertation on the Gout, and all Chronic Diseases, Jointly Considered, as Proceeding from the Same Causes; What those Causes Are; and a Rational and Natural Method of Cure Proposed. Addressed to all Invalids* (London, 1772), 14.

[37] Ibid.   [38] Ibid.

The physician should leave the body alone to right itself—'The judicious physician ... confides in nature'—or provide only minimal interference: 'The best physicians, in every age, were those who, attentively watching the operations of nature, restrained them when *inordinate*, stimulated them when *torpid*, and confined them when sallying from the safe and medium course.'[39] This was true for mild, short-term ailments such as a cold and for severe, chronic maladies like gout. Cadogan chastised the patient who expected too much from their physician:

> Did ... [they] think they might live as they did with impunity, expecting repeated remedy from art; or, did they know any thing of the nature of medicine, they would find that though fits of pain have been relieved, or sickness cured by it for a time, the establishment of health is a very different thing.[40]

It was foolish to think the doctor could do anything but guide and coax nature towards a chosen resolution.

None of that is to say that early modern medicine was impotent in the face of sickness. That Cadogan had to chastise the patient for expecting a cure meant that it must have been within the realms of possibility to cure. 'To cure' must have existed as a concept, even if it was an unlikely outcome in many cases. In response to the build-up in the body of an imbalance of 'peccant humours' (toxic fluids), physicians had an entire arsenal of interventions to encourage the body's own attempts to expel bad blood, vile bile, or indurated faeces. Patients purged, emitted, sweated, and bled; and these interventions could be effective. The eighteenth-century actor David Garrick wrote to his doctor about a purge he had prescribed to his wife, 'She finds herself much better ... she ... swears, that you will restore her status quo.'[41] The purge had resettled her equilibrium, and returned her to health. In 1782, Lord Herbert informed the Reverend William Coxe that such remedies had produced positive effects, 'Bleeding, purging and sweating has cleared me completely of all ailing.'[42] These therapies had returned the body to normalcy—they had reversed decline. Thus, a 'cure' was not impossible, but health was not strictly dependent on medical intervention and the doctor's role was to collaborate with nature rather than overrule her.

---

[39] James Johnson, *Practical Researches on the Nature, Cure, and Prevention of Gout, in all its Open and Concealed Forms; Partly Translated and Condensed from the French of Guilbert and Hallé; with a Critical Examination of some Celebrated Remedies and Modes of Treatment Employed in this Disease* (London, 1819), iv.

[40] Cadogan, *A Dissertation on the Gout*, 13.

[41] Quoted in Dorothy Porter and Roy Porter, *In Sickness and in Health: The English Experience 1650–1850* (London, 1988), 265; David M. Little and George M. Karhl (eds.), *The Letters of David Garrick* (London, 1963), 164.

[42] Quoted in Porter and Porter, *In Sickness and in Health*, 266; Lord Herbert (ed.), *Pembroke Papers (1790–1794): Letters and Diaries of Henry, Tenth Earl of Pembroke and his Circle* (London, 1950), 199.

However, cancer did not conform to this pattern of recurring intervention and recovery. While with other maladies the body might correct its own imbalances— or, in some cases, require gentle and collaborative treatment to help nature along her way—cancer could not resolve itself. In 1802 the Society and Institution for Investigating the Nature and Cure of Cancer asked 'Is Cancer, under any circumstances, susceptible of a natural cure?'[43] In a later reprint of the thirteen queries, the committee responded with a resounding 'no':

> Many diseases and accidents, to which the human body is liable, are cured or repaired by some process of the constitution peculiarly and admirably adapted to the kind of disease or accident. But in no instance has every occurred, or been recorded, of cancer being cured by any natural process of the constitution.[44]

Crucially, here, the committee refers not just to 'diseases' but also to 'accidents'. Surgical injuries, as well as medical maladies, might be 'cured by any natural process'. However, while nature was powerful, even she had her limits. This suggests that cancer was set apart in its extreme opposition to a 'natural cure'. Indeed, Hayle Walshe argued that cancer's very 'nature' was 'opposed to resolution'.[45]

While the curability of a diseases was, at the end of the eighteenth century, best described as a spectrum with plenty of shades of grey between, there was also an acknowledged dichotomy between cancer and other maladies. Cancer was repeatedly designated the 'crudele opprobrium medicorum'—the *cruellest* challenge to the medical faculty.[46] It was a 'pernicious disease', synonymous with death and decline and feared by doctor and patient.[47] It was, 'of all the ills to which the human frame is liable', the 'most poignant'.[48] In various ways, therefore, cancer was articulated as superlative—as the most extreme case on a spectrum—it was the 'most' and the 'cruellest'. Thomas Denman insisted, 'Of all diseases deemed *incurable*, that which is denominated *Cancer* has been most generally allowed to be so.'[49] Of course, many other ailments ended in death in this period, but few were set on that trajectory from the moment of diagnosis. Cancer had no hope of resolution, and its identification fixed the patient on an irreversible decline. Thus, cancer's identity as an intractable malady was dependent on an implicit comparison—if cancer was unresolvable then it must follow that there were other diseases that practitioners could arrest and erase. There were, after all,

---

[43] Schoenberg, 'Program for the Conquest of Cancer', 10–13.
[44] Bernard, 'Extract from an Account', 389.
[45] Hayle Walshe, *The Anatomy, Physiology, Pathology, and Treatment of Cancer*, 146.   [46] Ibid.
[47] Abernethy, *Surgical Observations on Tumours*, 74.
[48] Thomas Pope, 'On Cancer', *Association Medical Journal*, 3 (1855), 859.
[49] Thomas Denman, *Observations on the Cure of Cancer, with some Remarks upon Mr. Young's Treatment of that Disease* (London, 1816), 3.

instances where an intervention might entirely halt a malady or repair an injury. For example, practitioners might 'cure' an acute fever with a good diet, leeches, and ice; and surgeons might sometimes save a life—'cure'—by removing a bullet, fixing a fracture, or amputating a limb. Thomas Denman wrote about how 'means have been gradually discovered by which the diseases the human frame is liable to, may be often prevented, always alleviated, and generally cured'.[50]

Not only was the designation 'incurable' dependent on an implicit comparison with illnesses that might be susceptible to either a natural cure or to interventionist coaxing, but cancer was defined as an incurable *disease*, rather than an incurable *body*. While there had long been 'incurable people'—a category of the population with ailing constitutions, unable to function in society because of systemic bodily or moral weaknesses—cancer was an invasive malady that took over body and soul, irrespective of constitutional strength and intellectual resilience. The surgeon John Pearson wrote, 'Cancer is...a disease which triumphs alike over the powers of the constitution, and the virtues of medicines.'[51] Here, he implied a distinction between the 'disease' and the 'constitution'—suggesting that cancer was an identifiable disease separate, and with a degree of agency, from the host body. Thomas Denman wrote that cancer 'possess[ed] a life distinct from that of the general frame'; and Abernethy argued that tumours were 'such swellings as arise from some new production, which made no part of the original composition of the body'.[52] Medical literature described cancer as an invasive and malignant force, against which the body had only meagre defences. There was something troublingly 'non-natural' about cancer—it was neither entirely 'of' the body, nor entirely separate from it—and would not succumb to a 'natural cure'.[53]

These metaphorical allusions to cancer's character—its invasive malignancy and an inveterate commitment to consumption and growth—were encased within an explicit designation of incurability, and this incurability increasingly came to define cancer above all else. In the 1840s, Hayle Walshe reviewed the eighteenth-century work of Mr Hill of Chester, who operated on eighty-eight cancer patients. Two years later there were 'about forty patients alive and sound'.[54] Hayle Walshe dismissed this, arguing that he and Hill 'did not write of the same disease'. While Hill might have claimed that these cases were cancerous, he must have been wrong. Instead they were likely 'examples of simple mammary hypertrophy, of fibrous tumours, and other non-carcinomatous conditions'. Or, put more simply,

---

[50] Ibid., 2.
[51] John Pearson, *Practical Observations on Cancerous Complaints: With an Account of some Diseases which Have Been Confounded with the Cancer* (London, 1792), 2.
[52] Denman, *Observations on the Cure of Cancer*, 3; Abernethy, *Surgical Observations on Tumours*, 74.
[53] Robert A. Aronowitz alludes to this status in the title of his book: *Unnatural History: Breast Cancer and American Society* (Cambridge, UK, 2007), 7.
[54] Hayle Walshe, *The Anatomy, Physiology, Pathology, and Treatment of Cancer*, 149.

'The complaint could not have been cancerous, *because it was cured.*'[55] This implied that the only meaningful way to diagnose cancer was retrospectively—it was a cancer if it killed you, some other form of benign tumour if it did not. This diagnostic mechanism emphasized the supremacy of the clinic—the practitioner needed the whole person, for the duration of their disease from diagnosis through to death, to identify a 'true' (and therefore incurable) cancer. It followed that the hospital was a valuable place to study cancer, for it was only there that the disease's incurability could be observed, elaborated, and better understood.

Incurability and Medical Identity

The texts produced by and in conjunction with the two institutions suggests that 'incurability' was far more than just a biological concept: it was also a rhetorical device that enabled ambitious, improving medical men (primarily surgeons) to articulate and perform a collective identity that was grounded in their feelings for patients' suffering, their desire for their profession to be seen as humanitarian, and their optimism that, through the hospital, cancer could ultimately be made curable. The hospitalization of cancer was likely at least in part motivated by concern for unchecked suffering. The institutions' foundational documents and the tracts and treatises produced by the associated medical men are replete with affective commentaries on the sufferings inflicted by cancer in general and the miseries of individual cases. These men encountered cancer regularly, if not in the hospital then in their own private practice. They all attested to its frequency, and all lamented the pain it caused. Many wrote up their cases, and used them to codify their knowledge and to derive generalities. In and among these scientific endeavours, fragments of highly charged emotional language emerged. For example, Denman wrote in the introduction to his *Observations on the Cure of Cancer*, 'The frequency of this disease, and the dreadful sufferings of those who are afflicted with it, are universally known.'[56]

Indeed, confronted by cancer suffering, the surgical elite were frequently moved. Denman wrote about one woman he treated for breast cancer, 'No case I apprehend had ever more painful and terrifying appearances.'[57] The language used to describe cancer patients often called to mind both physical and emotional suffering—for example the repeated use of 'misery'. Denman wrote about another patient, 'I thought her not likely to live many weeks, and took it for granted that the time she had to live would be passed in extreme misery.'[58] Not only were these men concerned by cancer suffering, they were also anxious that the disease seemed to particularly affect the poor, many of whom lacked access to long-term medical

---

[55] Ibid., original emphasis.   [56] Denman, *Observations on the Cure of Cancer*, 3.
[57] Ibid., 99.   [58] Ibid.

support. It was, after all, 'a disease to which the rich, as well as the poor, are liable; but which seems to bear more hardly on the latter, as wanting that alleviation of pain, and that degree of attention and assistance, which an evil so hopeless, and so aggravated, must require'.[59]

The inclusion of an incurable disease into the hospital system had a powerful symbolic function that was representative of the medical community's increasing role in public, charitable, and civic life.[60] Cancer patients were, according to the Middlesex minutes, 'Objects of Charity'.[61] As argued, both institutions had explicitly charitable roots. The men involved deployed the incurability of cancer to suggest that medicine was a fundamentally humanitarian endeavour—an endeavour that formed a crucial part of the concurrent Enlightenment ideals of duty, honour, civility, and virtue. Denman articulated any investigation into the disease's causes, characteristics, and cures as an attempt 'towards lessening the mass of human misery'.[62] Denman saw himself—a medical professional—as having a social as well as a scientific role. Similarly, John Abernethy reflected on the current trend using emotive language that focused on cancer's human costs: 'The minds of medical men having of late been laudably excited to investigate the nature of cancer, in hopes of discovering something serviceable in that dreadful disease.'[63]

Cancer's identification with humanitarianism in this period suggests a continuity with the form and function of care in the eighteenth century. Intervention—of any description, whether it effected a cure or not—was valuable. It was the effort and intention that mattered more than the eventual outcome. Thus, in some ways, it mattered little (at least to the practitioners) that their therapeutics were ineffectual in curing cancer—because that was not the function of treatment. Rather, these interventions served a social role for the surgeon and physician. Cancer might be an incurable disease, but if medical practitioners could be seen to care for its sufferers, then systematic therapeutic 'failure' did little to dent their credibility.

To understand why the men involved in these two institutions wanted to project a humanitarian image we must reflect on the wider medical culture of the period. Historians have suggested that eighteenth-century medicine operated according to a 'medical marketplace' model.[64] This model was characterized by the large variety of people providing health care, both formally and informally, and on the ability of patients to freely select their practitioner according to their own standards or prior experience. This increased competition between doctors—orthodox and otherwise—and allowed the balance of power to rest with the

---

[59] Bernard, 'Extract from an Account', 355.   [60] Brown, *Performing Medicine*.

[61] UCLH Archive, London, 'Weekly Board Meeting', Middlesex Hospital Minutes, 10 January 1792.

[62] Denman, *Observations on the Cure of Cancer*, 3.

[63] Abernethy, *Surgical Observations on Tumours*, 2.

[64] Brown, *Performing Medicine*; Roy Porter, *Health for Sale: Quackery in England, 1660–1850* (Manchester, 1989).

patient rather than the physician.[65] It was a highly commercialized system: an unrestricted free market in which practitioners competed for patients who were increasingly aware of themselves as 'consumers' within a diverse economy.[66] However, the period between 1789 and c.1835 was a time of intense flux within the medical community. Successive legislation provided an increasingly professionalized medical structure. The members of the three traditional medical communities—the physicians, surgeons, and apothecaries—were generally criticized for placing 'more weight on social graces than on medical knowledge' and there were calls for reform from both within and without the profession.[67] Additionally, the conventional hierarchy of physicians, surgeons, and apothecaries (in declining degrees of power) was under threat. Not only were surgeons working to elevate their craft above that of physicians', both were endangered by the rise of the general practitioner.[68] In a review in 1822 it was noted that the elite physician was 'not of a very extensive utility or much in demand'.[69] Irvine Loudon claims that a great deal of surgery was, and would continue to be, carried out by general practitioners, and by 1858 the Medical Act had established and regulated the general practitioner as the dominant type of medical man.[70]

Against this turbulent backdrop of competition, surgeons were particularly concerned with elevating their own social, professional, and intellectual status. Both the Middlesex cancer ward and the Society and Institution for Investigating the Nature and Cure of Cancer provided ideal forums in which to articulate a coherent professional image and identity predicated on the 'values of humanity, benevolence and, above all, gentility'.[71] However, the writings produced by the surgeons involved in the two cancer-specific institutions also demonstrate a further range of professional concerns. The foundational documents of the hospital and ward, as well as Denman, Abernethy, and Home's published works, reveal an attempt to establish surgical practice as rigorous and scientifically sound and equivalent to the intellectual claims of the physicians. Not only did they project a charitable image outwards to the non-medical population, they also constructed an elite surgical identity and internal code of conduct based on the values of collaboration, humility, precision, and restraint.

Humanitarianism was not, therefore, the only attribute pertinent to professional identity in this period. Another crucial element of this image was the expression of intellectual humility and an acknowledgement of the limits of medical knowledge and surgical ability. This intellectual modesty with respect to cancer was a theme that ran throughout cancer discourse in this period. Along

---

[65] Brown, *Performing Medicine*, 4.   [66] Ibid.

[67] Irvine Loudon, *Medical Care and the General Practitioner 1750–1850* (Oxford, 1987), 270; Susan C. Lawrence, 'Private Enterprise and Public Interests: Medical Education and the Apothecaries' Act, 1780–1825', in R. French and A. Wear (eds.), *British Medicine in an Age of Reform* (London, 1991), 47.

[68] Loudon, *Medical Care and the General Practitioner*, 268.   [69] Ibid., 270.   [70] Ibid.

[71] Brown, *Performing Medicine*, 2.

these lines, the disease's incurability can be understood not just as a problem to be overcome, but a productive device that shaped and articulated a specific medical and surgical identity. Cancer allowed practitioners to present 'not knowing' as a virtue rather than a vice. Abernethy acknowledged the limits to his knowledge, 'In engaging in a new undertaking, I am likely to expose my own deficiencies of information.'[72] He admitted to not fully understanding his own natural history of cancer, 'Are such diseases as I have here described to be accounted carcinomatous? If not, what are the characters which discriminate between them and carcinoma? As I have no precise or satisfactory information to communicate I forbear to say anything on the subject.'[73] This notion of precision, or lack thereof, was central to an identification with intellectual nuance and dexterity. Rather than claiming certainty, physicians and surgeons working on cancer in this period emphasized the complexity of the disease. And, by implication, their skill in dealing with it.

Irish surgeon Richard Carmichael—geographically peripheral to the metropolitan 'cancer community'—was keen to establish his credentials along these lines, 'My own hopes were but moderate and I was careful that they should not wander far beyond the certainty of my experience.'[74] This rhetorical style was in direct contrast to those practitioners who claimed the absolute ability to cure. These men and women were labelled 'empirics' or 'quacks' (see Chapter 4 for more on 'quacks'). Denman wrote, 'the extirpation of a cancerous part is usually spoken of by empirics, as if they had cured *Cancer*; but this cannot be allowed to be a proper or just mode of expression, though it may answer the purpose of enhancing their merit. The amputation of a leg is not curing a compound fracture, or a diseased foot.'[75] Thomas Bernard was explicit about the connections between intellectual and ethical quality and incurable cancer:

> There is no physician, no any medical man of reputation, who would hesitate to admit that his knowledge of any method, by which this disease may be prevented, or even its progress retarded, is very defective; and that, when it is confirmed, he does not entertain even a hope of curing it.[76]

These men were constructing their version of medical etiquette and ethics. They articulated a schema of medical efficacy and affect through the brick-and-mortar façade of the hospital and the institution now acted as a vehicle for them to construct and display their professional identities, outline an internal 'code of conduct' that differentiated between practitioners of different 'quality', and dictate the limits to their craft.

---

[72] Abernethy, *Surgical Observations on Tumours*, 4.   [73] Ibid., 84.
[74] Carmichael, *An Essay on the Effects of Carbonate*, 1–2.
[75] Denman, *Observations on the Cure of Cancer*, 36; see Chapter 3.
[76] Bernard, 'Extract from an Account', 355.

Pessimism and Optimism

In the case of early nineteenth-century cancer, the future operated as a key discursive realm within which practitioners could interact and mediate their actions.[77] Cancer might currently guarantee the patient's final descent; however, its incurable status was not necessarily permanent. While the medical community could offer little more to their patients than the amelioration of suffering—easing their passage towards death—if there were some circumstances in which they *could* completely cure disease, then there was no reason to suggest that cancer might not, one day, be one of those maladies. Or rather, if some diseases could be cured, then early nineteenth-century practitioners might hope or anticipate that in the future cancer might be counted among their number. Thomas Bernard wrote:

> We ought, therefore, to hope that a remedy may at length be found out for cancer; and, with such hope, it is the duty of medical men to exert their faculties, for the investigation of the nature and cause of them, and for the discovery not only of the means of *relief,* but of *cure.*[78]

He drew an explicit distinction between the *care* ('relief') they were currently providing and the '*cure*' they would soon be able to administer.

Thus, early nineteenth-century cancer discourse made use of a medical chronology that expressed a professional past, present, and future. Surgeons in particular decried their predecessors' 'barbarity', and narrated a 'rags-to-riches' tale from miserable butchery to scientific surgery.[79] Practitioners' institutional neglect of cancer sufferers in the eighteenth century fit neatly within this narrative and Denman, Abernethy, and Home could easily contrast their own humanitarianism with their forerunners' brutalism. Unlike their eighteenth-century predecessors, the medical men involved in both hospitals brought death, dying, and fatal disease closer—sharing in their patients' experiences of suffering and encountering the incurability of cancer on a new scale. These expressions of emotional engagement with their patients also worked in support of their belief that the early nineteenth century was an edified era—'the present enlightened state of medicine'—one

---

[77] Much has been written about how practitioners used their own histories to set out a sense of surgical and medical identity and various scholars have attended to conceptualizations of the 'past and present' of surgery and medicine. See Christopher Lawrence, 'Democratic, Divine and Heroic: The History and Historiography of Surgery', in Christopher Lawrence (ed.), *Medical Theory, Surgical Practice: Essays in the History of Surgery* (London, 1992); Peter Stanley, *For Fear of Pain: British Surgery, 1790–1850* (Amsterdam, 2003). Delia Gavrus makes similar arguments about neurologists and neurosurgeons in the mid-twentieth century: 'Men of Dreams and Men of Action: Neurologists, Neurosurgeons, and the Performance of Professional Identity, 1920–1950', *Bulletin of the History of Medicine*, 85 (2011), 57–92.

[78] Bernard, 'Extract from an Account', 355.   [79] Lawrence, 'Democratic, Divine and Heroic'.

markedly different to that of their fathers and forebears.[80] Various practitioners contrasted the cruelty of the past with the 'perfection' of the present; part of this 'perfection' was the contribution to society and humanity by medicine and its practitioners.

Indeed, while early nineteenth-century cancer discourse was frequently melo-dramatic and emotive, it also was paradoxically positive. The present was humani-tarian, but the future might be curative. The language of the investigative project as a whole—contained in tracts, treatises, and the thirteen queries—suggests that complete curability was the planned or ideal destination. Indeed, despite frequent recourse to lamentations and despair, practitioners were broadly optimistic. In his tract, *Observations on the Cure of Cancer*, Thomas Denman responded to the thirteenth query. He argued that, 'the acknowledgment of ignorance ought not to be considered as a sanction for negligence or indifference, or as a screen from censure'.[81] Cancer might be incurable, but that should not be an excuse for inaction.

Denman did not think that cancer was inherently incurable; rather that medical art had not yet been able to find an effective treatment. In his preface, he was sanguine, 'those who have seen many instances of Cancer, must rejoice at the prospect before us, of a method of cure being at length discovered and estab-lished'.[82] He was confident in the ultimate ability of the medical community:

> It appears...from the earliest records of medicine, that notwithstanding their utmost endeavours, there ever remained a certain number of diseases, which were acknowledged to be *incurable*... By this term, it may be presumed, was only meant, that they were not to be cured by any means or methods with which the ancients were then acquainted. They, especially professional men, seeing what had been already done, were too wise to limit or circumscribe what, at some future time, might be accomplished by the continued efforts of enlightened men, separate or conjoined.[83]

In general, the medical men involved in the investigation of cancer believed emphatically in the perfectibility of surgery and medicine, and they saw that process of improvement as a duty or calling. They articulated their role as instrumental in lessening 'the mass of human misery' and conceptualized it as collaborative and necessitating 'the assistance of others'.[84] For while, 'all medicines and methods of treatments hitherto proposed and tried have been unavailing', they would soon 'obtain a remedy for a most painful and dreadful disease'.[85]

---

[80] Bernard, 'Extract from an Account', 355.
[81] Denman, *Observations on the Cure of Cancer*, iv.   [82] Ibid.   [83] Ibid., 2.
[84] 'Institution for Investigating the Nature and Cure of Cancer', *Edinburgh Medical and Surgical Journal*, 2 (1802), 382–9, at 389.
[85] Ibid.

Indeed, this curative project was divinely ordained, 'It has, however, pleased God that means should be discovered for the cure of diseases, which once thought incurable.'[86]

Thus, while institutions were key to the future of the disease, the rhetoric that surrounded them was as much about an 'imagined community' of practitioners as it was about the strategic role of the hospital in cancer investigation.[87] The very name of the Society and Institution for Investigating the Nature and Cure of Cancer was optimistic; it suggests that the practitioners involved thought a cure might be within the grasp of future medical men. Their investigative project was designed to produce information that would accumulate to furnish later generations with sufficient knowledge to erase cancer entirely. John Abernethy called his *Surgical Observations on Tumours* 'an attempt to form a Classification'.[88] He went on to say in his introduction,

> It appears to me, that, in order fully to investigate any subject with advantage, a great deal of collateral knowledge is required, which serves, like light shining from various places, to illuminate the object of our researches. I am not without hopes that this paper will tend to point out the required distinctions, and furnish such collateral knowledge.[89]

Thomas Denman described the expansion of cancer knowledge as a 'duty', and saw himself and his co-practitioners as driven by an investigative zeal.

Both The Middlesex Hospital and the Society and Institution were explicit about the role of hospitalization in knowledge-gathering. The Society and Institution wrote, 'Measures should be taken for the establishment of a Charity, or institution, for the express purpose of investigating the nature of *Cancer*, and of making experiments, for the discovery of a method of curing that disease.'[90] After all, the Institution was 'formed, not merely with a design of affording an asylum for the distressed, but professedly for the purpose of experiment and discovery'.[91] The Society and Institution saw their activities as a collaborative effort to improve cancer knowledge, so as to bring about more effective treatments, 'If any progress in the investigation of the nature and cure of cancer be made...it will, without

---

[86] Bernard, 'Extract from an Account', 355.

[87] Michael Brown applied Benedict Anderson's phrase—'imagined community'—to nineteenth-century medicine. Benedict Anderson, *Imagined Communities: Reflections on the Origin and Spread of Nationalism* (London, 1991); Brown, 'Medicine, Reform and the "End" of Charity'. Brown also observed that while Ludmilla Jordanova applied Anderson's ideas to an examination of the construction of the 'scientific community', few have followed her lead. Ludmilla Jordanova, 'Science and National Identity', in R. Chartier and P. Corsi (eds.), *Science et Langues en Europe* (Paris, 1996); Ludmilla Jordanova, 'Science and Nationhood: Cultures of Imagined Communities', in G. Cubitt (ed.), *Imagining Nations* (Manchester, 1998).

[88] Abernethy, *Surgical Observations on Tumours*, x.   [89] Ibid.

[90] Denman, *Observations on the Cure of Cancer*, 87.

[91] Bernard, 'Extract from an Account', 355.

delay, be laid before the public by the Medical Committee.'[92] The founders were enemies of jealousy, and conceptualized their investigations as in aid of a civic, humanitarian good rather than individual advancement.

The Middlesex had parallel investigative goals. Mr Howard declared a twofold objective: 'I take the liberty to observe that two principal objects present them-selves to my Mind on this occasion ... the relief of Persons afflicted with Cancer, and the Investigation of a Complaint.' He framed the investigation in Baconian terms:

> Lord Bacon has observed that Medical People should make themselves Proficient in Physic by studying one disease at a time ... By confining one or more Wards to Cancers only the attention of Pupils and others will be directed very strictly to the study of this Disease, they will see facts as they arise in the aggregate from a large number of Patients, new lights will appear and new discoveries will probably be made.[93]

As part of his investigation, Howard advocated the keeping of a detailed case history for every patient admitted, 'In order to improve a subject ... I propose, that a faithful account of the history and circumstances of every case be kept, its antecedents and consequences should be marked, the effects of medicines and of Operations, when necessary, noted, together with all the collateral details.'[94] The Middlesex minutes recorded, 'If I knew accurately the natural history of any disease, I should never be at a loss for a proper method of treating it.'[95] Howard believed that 'much useful knowledge may be disseminated, and that we may in no great length of time be furnished with documents on the Disease and its cure, much more authentic than any we are at this time in possession of'.[96] Similarly, Denman reflected approvingly on his friends' habit of keeping case notes, 'Much credit is due to men of distinguished scientific abilities, and of high professional rank and character, who, whilst they are engaged in the active business of life, accustom themselves to keep regular accounts of cases ... for the purpose of improving their profession.'[97] Thus, Abernethy, Denman, and Howard saw their endeavours as preparing the ground for future discovery, and conceptualized themselves as within a broader community of scholars that was both geograph-ically and chronologically diverse. In other words, they imagined themselves to be working in concert with surgeons and physicians from prior and subsequent generations.

Denman, Abernethy, Home, and company were positioning themselves at the beginning of a progressive teleology. They might not have had the answers then,

[92] 'Institution for Investigating the Nature and Cure of Cancer', 389.
[93] UCLH Archive, 'Weekly Board Meeting', 10 January 1792.   [94] Ibid.   [95] Ibid.
[96] Ibid.   [97] Denman, *Observations on the Cure of Cancer*, 21.

but they were convinced that they would solve the 'cancer problem' at some point in the not-too-distant future. The board of the Middlesex was also confident, 'If such an Institution be fairly set on foot, it cannot fail of producing beneficial consequences to all descriptions of Persons labouring under this dreadful Malady'—a cure was inevitable.[98] Indeed, there was a boldness—an optimism— to early nineteenth-century medicine that allowed for conviction in the future curative powers of intervention. Professor of the Institute of Medicine at the University of Edinburgh, William Pulteney Alison, wrote in his 1834 survey of the recent history of medicine that there was 'nothing irrational, or Utopian' in his view of surgical progress—the proponents of scientific medicine would, he predicted, gradually but surely extend their knowledge of the nature of disease and would ultimately be able to prevent or relieve 'all the sufferings, which we now regard as necessarily attendant on our physical constitution'.[99]

Conclusion

The two cancer-specific institutions confirmed and constructed cancer as a disease identifiable through surgical touch and skilled observation; as a malady with an implacable tendency towards growth and spread; and as an incurable illness that wreaked havoc on life and limb. However, this incurable identity was not just a biological observation, but also a flexible category that could be deployed to various professional and personal ends. An interrogation of incurability in early nineteenth-century London reveals that while much of medicine was about the management of suffering and decline—about the shades of grey between life and death—cancer was far more binary. Death was inevitable with cancer—the patient moved in only one direction. However, this narrative was not just melancholic— and while the practitioners involved in both institutions frequently expressed affective engagement with their patients, and waxed lyrical on the subject of suffering, they were not overwhelmingly pessimistic. Instead, they used cancer's incurability to articulate a coherent identity predicated on the values of humanity, humility, and restraint. They also used the disease's intractability to reflect on the 'futurority' of their profession and to situate their current practices—the at-present inability to cure—against a progressive teleology in which all maladies might be overcome. They also articulated a different sort of cure: whereas the interventions of the eighteenth century were about returning the body to balance and achieving a healthful equilibrium, the cancer cure would be far more decisive.

---

[98] UCLH Archive, 'Weekly Board Meeting', 10 January 1792.
[99] William Pulteney Alison, *Dissertation on the State of Medical Science: From the Termination of the Eighteenth Century to the Present Time* (London, 1834), 38.

If cancer was a 'disease-object' then a cure would effect that object's complete destruction.

However, the authoritative optimism that mapped out the upcoming age as a period of advancement and medical perfection was shadowed by doubt and insecurity. Nestled within bombastic optimism, were kernels of anxiety. Abernethy recalled how having to operate ought to be 'an [sic] humiliating reflection...a confession that our art is inadequate to the cure of disease'.[100] Similarly, Charles Bell mused, 'The conviction comes tardily on the surgeons' mind that there is a limit to his boldness and ingenuity.'[101] And, finally, another surgeon lamented how 'every failure...does harm to our art'.[102] Cancer exposed vulnerabilities in early nineteenth-century medical knowledge, and as Chapter 3 will show, in surgical practice as well. While practitioners could be enthusiastic about the medical future, success was by no means guaranteed. Thus, while medical and surgical identity in the early nineteenth century was woven with optimism, cancer's present and presence maintained a thread of pessimism; and the next one hundred years were dominated by the tensions between these two professional emotions. Chapter 3 explores the first tentative steps along the therapeutic journey and the contested efforts to redefine cancer as a curable disease.

---

[100] Quoted in Stanley, *For Fear of Pain*, 68.   [101] Ibid.   [102] Ibid., 69.

3

Cancer Therapeutics

In 1859, the Scottish writer, Dr John Brown, published his short story *Rab and his Friends*.[1] Set in Edinburgh, the title character Rab was an 'old, grey, brindled' mastiff, as 'big as a Highland bull'. The dog's owner, James Noble, was a carter or carrier by trade and had an ailing and appropriately named wife, Ailie, who had some 'kind o' trouble in her breast'.[2] Over the course of the tale, Noble befriended the young Dr John Brown, an assistant surgeon at the local hospital, and asked him to inspect his wife's troubled breast:

> I looked at and examined it carefully,—she and James watching me, and Rab eying all three. What could I say? There it was, that had once been so soft, so shapely, so white, so gracious and bountiful, so 'full of all blessed conditions',— hard as a stone, a centre of horrid pain, making that pale face, with its grey, lucid, reasonable eyes, and its sweet resolved mouth, express the full measure of suffering overcome.[3]

Cancer had converted Ailie's soft, feminine flesh into the hardness of a malignant tumour. The next day, Brown's master, the surgeon, examined the tumour for himself. In accordance with prevalent ideas about cancer and its incurability, he declared that, 'There was no doubt it must kill her, and soon.' However, there was a kernel of hope, 'It could be removed; it might never return; it would give her speedy relief: she should have it done.'[4] While Brown was writing in 1859, his story was set several decades earlier, before the widespread adoption of chloroform. As a result, the operation—which was to take place the following day— would be performed without anaesthesia. Ailie bore the surgery well and the wound healed 'by the first intention'.[5] So far so good, but four days after the operation the patient became restless, 'her eyes were too bright, her cheek coloured ... mischief had begun'.[6] Her pulse became rapid, her breathing quick, and a few days later she died.

While fictional, Brown's tale tracks a broader narrative about cancer treatment in the nineteenth century. It gestures towards a range of questions, including how best to treat a disease that seemed to have no effective cure; what practitioners

---

[1] John Brown, *Rab and his Friends* (Edinburgh, 1859). See also Peter Stanley, *For Fear of Pain: British Surgery, 1790–1850* (Amsterdam, 2003), 7–9.
[2] Ibid., 13. [3] Ibid., 15. [4] Ibid., 18. [5] Ibid., 22. [6] Ibid.

The Cancer Problem: Malignancy in Nineteenth-Century Britain. Agnes Arnold-Forster, Oxford University Press (2021).
© Agnes Arnold-Forster. DOI: 10.1093/oso/9780198866145.003.0004

could offer desperate and suffering patients; and how did the fortunes and meanings of different interventions change over time—before and after the introduction of anaesthesia, for example. The surgeon had been cautious but optimistic about the curative potential of an operation to remove Ailie's breast. The tumour 'might never return' and at the very least the surgery would provide 'speedy relief' from the 'horrid pain'. Recovery was deemed possible and her eventual death was a disappointment to doctors and dog alike.

There was a diverse array of treatments on offer to the cancer sufferer in the nineteenth century—and the knife was but one of the many tools at the surgeon's disposal. However, in the first few decades of the century—against a backdrop of shifting professional, intellectual, and social concerns, and according to elite practitioners—surgeons and surgery superseded physicians and internal medicaments as the *ideal* response to malignancy. Indeed, while the medical men who orbited around the various institutions dedicated to the care and investigation of cancer in the early nineteenth century may have derived social and professional capital from lamentations and doubt, they were also optimistic. Not only did they contrast the current incurability of cancer with future, almost inevitable, mastery over the disease, they also believed that in some cases surgery might delay or even avert death.

Surgery's 'ideal' and potentially curative status was, however, short-lived. The initial enthusiasm that surrounded operative excision of the malignant tumour rapidly gave way to a more restricted realism. Elites' optimism about their capacity to cure cancer faded, and surgery's status was increasingly contested. And yet surgeons were unwilling to give up their newly acquired and hard-fought status as the medical men most likely to offer support and relief to cancer patients. Thus, rather than promising a cure, elite practitioners renegotiated surgical intervention as a palliative enterprise—something that ameliorated suffering without addressing the underlying malady—and in doing so salvaged an element of effectiveness and prestige for a practice that was otherwise impotent in the face of the 'dread disease'.[7] In this way, cancer's incurability prompted the medical community to construct a new category of intervention—a kind of palliative surgery that was adversarial, energetic, violent, and predicated on an affective engagement between practitioner and patient. After all, operating to lessen suffering and lengthen life required a different kind of assessment of whether an intervention 'worked' or not. In this way, palliative surgery complicated ideas of therapeutic efficacy and redefined what it meant to provide 'successful' clinical intervention. Thus, while the

---

[7] 'Palliative', 'palliation', and 'palliate' were used throughout the nineteenth century and before, and I borrow my actors' phrasing in describing their theory and practice.

nineteenth-century medical community had yet to overcome cancer's intractability, the disease's incurability produced new surgical categories and practices.[8]

This chapter will, therefore, look at the application, assessment, and justification of palliative surgery in practice, particularly through the work of two practitioners: Charles Bell (1774–1842) and James Young Simpson (1811–1970). Bell was a Scottish surgeon, anatomist, neurologist, and philosophical theologian. He received his medical degree from Edinburgh in 1798, before moving to London.[9] Simpson was also Scottish but based in Edinburgh. He was an obstetrician, surgeon, and the first to demonstrate the anaesthetic properties of chloroform on humans.[10] Bell and Simpson were elite practitioners, working in large, prestigious hospitals, with extensive and profitable private practices, and both were based in metropolitan centres. However, when read alongside other surgeons' responses to the disease—such as those collated by Walter Hayle Walshe (1812–1892)—their works were broadly representative of the profession's attitudes towards surgical palliation.[11]

As this chapter will show, close attention to patient pain and suffering was essential to surgeons' assessments of the efficacy of palliative surgery. Bell and Simpson performed palliative procedures partly because they were concerned by their patients' suffering and, as suggested in Chapter 2, partly because they wanted to present themselves as enlightened, improving gentlemen. However, surgeons also saw their patients' pain and anguish as useful. While practitioners might see affective patient responses—screams, moans, and complaints—during supposedly curative surgery as frustrating obstacles to effective treatment, in the aftermath of palliative operations, patient feeling and physical well-being were key to the surgeon's assessment of whether their interventions had worked or not. If the goal was to reduce suffering, then the patient's account of their pain and distress before, during, and after surgery was a useful mechanism by which practitioners could assess their intervention. Indeed, the texts analysed here—and the promotion of palliative surgery more generally—provide an alternative portrayal to that of the crude and dispassionate Victorian practitioner and my argument

---

[8] This chapter draws on Martin S. Pernick's ideas of a 'calculus of suffering'. Martin S. Pernick, *A Calculus of Suffering: Pain, Professionalism, and Anesthesia in Nineteenth-Century America* (New York, 1985).

[9] Charles Bell, *Surgical Observations; Being a Quarterly Report of Cases in Surgery; Treated in the Middlesex Hospital, in the Cancer Establishment, and in Private Practice* (London, 1816); L. S. Jacyna, 'Bell, Sir Charles (1774–1842)', in *Oxford Dictionary of National Biography* (Oxford, 2004). For more on Charles Bell see Carin Berkowitz, 'Charles Bell's Seeing Hand: Teaching Anatomy to the Senses in Britain, 1750–1840', *History of Science*, 52 (2014), 377–400, and *Charles Bell and the Anatomy of Reform* (Chicago, 2015).

[10] Malcolm Nicolson, 'Simpson, Sir James Young, First Baronet (1811–1870)', in *Oxford Dictionary of National Biography* (Oxford, 2004).

[11] Walter Hayle Walshe, *The Nature and Treatment of Cancer* (London, 1844).

owes much to historians who have recently problematized the unfeeling nineteenth-century surgeon.[12]

Finally, this chapter's expansive geographical and chronological scope tracks the continuing contestation of cancer's incurability right up to the turn of the twentieth century, focusing particularly on William Halsted and his reception in Britain. Halsted is a well-studied character in the history of cancer. He pioneered and popularized the radical mastectomy (although did not invent it). He was trained in Europe and practised at Johns Hopkins Hospital in Baltimore, United States of America.[13] Improved surgical survival rates in the late century—after the introduction of anaesthesia and asepsis—prompted a reconsideration of cancer's incurability. Crucially, however, these innovations did not fundamentally affect the climate of pessimism and dread among the medical profession, nor alter the rationality of palliative intervention. Indeed, the construction of cancer treatments as palliative rather than curative has had a lasting impact on conceptualizations of the disease, and it continues to shape understandings of interventions designed to slow rather than stop cancer's progress through organs and tissues.

Internal or External Treatments

There were various remedies available to the nineteenth-century cancer sufferer. These could be broadly divided into two categories: internal or external. Internal treatments were anything ingested by the patient—ranging from pills, potions, and tonics, to strict diets and powerful purges. Internal remedies were diverse but included belladonna, hydrocyanic acid, oxide of gold, copper salts, chloride of barium, mercury, and iodine. Walter Hayle Walshe reported a patient who, 'affected with a cancerous tumour in the face, swallowed upwards of four hundred grey lizards in the course of two months'.[14] Unfortunately (not least for the lizards), this treatment was met 'without obvious effect of any kind'.[15] These plants, animals, and chemicals were popular but controversial in early modern Britain because they could have extreme effects on the body and were hazardous

---

[12] Christopher Lawrence, 'Medical Minds, Surgical Bodies: Corporeality and the Doctors', in Christopher Lawrence and Steven Shapin (eds.), *Science Incarnate: Historical Embodiments of Natural Knowledge* (Chicago, 1998), 194. See the work of Michael Brown, whose recent project 'A Theatre of Emotions: The Affective Landscape of Nineteenth-Century British Surgery' explores the place of emotion in the practice, politics, and representation of nineteenth-century surgery. Michael Brown, 'Surgery and Emotion: The Era before Anaesthesia', in Thomas Schlich (ed.), *The Palgrave Handbook of the History of Surgery* (Basingstoke, 2017). See, too, Joanna Bourke, *The Story of Pain* (Oxford, 2014); Peter Stanley, *For Fear of Pain: British Surgery, 1790–1850* (Amsterdam, 2003); and Peter Stanley, 'How did Civil War Surgeons Cope?', *Surgeon's Call*, 19 (2014), 3–5.

[13] Barron H. Lerner, *The Breast Cancer Wars: Fear, Hope, and the Pursuit of a Cure in Twentieth-Century America* (Oxford, 2001), 16.

[14] Hayle Walshe, *The Nature and Treatment of Cancer*, 203.   [15] Ibid.

to ingest.[16] They caused bizarre delirium, hallucinations, headaches, dizziness, rapid heart rate, shortness of breath, and vomiting. These symptoms could be followed by a slowing of the pulse, lowered blood pressure, loss of consciousness, and cardiac arrest. Practitioners and patients justified the consumption of these remedies partly because the damage inflicted matched the threat of the disease itself. 1Hayle Walshe concluded in 1846 that, 'the more powerfully alterative a medicine is, the greater the chance...of its proving beneficial in that disease'.[17] Alanna Skuse has described this as an 'adversarial therapeutic approach', in which only a poison (the therapy) could sufficiently counter a poison (the cancer).[18]

External (or surgical) treatments, on the other hand, were anything that removed the tumour from the body. These methods were equally diverse as internal remedies and equally 'adversarial'—involving the use of the knife, cautery, compression, or caustic applications. While later generations of medical men excluded the latter three techniques from the roster of orthodox and 'respectable' surgical practice—consigning caustics in particular to the preserve of quackery— in the first half of the nineteenth century all were easily incorporated into the elite's surgeon's therapeutic arsenal. That is not to so say, however, that these methods were consistently understood as equal in ease of use and effectiveness. Each had its own champions and the various techniques waxed and waned in popularity among hospital-based practitioners. However, it would be anachronistic to equate 'surgery' with 'the knife' alone—and the practice and its practitioners were more accurately delineated by their attendance to the local, physical mass than by the tools they used to divorce cancerous tumours from healthy flesh.

Descriptions of surgical practice are hard to come by and in hospital case notes operations are denoted by single-word entries: 'removal', 'excision', and 'enucleation'.[19] It is also difficult to identify the proportion of patients operated on and how common surgeries were. From 1805 to 1838, only 20 per cent of the women on The Middlesex Hospital cancer ward had their tumours removed.[20] We know, however, that enough operations for cancer were performed for it to feature in the popular press without excessive commentary or alarm. In 1801, *The Times* ran an obituary for the Countess of Holderness, who had died 'at the advanced age of seventy-six'. Her 'complaint' was a cancerous tumour in her mouth, 'which had destroyed the upper jaw, and part of the tongue'. The disease had originated in her left breast, and required an 'amputation' three years before her death. *The Times* reported that she 'bore the painful operation with uncommon fortitude'.[21] Skuse

---

[16] Belladonna is also known as deadly nightshade, the most toxic plant in the eastern hemisphere; and hydrocyanic acid is a solution of hydrogen cyanide which was the Zyklon B used in Nazi extermination camps to facilitate the 'Final Solution' during the Second World War.

[17] Hayle Walshe, *The Nature and Treatment of Cancer*, 201.

[18] Alanna Skuse, *Constructions of Cancer in Early Modern England: Ravenous Natures* (Basingstoke, 2015), 19.

[19] UCLH Archive, Case Notes from the Cancer Ward at the Middlesex Hospital (1805–1838).

[20] Ibid.   [21] 'Obituaries', *The Times*, 16 October 1801, 3.

makes a similar observation about the seventeenth century: 'In May 1665, Samuel Pepys remarked upon the mastectomy of his "poor aunt James" with sympathy but without much surprise.'[22]

Apart from newspaper articles, and published and unpublished case histories, most of our evidence for how surgery was practised comes from books of reference and pedagogical texts such as Samuel Cooper's *The First Lines of the Practice of Surgery*, which was designed as an 'introduction for students'.[23] In 1819, Cooper insisted in relation to cancer that, 'without an entire removal of all the diseased parts, there is no chance of success'.[24] His 663-page volume included references for how to remove cancerous breasts, lips, eyes, and tongues. The operation for breasts was 'usually performed as the patient is in a sitting posture, well supported by pillows and assistants'.[25] His descriptions of operations make clear the radical nature of cancer surgery and its disfiguring effects. He narrated how the surgeon was to wield the knife (see Figure 3.1):

> The portion of the skin, intended to be taken away, must be included in two semi-circular incisions; which meet thus () at their extremities; and when the base of the tumour is to be detached, the surface of the pectoral muscle, wherever it is adherent to the tumour, is also to be removed. The advantage of making the incision in the preceding manner obviously consists in enabling the surgeon to bring the edges of the wound together after the operation, so as to form a straight line, and be capable of uniting by the first intention [meaning the edges of the skin would meet together at the first try].[26]

Tracking the changes and continuities contained within these practical volumes suggests that the techniques, radical nature, and disfiguring effects of cancer surgery changed little throughout the nineteenth century. Cooper did not include images in his own book. Other writers, however, did, and while Figure 3.1 was published in 1856 after the widespread adoption of anaesthesia, it seems to illustrate the technique Cooper described. It mimics the elliptical incisions and draws the skin together after the removal of the breast tissue. Moreover, this image was also used to illustrate an 1841 volume, suggesting that surgical techniques for the removal of the breast did not alter dramatically in the years following the introduction of anaesthesia in c.1846.[27] There would, of course, be practical differences between operating on a sensible or insensible patient—a distinction

[22] Skuse, *Constructions of Cancer*, 126.
[23] Samuel Cooper, *The First Lines of the Practice of Surgery: Designed as an Introduction for Students and a Concise Book of Reference for Practitioners*, vol. 1, 4th edn (London, 1819).
[24] Ibid., 280.   [25] Ibid., 587.   [26] Ibid., 587–8.
[27] J. M. Bourgery, *Iconografia d'Anatomia Chirurgica e di Medicina Operatoria* (Florence, 1841), plate 27.

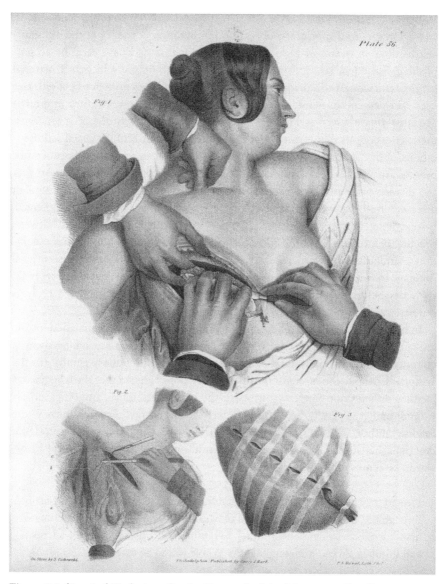

Figure 3.1 'Surgical Technique for the Removal of the Mammary Gland'

Source: From Joseph Pancoast, *A Treatise on Operative Surgery Comprising a Description of the Various Processes of the Art, Including all the New Operations; Exhibiting the State of Surgical Science in its Present Advanced Condition* (Philadelphia, PA, 1856), plate LVI. Wellcome Images.

William Fergusson, Professor of Surgery at King's College London, alluded to in 1846, 'On the dead subject the operation [amputation of the leg at the hip joint] can be done in twelve or twenty seconds, and it may as I have seen, be accomplished with equal celerity on the living.'[28] A writhing body in pain frustrated surgical efficiency. Indeed, it is likely that Figure 3.1 represents a dead patient. Her eyes are open and fixed and she is shrouded in white. This was a convention that predated anaesthesia—as Figure 3.2 demonstrates—and was one of several aesthetic conventions that formed part of many nineteenth-century visual representations of breast cancer and its treatment.[29] The patient's supposedly cancerous breasts are youthful (in contrast to the prevailing contemporary opinion that the disease primarily affected post-menopausal women) and show no sign of disease.[30] Both breasts are exposed, and the patient's hair is elegantly arranged. Instructional illustrations idealized surgery and flattened distinctions between practice before and after the introduction of anaesthesia. Note the representational similarities between Figure 3.1 and Figure 3.2—the latter depicts surgical drainage to treat empyema (an accumulation of pus), and was published in 1841, six years before the first use of chloroform in Britain. The patient's body is unrestrained and his gaze is fixed.

In his description of the removal of the breast, Cooper also campaigned for the 'free removal of the skin covering and adjoining a scirrhus...taking away a quantity of the surrounding fat', and the excision of the 'axillary glands' (in the armpit).[31] Despite the extent of the operation, Cooper argued that the surgery was 'neither difficult nor dangerous in itself; the wound resembles any other simple wound; and it generally heals up very well'.[32] In contrast, Frances Burney, the English author who was operated on for a suspected breast cancer in 1811, described her horror when she realized—mid-operation—that her entire breast was to be removed:

> I feared they imagined the whole breast infected—feared it too justly,—for, again through the Cambric, I saw the hand of M. Dubois held up, while his forefinger first described a straight line from top to bottom of the breast, secondly a Cross, and thirdly a circle; intimating that the Whole was to be taken off.[33]

---

[28] William Fergusson, *A System of Practical Surgery* (London, 1846), 413.

[29] See Bridget L. Goodbody, '"The Present Opprobrium of Surgery": "The Agnew Clinic" and Nineteenth-Century Representations of Cancerous Female Breasts', *American Art*, 8 (1994), 32–51.

[30] See Chapter 1. Also, 'There has been no little difficulty in determining what is the earliest period of life at which Cancer has appeared, and at what period we are most liable to it. To the latter, I believe, may be answered, without much hesitation, in advanced life': Thomas Denman, *Observations on the Cure of Cancer; with some Remarks upon Mr Young's Treatment of that Disease* (London, 1816), 43.

[31] Cooper, *The First Lines of the Practice of Surgery*, 280.   [32] Ibid., 277.

[33] Frances Burney, 'Account from Paris of a Terrible Operation', in *Journal Letter to Esther Burney* (London, 1812). For more on Frances Burney see J. E. Epstein, 'Writing the Unspeakable: Fanny Burney's Mastectomy and the Fictive Body', *Representations*, 16 (1986), 131–66; and S. Mediratta,

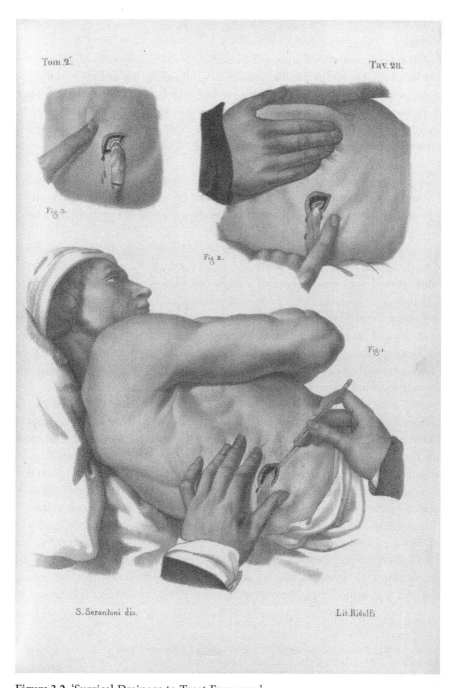

Figure 3.2 'Surgical Drainage to Treat Empyema'

Source: From J. M. Bourgery, *Iconografia d'Anatomia Chirurgica e di Medicina Operatoria* (Florence, 1841), plate 28. Wellcome Images.

A mundane operative necessity for the surgeon was met with dismay by the patient.

Other body parts posed greater challenges for both practitioner and patient. For cancer of the lip, and when the tumour was still small, 'the operation should be done as for the hare-lip, making the wound of such a shape as will allow its edges to be evenly united by adhesion, and taking care to extirpate every portion of the morbid part'. However, when the 'affection is extensive', the surgeon needed to remove the whole lip,

> A most unpleasant occurrence, as the patient's saliva can then only be prevented from continually running over his chin by some artificial mechanical contrivance; the deformity is very great; and swallowing, and the pronunciation of words, can only be imperfectly performed.[34]

This operation would cause lifelong difficulties for the unhappy sufferer. Similarly, with operations to remove parts of a cancerous tongue, speech would be affected and the surgery was attended by the risk of haemorrhage (Figure 3.3). Operations to remove a malignant eye were perhaps the riskiest as they carried with them the possibility of brain damage: 'In the performance of the operation, there are two important circumstances to which attention ought to be paid. The first is to remove every particle of the disease . . . The second is to avoid piercing or injuring the orbit, behind which the dura mater is immediately situated.'[35]

As I have suggested, the knife was not the only instrument deployed by the surgeon and the early nineteenth century witnessed what one practitioner described as a 'catalogue of surgical novelties' in response to cancer.[36] In 1810, for example, the Bedford surgeon Samuel Young suggested 'compression' as an effective external treatment for cancer. In this system, pressure was applied to a tumour with an air-pad and spring, or by layering plaster of Paris sheets over linen placed on the mass and then progressively increasing the pressure with straps.[37] This practice was dependent on a long-standing idea that prolonged compression of a tissue could provoke atrophy, even of bones. In his book, *Lectures on the Principles of Surgery*, John Hunter mentioned that compression could prevent the development of tumours and in some cases destroy them entirely.[38] Young believed that sufficient pressure would cause the body to absorb the tumour and

'Beauty and the Breast: The Poetics of Physical Absence and Narrative Presence in Frances Burney's Mastectomy Letter (1811)', *Women: A Cultural Review*, 19 (2008), 188–207.

[34] Cooper, *The First Lines of the Practice of Surgery*, 423.   [35] Ibid., 484.

[36] Langston Parker, *The Treatment of Cancer Diseases by Caustics* (London, 1856), 3.

[37] Samuel Whitbread, 'Prefatory Letter Addressed to the Governors of the Middlesex Hospital', in Samuel Young, *Minutes of Cases of Cancer and Cancerous Tendency, Successfully Treated by Samuel Young* (London, 1815), xiv.

[38] John Hunter, *Lectures on the Principles of Surgery* (Philadelphia, PA, 1839), 198.

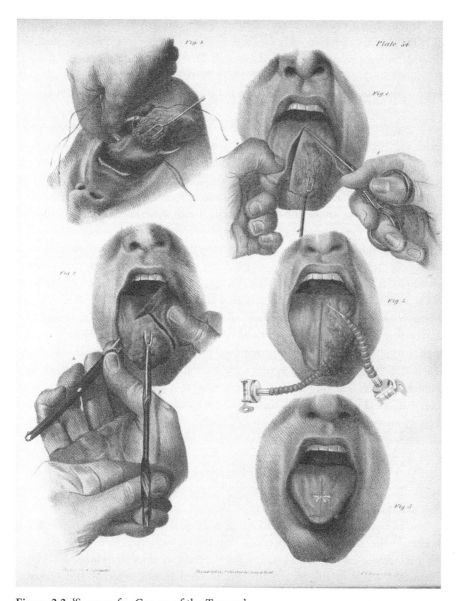

Figure 3.3 'Surgery for Cancer of the Tongue'

Source: From Joseph Pancoast, *A Treatise on Operative Surgery Comprising a Description of the Various Processes of the Art, Including all the New Operations; Exhibiting the State of Surgical Science in its Present Advanced Condition* (Philadelphia, PA, 1856), plate LIV. Wellcome Images.

return the patient to comfort and health.[39] The treatment had powerful support. In 1815, Thomas Denman addressed a pamphlet to Sir Benjamin Brodie, strongly advocating compression in cases of cancer.[40] That same year, Samuel Whitbread, the anonymous financial backer of The Middlesex Hospital's cancer ward, wrote a letter to the institution's governors campaigning for the intervention's incorporation into their clinical arsenal.[41]

Caustic treatments were popular in the eighteenth and early nineteenth centuries and involved the application of corrosive substances to the surface of cancerous tumours. These substances included arsenical pastes, chloride of zinc pastes, concentrated mineral acids, chloride of bromine, used either alone or in combination with the chlorides of zinc, antimony, or gold. In contact with the skin or malignant mass these substances would burn through flesh and could be reapplied until the tumour had been completely eaten away. Caustic treatments provided the dual benefit of not only removing the cancer from the body, but also sealing off the offensive sore. Surgeon Spencer Wells described a case of a woman whose breast cancer tumour was so foetid that 'the odour of her room, and indeed of the whole house, was so overpowering that the comfort of the inmates was destroyed; servants could not be kept; and even nurses could only be induced to stay by high wages and an almost unlimited allowance of brandy'. The, 'very first application of the chloride of zinc' removed and 'completely destroyed' all 'offensive odour'.[42] These chemical agents were often mixed with herbal elements, like liquorice root or saffron, which were supposed to effect a more permanent cure than the acid alone. Sometimes these herbal additions derived special power from their exotic origins.[43]

From Internal to External Interventions

The therapeutic landscape of cancer at the turn of the nineteenth century was diverse and patients frequently underwent a series of different treatments for their disease—either one after the other or in tandem. However, in its first few decades the nineteenth century witnessed a subtle shift in understandings of cancer treatment. While in the eighteenth century and before, internal and external remedies for cancer shared space, prestige, and theoretical legitimacy, by the middle of the nineteenth century—and particularly among elite, orthodox, and hospital-based practitioners—internal medicaments for cancer ceded therapeutic ground to external treatments for the disease. In 1848, an American surgeon called

---

[39] Whitbread, 'Prefatory Letter', ixx.   [40] Denman, *Observations on the Cure of Cancer*.
[41] Whitbread, 'Prefatory Letter'.
[42] Spencer Wells, *Cancer Cures and Cancer Curers* (London, 1860), 55.
[43] J. Weldon Fell, *A Treatise on Cancer, and Its Treatment* (London, 1857), 40.

Usher Parsons wrote, 'No medicine, yet discovered, possesses the power of resolving or otherwise curing cancerous tumours...Extirpation, then, with the knife...is the chief if not the only measure that promises to effect a cure.'[44] In arguing that surgery was the pre-eminent, if not guaranteed, treatment for cancer, Parsons was echoing his co-professionals across the Atlantic. Moreover, and as Parsons' quotation demonstrates, this shift took place *before* the widespread adoption of anaesthetics or asepsis.

Parsons was part of a loud and harmonious chorus of voices who increasingly insisted that internal medicaments were futile and that the only possible recourse in cases of cancer was surgery, irrespective of specific method or instrument (the knife, caustics, etc.). The tumour had to be removed and ingested pills, potions, and tonics were deemed ineffectual at best and harmful at worst. In an 1856 translation of his work, *A Treatise on Cancer of the Breast and of the Mammary Region*, the French anatomist and surgeon Alfred-Armand Velpeau wrote, 'To express it in two words, the cancerous nature of the disease being fully established, no remedy, no internal treatment has been discovered equal to its cure.'[45] A year later, Manchester surgeon George Southam argued along similar lines in his *Address in Surgery* read before the British Medical Association, 'Cancerous deposit is considered, under ordinary circumstance, not to be capable of undergoing absorption. Its removal can, therefore, only be effected either by the knife, by caustics, or by the ligature.'[46]

In the early nineteenth century, therefore, various theoretical and professional transformations secured surgery as the most rational of cancer remedies. Crucially, as this took place before the adoption of anaesthesia after *c*.1850, the ability to immobilize the patient was not in itself responsible for the rising popularity of surgical intervention in cases of cancer. Rather, this new consensus relied on a shift in the way the disease was conceptualized.[47] As shown in Chapter 1, while cancer was broadly understood as a 'systemic', 'general', or 'constitutional' disease in early modern cosmologies, in the first few decades of the nineteenth century and against a backdrop of a decline in humoral theories, increasing hospitalization, and the rising status of surgeons as compared to physicians and apothecaries, it was reconstructed as a 'local' disease—a physical and tangible entity that was at its outset confined to a single bodily location.

This altered conceptualization was tracked by a broader shift in therapeutic regimes. If, in the eighteenth century, treatments were highly individualized

---

[44] Usher Parsons, *Cancer of the Breast* (Providence, RI, 1849), 181–2.

[45] Alfred-Armand Velpeau, *A Treatise on Cancer of the Breast and of the Mammary Region*, trans. W. Marsden (London, 1856), 142.

[46] George Southam, *The Nature and Treatment of Cancer: Being the Address in Surgery Read before the 25th Meeting of the British Medical Association, Held at Nottingham July 1857* (London, 1858), 30.

[47] For more on the introduction of anaesthesia into British surgery see, Stephanie J. Snow, *Operations without Pain: The Practice and Science of Anaesthesia in Victorian Britain* (Basingstoke, 2006).

according to the sufferer's unique physiology and pathology, by the middle of the nineteenth century, medical and surgical practice attended to specific disease entities.[48] Or, in other words, from the beginning of the nineteenth century onwards, rather than tailoring treatments to the patient's body and soul, interventions were targeted towards 'specific' or particular maladies.[49] This was true for cancer too. Hayle Walshe repeatedly criticized one internal remedy or another for not having a 'specific' influence on malignancy. Hydrocyanic acid, for example, 'may be doubtless useful as a sedative, but is utterly devoid of specific action in this disease'.[50] He went on to say, 'There is no medicine known having claims to the character of a specific in cancerous diseases, nor even endowed with the special attribute of invariably modifying the course of the affection.'[51] The reconfiguration of surgery as an appropriate and potentially curative response to cancer thus relied on the disease's reinterpretation as a local, rather than general, affliction. If cancer could be confined to a singular spot in the body, then surgical removal could now remove not just the sign and symptom, but the underlying malady as well.

Surgery Contested

It might be tempting to write a history of nineteenth-century cancer treatment that reveals a progressive replacement of internal medicaments with increasingly pain-free, safe, and effective surgery. However, while excision was increasingly deemed the *ideal* response to the disease, in practice its status as the superlative intervention was contested. Indeed, cancer treatment was the subject of 'warm controversy' in the first half of the nineteenth century, and while elite practitioners may have reached an uneasy consensus over the *medical* incurability of cancer, they had not achieved parallel unity over the curative nature of *surgery*.[52] Hayle Walshe wrote, 'in respect of the possibility of eradicating it from the system by operation there is no such unanimity'.[53]

By the second half of the century, early optimism over the curative effects of cancer surgery had faded and elite practitioners who advised operation did so with multiple caveats. Hayle Walshe provided a five-part list of circumstances in which 'prudent surgeons' should not 'advise removal of carcinoma', which included, 'when such adhesions or local extensions of the primary disease exist, as would

---

[48] See Mary E. Fissell, 'The Disappearance of the Patient's Narrative and the Invention of Hospital Medicine', in R. French and A. Wear (eds.), *British Medicine in an Age of Reform* (London, 1991); Michel Foucault, *The Birth of the Clinic: An Archaeology of Medical Perception* (London, 1973).
[49] See Nicholas D. Jewson, 'The Disappearance of the Sick-Man from Medical Cosmology, 1770–1870', *Sociology*, 10 (1976), 225–44; and John Harley Warner, *The Therapeutic Perspective: Medical Practice, Knowledge, and Identity in America, 1820–1885* (Princeton, NJ, 1997).
[50] Hayle Walshe, *The Nature and Treatment of Cancer*, 196.   [51] Ibid., 225.
[52] Ibid., 146.   [53] Ibid., 148.

render it impossible to remove the mass completely either by excision or by amputation of a limb'; 'when the disease is manifestly spreading or in a state of active growth'; and 'when the existence of internal carcinoma is even probable'.[54] He argued that the surgeon had to 'balance the dangers of the operation against the degree of strength and vital energy of the patient, and act accordingly'.[55] The scale more frequently tipped in favour of non-intervention, and operations for cancer were infrequently performed and always attended by anxiety and uncertainty. George Southam wrote, 'Even these means [the knife, caustics, ligature] are regarded by many as of doubtful efficacy; and certainly, when they are undertaken without due discrimination, they do not appear to increase the chances of life.'[56]

Critiques of, and ambivalence about, surgery partly oscillated around general anxieties over operations in an era before anaesthesia and asepsis. Practitioners and patients alike expressed concern about pain, haemorrhage, and infection. Pre-anaesthesia surgery was frequently represented as acutely painful. Frances Burney narrated an episode of intense pain:

Yet—when the dreadful steel was plunged into the breast—cutting through veins—arteries—flesh—nerves—I needed no injunctions not to restrain my cries. I began a scream that lasted unintermittingly during the whole time of the incision—and I almost marvel that it rings not in my Ears still! So excruciating was the agony.[57]

Denunciations of corrosive applications often centred on the pain caused. Langston Parker, surgeon to the Queen's Hospital, Birmingham, argued in 1856 that caustic treatments were 'valuable, effective, and safe'.[58] Yet even he acknowledged that a key drawback to these applications was the 'pain occasioned by the prolonged contact of the caustics with the disease, which varies from a period of twelve to forty-eight hours'.[59] Chloride of zinc was supposed to be 'one of the most painful of caustics'. Velpeau wrote, 'The majority of patients on whom I have used it complained so greatly that they had no hesitation in submitting to the use of the knife rather than re-commence its application.'[60] However, caustic applications were not without their comparative merits. They were understood as preferable to the knife in some cases, because they were supposed to lessen the risk of haemorrhage and reduce what we would term post-operative infection. Parker suggested that they were particularly useful in 'large, fetid, bleeding cancerous or cancroid ulcers where the knife is utterly out of the question, and where the patient is sinking from local irritation and haemorrhage'.[61]

---

[54] Ibid., 169.   [55] Ibid.   [56] Southam, *The Nature and Treatment of Cancer*, 30.
[57] Burney, 'Account from Paris of a Terrible Operation'.
[58] Parker, *The Treatment of Cancer Diseases by Caustics*, 16.   [59] Ibid.
[60] Quoted in Fell, *A Treatise on Cancer*, 51.
[61] Parker, *The Treatment of Cancer Diseases by Caustics*, 15.

The Tumour Returns

However, barely any space in pre-anaesthesia surgical texts (those that dealt with the knife) was devoted to discussions of haemorrhage, infection, and surgical pain. Rather, surgeons were increasingly insisting on the safety of excision, 'It is probable that not one in five hundred die of the operation.'[62] However, what constituted 'safe' depended on the procedure performed. According to Professor of Surgery at King's College London, Sir William Fergusson, only about a third of patients survived amputation of the leg at the hip joint.[63] Nonetheless, the most prominent anxiety that contributed to the pervasive ambivalence over surgical efficacy was one peculiar to cancer—the threat of relapse and the inability to guarantee the complete removal of the disease from the body. Surgeons were profoundly troubled by the likelihood of recurrence, and already at the beginning of the nineteenth century practitioners were speaking of their cancer patients in terms of years gained, rather than complete cures procured. Sufferers might still be living six months later, one year, or two, but only very rarely was this cancer-free life permanent. Hayle Walshe discussed in detail the rate of relapse after cancer surgery, collating the evidence from various practitioners. Overall, the picture was dire. Of the sixty people the Scottish surgeon Alexander Munro operated on, only four remained free from disease at the end of two years.[64] Similarly, throughout Italian surgeon Antonio Scarpa's long career, he only observed 'three cases of extirpation of true scirrhus permanently successful'.[65]

Even after the most radical and extensive operations cancer was likely to return. For while malignancy was a local disease, that identity was only temporary. As shown in Chapter 1, cancer was defined by its capacity for spread. Or, as Hayle Walshe termed it, 'malignity', which was, 'the power of a morbid growth at once to assimilate different tissues to its own substance, to produce similar disease in distant parts, to reappear after destruction and give rise to a peculiar cachexia'.[66] He thus stressed 'the absolute necessity of removing every particle of diseased mater; and in order to ensure this result, a stratum of healthy tissue should if possible be removed along with the morbid growth'.[67] Those surgeons who felt surface cancer with their hands were well aware that these masses could be later-stage manifestations of an internal disease, or that breast cancer, for example, could spread to the liver or lungs. They knew that cancer could and would affect the internal organs, even if its presence there could only be verified after the person had died.

---

[62] Parsons, *Cancer of the Breast*, 184.   [63] Fergusson, *A System of Practical Surgery*, 413.
[64] Walter Hayle Walshe, *The Anatomy, Physiology, Pathology, and Treatment of Cancer* (Boston, MA, 1844), 148.
[65] Ibid.   [66] Ibid., 183.   [67] Ibid., 172.

This notion of recurrence supported ideas about cancer's incurability, and, as discussed in Chapter 1, only became widely agreed upon in the nineteenth century. After the hospitalization of the disease, surgeons were newly able to compile data and statistics, and view their patients in aggregate. Hospitalization was framed as an opportunity to derive new knowledge from expansive cohorts of patients, systematically studied. The foundational documents of The Middlesex Hospital cancer ward stated:

> By confining one or more Wards to Cancers only the attention of Pupils and others will be directed very strictly to the study of this Disease, they will see facts as they arise in the aggregate from a large number of Patients, new lights will appear and new discoveries will probably be made.[68]

Moreover, the early nineteenth century saw the British populace increasingly quantified—at multiple different scales. This practice derived in part from the development of statistical methods and epidemiology, and grew alongside a quantitative study of people and their activities more generally.[69]

For example, while it initially received influential medical and lay support, compression soon fell out of favour because, by mid-century, it had been deemed ineffective. Usher Parsons compiled 'statistical tables' to come to this conclusion, a practice only possible in a context where large numbers of patients were being treated and the outcomes recorded.[70] In evidencing his claims over surgical inefficacy, George Southam wrote, 'numerous statistical tables have been prepared on this subject, from which various results have been deduced'.[71] These 'extensive statistical inquiries' demonstrated that the knife obtained 'a very little advantage' for cancer sufferers. Velpeau spoke of subjecting cancer treatments to 'a rigorous proof in a great number of patients'.[72] Thus, and as argued in Chapters 1 and 2, the institutionalization of cancer turned incurability from an incidental detail into a defining characteristic.[73]

Additionally, while these surgeons had all observed patients apparently cured by the removal of their cancerous tumours, these were occasional minorities that cast doubt on the initial diagnosis. If surgery had cured the disease, then perhaps the tumour had been benign rather than malignant. Velpeau wrote, 'Some believe

---

[68] UCLH Archive, London, 'Weekly Board Meeting', Middlesex Hospital Minutes, 10 January 1792.

[69] See John M. Eyler, 'The Conceptual Origins of William Farr's Epidemiology: Numerical Methods and Social Thought in the 1830s', in Abraham M. Lilienfeld (ed.), *Times, Places, and Persons* (Baltimore, MD, 1980); Ian Hacking, *The Taming of Chance* (Cambridge, UK, 1990); Eileen Magnello and Anne Hardy (eds.), *The Road to Medical Statistics* (Amsterdam, 2002).

[70] Parsons, *Cancer of the Breast*, 189.   [71] Southam, *The Nature and Treatment of Cancer*, 31.

[72] Velpeau, *A Treatise on Cancer of the Breast*, 136.   [73] See Chapter 1.

they have cured cancers, simply because they have at first mistaken harmless tumours for malignant ones.'[74] He argued that any opinion contrary to the practical incurability of cancer 'rests merely on errors in diagnostics'.[75] This process of retroactive diagnosis—identifying the disease only once it had killed the patient—reveals the inextricable and practical connection between cancer and incurability. In some ways, this was the only predictable and therefore only manageable feature of malignancy, and it provided a form of paradoxical stability in clinical interactions otherwise marked by material disorder and therapeutic failure.

In theory, too, cancers could be cured by the knife if caught very early—before they had spread to other organs and into the constitution. Hayle Walshe suggested that 'the earlier the morbid mass is removed the stronger are the chances of ultimate recovery'.[76] If the surgeon could intervene when the tumour was still small, still local, then they might be able to entirely prevent relapse. Italian surgeon Antonio Scarpa argued that as long as the 'morbid seed' remained 'latent and inert', the disease would be 'purely local', and as a result could be 'susceptible of a favourable and permanent cure by extirpation'.[77] Larger, ulcerating masses were likely to have already spread to distant or internal organs, rendering surgery futile and the body prone to recurrence. Moscucci describes this as an idea of 'relative' incurability—in which cancer was thought to 'progress' through various stages of intractability.[78]

However, this transition from phase to phase—from local to general—was unpredictable and difficult to identify from physical examination or narrative histories. While surgeons could assume that foetid tumours had already spread— 'once the cancerous degeneration has set in, the operation . . . is quite useless'[79]— smaller lumps still buried in the flesh were less predictable, and surgeons bemoaned the disease's erratic trajectory. In these cases, the surgeon had to use his judgement, take the disease on a 'case-by-case' basis, and deploy a wide variety of metrics to decide what to do when. However, even if easily identifiable, these early cases rarely presented themselves. Frustratingly for practitioners, they were dependent on the decision of their patients as to when they could access the diseased body. As argued in Chapter 1, most cancer patients only sought medical advice when the tumour had become impossible to live with and surgeons argued that cancer's high rate of recurrence was the result of what we now term 'late presentation'. Thus, and as Ilana Löwy has argued, those who advocated surgical

---

[74] Ibid.   [75] Ibid.

[76] Hayle Walshe, *The Anatomy, Physiology, Pathology, and Treatment of Cancer*, 151.

[77] Antonio Scarpa, *Remarks and Practical Results of Observation on Scirrhus and Cancer*, trans. James Briggs (London, 1822), 29.

[78] Ornella Moscucci, *Gender and Cancer in England, 1860–1948* (London, 2017), 50.

[79] Bransby Blake Cooper, *Lectures on the Principles and Practice of Surgery* (London, 1851), 217.

intervention for suspected uterine cancer in the early nineteenth century campaigned strongly for an early operation.[80] Surgical dictionaries and domestic medicine manuals implored their readership to seek advice quickly. *The Female's Medical Guide and Married Woman's Adviser* told its readers in 1849, 'Were proper means used in due time, a cancer might often be prevented; but after the disorder has arrived at a certain height it generally sets all medicine at defiance.'[81]

Thus, while cancer might be permanently cured by surgical intervention in theory, in practice such a case almost never arrived in the clinic on time. These observers were all grappling with the same question: what was the use of subjecting a patient to a protracted, painful and potentially lethal operation if the body was already under threat elsewhere? Should surgeons, therefore, refuse to operate except in only very rare cases where they thought it might result in a complete cure? And, if so, what was a surgeon's responsibility to a patient with late-stage cancer? In a rhetorical device, Hayle Walshe put words to a nineteenth-century shift in emphasis with respect to cancer surgery:

So far we have spoken of the operation as a means of radical cure; but it may perhaps become allowable as a palliative,—as likely to prolong life and conduce to a comparative *euthanasia*, in certain cases, where the agony endured and the abundance of the haemorrhage are rapidly wearing out the existence of the sufferer.[82]

Thus, while elite practitioners at the beginning of the century had hoped that surgery might be a curative intervention, as we move forward into the 'future' discussed in Chapter 2, the operation's apparent limitations only reconfirmed cancer's incurable status. The early nineteenth-century practitioners that appeared in Chapter 2 mapped out the upcoming age as a period of advancement and medical perfection—a period that would witness the removal of cancer from the roster of 'dread diseases'. However, as the years marched on, this initial optimism gave way to a more restrictive realism that found expression in the increasing practice and justification of *palliative* surgery.

---

[80] Ilana Löwy, ' "Because of their Praiseworthy Modesty, They Consult Too Late": Regime of Hope and Cancer of the Womb, 1800–1910', *Bulletin of the History of Medicine*, 85 (2011), 356–83.

[81] Henry Burchstead Skinner, *The Female's Medical Guide and Married Woman's Adviser: Containing a Description of the Causes, Symptoms and Cure of Diseases Peculiar to Females, whether Married or Single, from Early Childhood to Old Age, such as Retention, Suppression and Cessation of Menses, Difficult and Irregular Menstruation, Pregnancy, its Indications and Attendant Diseases, Miscarriage or Abortion, Midwifery, the Turn of Life, Causes and Cure of Barrenness, and Female Complaints Generally. The Whole Adapted to the Private Use of Families* (Boston, MA, 1849), 78.

[82] Hayle Walshe, *The Anatomy, Physiology, Pathology, and Treatment of Cancer*, 170–1.

Palliative Surgery

Cancer surgery had, therefore, multiple purposes in the nineteenth century. 'To cure' was only one of many. In the 1850s, Hayle Walshe wrote, 'The extirpation of cancer may be undertaken with the following various intentions: To cure the disease; To prolong life; To relieve urgent symptoms; To procure a comparatively easy death for the sufferer; To satisfy the importunate desires of patients.'[83] Some variety of palliation (ameliorating pain and easing the passage towards death) had long been a basic element of intervention in cases of cancer, and the alleviation of suffering was key to the periodic interaction between doctor and patient in all varieties of health and ill-health. However, the first half of the nineteenth century witnessed an increasing use of the terms 'palliative', 'palliate', and 'palliation' in surgical texts that dealt with the problem of cancer. In 1790, the physician William Rowley wrote, 'In this hopeless state...all medical endeavours should be directed to the palliation of symptoms.'[84] This might involve laudanum, alterations to diet, alcohol, and other non-surgical interventions to sooth. In the decades following the institutionalization of cancer, however, practitioners renegotiated *surgical* intervention (rather than Rowley's 'medical endeavours') as a palliative enterprise—salvaging an element of effectiveness and prestige for a procedure that was otherwise practically impotent in the face of the 'dread disease'.

Palliative surgery's main novelty lay in the explicit intention to relieve suffering, rather than effect a cure. Its sole aim was to relieve the *symptoms* of cancer, rather than the underlying disease—predicated on the belief that there was little that surgeons could do to access, let alone reverse, constitutional malignancy. In cases of late-stage or degenerated cancer, palliative surgery worked to achieve three things: to 'relieve pain', 'remove foetor', and provide an at least partial return to physical and social function. Deciding whether to perform or undergo palliative surgery involved strategic calculations by both doctor and patient. It was a comparative exercise—contrasting suffering from unchecked cancer (disease allowed to follow its own, unimpeded trajectory)—to the pain and risk associated with surgical intervention. Doctors needed to decide how much agony they could inflict—or how much pain patients were willing to bear—to (only) temporarily alleviate the cancer symptoms. The agony inflicted by the untrammelled tumour was compared with the suffering provoked by the operation. Consequently, even before the introduction of anaesthesia—and in contrast to doctors' assessments of surgery as a curative enterprise—conversations over the palliative utility of surgery made frequent reference to the pain, suffering, and abjection it caused.

---

[83]   Hayle Walshe, *The Nature and Treatment of Cancer*, 231.
[84]   William Rowley, *A Treatise on the Management of Female Breasts during Childbed; and Several New Observations on Cancerous Diseases*, 2nd edn (London, 1790), 50.

This comparative exercise drew on extensive clinical observation and on a vibrant public literature that emphasized the pain and abjection that accompanied dying from cancer. Late-stage cancer was known to be intensely painful. Sufferers described the pain by analogy to 'the prodding of knives, incision with lancets'.[85] It was supposed to be 'most severely felt at night', and an advert posted in the *Leeds Mercury* in 1844 included a testimony from Elizabeth Crowther, who had been suffering 'under extreme pain' from cancer of the breast.[86] However, pain was not the only consequence of dying from cancer though histories and public health commentaries on palliative care focus on pain, to the exclusion of other effects.[87] Cancer pain was almost invariably accompanied by foetid flesh. As a result, palliative surgery worked to re-control the body's boundaries and return integrity to its surface. The cancerous body was increasingly abject, 'the fact of a sanies of fetid odor and peculiarly acrid qualities being more or less abundantly thrown out by the disorganised surface'.[88] This description by Hayle Walshe was in part metaphorical, alluding to the anxieties provoked by the diseased state. The surface was 'disorganised'—no longer in its proper order, no longer aligning with what we expect and can predict. One writer reflected on the benefits conferred by dying from a cancer of the internal organs rather than from a tumour on the skin's surface—they were saved from the 'painful and disgusting' death that attends cancer, 'when allowed to proceed in its natural course to a fatal termination'.[89] These ulcerations and suppurations were no doubt unpleasant, but they also prevented sufferers from performing day-to-day duties and pleasures. As noted in Chapters 1 and 2, people sought hospital care and surgical consult when they could no longer remain at home and in their communities—likely either because their foetid flesh made society shun them or because they became a burden on household economies.

In justifying palliative surgery, practitioners often drew on the horrors of late-stage cancer and compared surgery favourably to this suffering. Charles Bell and James Young Simpson both published case histories of their patients and their texts constitute the period's most extensive and descriptive record of cancer surgery. Charles Bell was a Scottish surgeon, anatomist, neurologist, and philosophical theologian. He was admitted to the Royal College of Surgeons of Edinburgh, moved to London in 1804, was instrumental in the creation of The Middlesex Hospital Medical School, worked on the institution's cancer ward, and published various texts on his surgical experiences of the disease.[90] From c.1816 he published a 'quarterly report of cases in surgery; treated in the Middlesex Hospital', and regularly included accounts of cancer patients. James Young

[85] Hayle Walshe, *The Anatomy, Physiology, Pathology, and Treatment of Cancer*, 136.
[86] Ibid.; see also 'Advertisements & Notices', *Leeds Mercury*, 24 February 1844.
[87] Julia Lawton, *The Dying Process: Patients' Experiences of Palliative Care* (London, 2000).
[88] Hayle Walshe, *The Nature and Treatment of Cancer*, 124.   [89] Ibid., 245–6.
[90] Bell, *Surgical Observations*; Jacyna, 'Bell, Sir Charles(1774–1842)'.

Simpson was a Scottish obstetrician, surgeon, and the first to demonstrate the anaesthetic properties of chloroform on humans.[91] He encountered cancer when it interfered with female reproductive organs. Simpson published his *Cases of Excision of the Cervix Uteri for Carcinomatous Disease* in 1846.[92] As elite urban surgeons, these men were part of a narrow and not necessarily representative stratum of medical society. Moreover, both showed a perhaps unusual career-long commitment to their patients' feelings. Bell published studies on emotional expression and was an anti-vivisectionist. Simpson was an early advocate of pain relief during surgery.[93] However, when read alongside contemporaries such as Hayle Walshe and his textbook, *On the Nature and Treatment of Cancer*, the works by these men were clearly typical of broadly held contemporary attitudes to surgical palliation.

Charles Bell invoked the suffering caused by cancer to offset the pain inflicted by his knife. He wrote, 'In some of these cases... the pain of the tumour in the latter period was so great, that the suffering of amputation was considered as the lesser evil.'[94] For Bell, the 'ulceration and self-destroying process of cancer [were] so horrible' that this constituted an 'argument for the operation'.[95] Death would be 'easier' if the mass was removed by the knife, rather than 'suffering it to proceed its natural course'.[96] Bell included the testimonials of past patients whose symptoms had been ameliorated and who compared the knife favourably with the disease. For example, one of Bell's patients, William Phineas, claimed that the pains during surgery 'were nothing to the agony of the disease'.[97] Hayle Walshe agreed, and concluded that the agony caused by tumours was 'infinitely greater than that produced by the knife'.[98] A subtle distinction between the 'pain' of surgery and the 'suffering' caused by unchecked cancer illustrates the difference between the two and helps explain why the former was bearable and the latter was intolerable. 'Pain' was perceived as a physical sensation whereas 'suffering' was a matrix of emotions caused, in part, by pain, but also by fear, anxiety, and grief. Or, in other words, the pain during surgery was deemed productive, because it would ameliorate suffering in the long term. The 'suffering' of late-stage cancer produced nothing but death and decline.

The removal of foetid flesh was more ambiguous territory than the relief of pain as the sensation inflicted by the knife was not directly comparable to the distress caused by an unsociable or intolerant body. Again, however, surgeons emphasized the unstable nature of the cancerous body in their defence of radical, palliative

[91] Nicolson, 'Simpson, Sir James Young'.
[92] James Young Simpson, *Cases of Excision of the Cervix Uteri for Carcinomatous Disease* (Dublin, 1846).
[93] Jacyna, 'Bell, Sir Charles (1774–1842)'; Nicolson, 'Simpson, Sir James Young'.
[94] Bell, *Surgical Observations*, 369.   [95] Ibid.   [96] Ibid., 379.   [97] Ibid.
[98] Hayle Walshe, *The Anatomy, Physiology, Pathology, and Treatment of Cancer*, 164.

intervention. In one of Simpson's cases he described the patient's experience of suffering in detail and quoted her in his narrative account:

> The discharge then assumed a more watery character, and imparted an excoriating burning feeling to the parts as it passed...After this watery 'boiling discharge' (as the patient herself termed it) had lasted profusely for about a fortnight, severe haemorrhage came on. It was kept under imperfect restraint by the supine posture.[99]

The surgeon's intervention palliated this suffering by removing the source of haemorrhage. It returned stability and integrity to the body, albeit without addressing the underlying cause of the patient's distress and decline.

Bell, too, often laced his descriptions with graphic imagery and grotesque language to make clear to his readership the multifaceted suffering of his patients and thus to justify operation. A farmer applied to him for advice about a 'large tumour which disfigured his face in an extraordinary degree'.[100] This physicality was invoked to vindicate the lengths surgeons would go to re-establish the integrity of flesh and contain the cancer within reasonable proportions, at least for a while. In this case, Bell's response was particularly violent, 'I crushed through the jaw, and brought away the whole mass.'[101] He implored his reader to understand his compassionate motives for this particularly destructive intervention and insisted on the appropriateness of his decision, 'If this be thought a severe operation, I must affirm that it is not equal to what I should now think myself authorised to perform in a similar case.'[102]

Once practitioners had convinced their readers of the comparative rationale that justified their palliative interventions, they turned their attention to assessing the success of their operations. While the suffering inflicted by the knife might pale in comparison to that caused by unchecked cancer, palliative surgery was still ineffectual if it did not actually lessen distress before dying or prolong life in a productive and enjoyable way. While surgery in other contexts might be judged according to whether the patient lived or died, palliative operations needed to take a more expansive view of what constituted 'success'. Or, in other words, while assessments of curative practices could be done with the patient's *bodies*, judgements over the palliative effectiveness of operations required the patient's *words*. The patient narrative was important, even in an age when historians have argued its clinical value diminished.[103] Assessments of palliative surgery could only be done with the help of testimonials from cancer sufferers and surgeons reproduced extensive case histories that narrated the sufferer's life before, during, and after treatment. Cancer's specific profile thus structured a different kind of surgical

---

[99] Simpson, *Cases of Excision*, 6.   [100] Bell, *Surgical Observations*, 416.   [101] Ibid., 418.
[102] Ibid.   [103] See Fissell, 'The Disappearance of the Patient's Narrative'.

environment and script, with its own internal logic and rationale. Simpson reflected on this very question. He presented his own successes, and wrote up his cases to illustrate and emphasize his competent and compassionate decision-making. With one patient, he argued that 'immediately after the operation was performed...[her]...health and strength have been in the meantime restored to her'.[104] But equally, he caveated his own achievements and willingly acknowledged the limits of what he could offer his patients: 'the morbid characters of the diseased structures that I removed, are such, certainly, as to render its future regeneration not at all improbable'.[105] Yet, he had alleviated the patient's suffering, re-controlled the body's integrity, and allowed her to return to a form of function: 'there seems to be no reasonable doubt but that the operation has restored the bodily comfort, and prolonged the life of the patient, if it has not entirely freed her from the risk of a future return of the disease'.[106] Thus, Simpson was arguing that surgical palliation worked to return patients' bodies to relative, albeit temporary, function.

Both Bell and Simpson included quotidian details in their case histories and revealed a commitment to a pluralistic understanding of health and therapeutic efficacy. Their remit for 'success' was broad, and suggests that they considered their patient's happiness alongside their physical condition. Simpson wrote about the recovery of another patient with cervical cancer: 'After the excision of the diseased structures the lumbar pains and local watery and haemorrhage discharges entirely ceased...The patient rallied so speedily in health and strength, that within a fortnight she was able to be taken into the garden.'[107] This mundane detail about the woman's leisure possibilities emphasized the very human relationship between patient and practitioner. In another case, J. Argyll Robertson from University College London detailed the return to health of one of his patients after the removal of a cancerous eye. Robertson quotes his patient as being, 'able to do a good day's work yet at his trade of weaving'.[108] Palliation meant not only a reduction in pain, but an ability to return to work. This focus on people's leisure and labour suggests efforts to put across an image of comprehensive compassion. Moreover, this preoccupation with the whole person, not just the malady or tumour, reveals that while cancer may have been conceptualized as a 'local' or 'surgical' disease, it was still understood along very individual lines. Practitioners considered cancer in terms of its effects on the life of that particular patient.

Both Bell and Simpson portrayed sympathy as a key—if not the only—motivation for operating. Their writings reinforce the argument made in Chapter 2 about compassionate, emotional surgeons rather than dispassionate automatons. They presented themselves as emotionally affected by their patients'

---

[104] Simpson, *Cases of Excision*, 5.   [105] Ibid.   [106] Ibid.   [107] Ibid., 7.
[108] J. Argyll Robertson, *Excision of the Eyeball in Cases of Melanosis, Medullary Carcinoma, and Carcinoma: With Remarks* (London, 1844), 8.

suffering. Bell wrote of feeling 'anxiety' for James Lewsley, a seventeen-year-old boy with a tumour on his thigh.[109] Similarly, Simpson inserted a comment that signalled the surgeon's emotional engagement with his patient's distress in an account of someone who was treated by two other practitioners: 'I am principally indebted for the notes of it to Dr Jackson, who, along with Dr Paterson, watched over the poor woman with great care and kindness.'[110] Bell made much of the emotional costs of surgery for the practitioner as well as the sufferer. He wrote about his 'gloomy presage' on diagnosing cancer, and how he always had 'the liveliest apprehensions' when treating someone with an incurable tumour.[111] In opting to promote the physical and emotional worlds of both them and their patients these surgeons presented an affective justification as much as intellectual rationalization.

Surgical texts that foreground evocative descriptions of pain and suffering can thus be read in multiple ways. They can be interpreted as descriptions, explanations, or justifications. They are sites of ambiguity and acted as fora through which practitioners could work through their reservations about the utility and humanity of surgery and justify their interventions. Building on the arguments of Chapter 2, these texts were performative, and used cancer's incurability to construct an identity predicated on restraint and emotional nuance. Both surgeons made clear to the reader that they appreciated that they might make the wrong decision about whether to operate or not. They emphasized their own caution. For example, Simpson was pessimistic about cancer's prognosis: 'I believe that in forty-nine instances out of every fifty in which we find the uterus or any part of it, the seat of true carcinomatous deposit, the disease inevitably leads, sooner or later, to a fatal termination.'[112] Likewise, Bell's texts were replete with rhetorical questions—as though he is asking himself as much as calling on the reader to reflect: 'Do these circumstances warrant amputation?', 'what is the chance of saving the life?', and 'could the patient bear such violence as would be necessary in the performance?'[113] Simpson wrote of his 'strong doubts' but was reassured by the perceived likelihood that his patient would soon have 'sunk under' her symptoms without his intervention.[114] He turned the tragedy of a women whose 'peace of mind was broken', whose 'constitution was so rapidly giving way under the constant, profuse, and weakening discharges which afflicted her', into a surgical achievement, albeit within strict parameters.[115]

Together, the portrayals of professional insecurity, affective engagement, and doubt complicate narratives of surgical heroism that position nineteenth-century surgeons as self-assured and disinterested in their patients' suffering. Rather than presenting themselves as insensitive and scientific practitioners—who were

[109] Bell, *Surgical Observations*, 390.   [110] Simpson, *Cases of Excision*, 8.
[111] Bell, *Surgical Observations*, 409–10.   [112] Simpson, *Cases of Excision*, 19.
[113] Bell, *Surgical Observations*, 396, 427.   [114] Simpson, *Cases of Excision*, 5.   [115] Ibid.

focused on a narrow definition of therapeutic efficacy (a complete cure)—instead, these practitioners painted textured self-portraits replete with emotional complexity. While we cannot see these texts as unmediated insights into the emotional landscapes of their authors, neither publication was widely disseminated. Both are brief collections of relatively unembellished case notes, and likely functioned more as records or instructive manuals than expositions on surgical ethics and identity. Moreover, I would like to suggest that while deliberate and instrumental 'uses' of emotional rhetoric played a part, we must also take a degree of expressed distress and sympathy at face value. It is possible for surgeons to have simultaneously cared deeply about their patients, but also have recognized the social and professional utility of framing their practice in such terms.

There is also evidence to suggest that these operations took place at the patient's request. Bell, Simpson, and many of their contemporaries suggested—implicitly or otherwise—that palliative surgery was more often demanded by sufferers than imposed by surgeons. It is possible that in emphasizing this, surgeons were working to shift responsibility of potential failure onto the shoulders of their patients. However, because we know that the suffering inflicted by late-stage cancer can be unbearable, it is not difficult to image that men and women sought out extreme means to limit their distress. Frances Burney reflected that she 'would far rather suffer a quick end without, than a lingering life with this dreadfullest of maladies'.[116] Thomas Denman treated a woman whose 'mind was so distressed on the occasion that she earnestly requested the breast might be taken off'.[117] Similarly, Bell observed that the suffering of his patient, William Phineas, 'must be great in degree, since he expresses a desire to lose the limb'.[118] Hayle Walshe made this aspect of patient demand explicit. He wrote that palliative surgery ought not to be performed, 'unless the patient be *determined* to submit to the knife with a full consciousness of the comparatively slight benefit he is entitled to expect from his submission'.[119] Rather, while the surgeon 'may *yield* to the entreaty of the patient', he must not 'advise removal'.[120]

Moreover, the suffering need not be physical to provoke radical solutions. Indeed, the anxiety and ambivalence expressed by Bell and Simpson was not just over the tenuous status of palliative surgery, but also over cancer, the disease itself. It was the 'dread and excruciating disease', synonymous with death and decline and feared by doctor and patient.[121] It was, 'of all the ills to which the human frame is liable', the most 'poignant'.[122] Key to cancer's peculiar threat was its incurability. However, the malady had also acquired a litany of meanings that extended beyond its intractable nature. Cancer was conceptualized as an entity

---

[116] Burney, 'Account from Paris of a Terrible Operation'.
[117] Denman, *Observations on the Cure of Cancer*, 69.   [118] Bell, *Surgical Observations*, 392.
[119] Hayle Walshe, *The Nature and Treatment of Cancer*, 245; emphasis added.   [120] Ibid.
[121] 'The Increasing Fatality of Cancer', *BMJ*, 1 (1883), 970.
[122] Thomas Pope, 'On Cancer', *Association Medical Journal*, 3 (1855), 859–60, at 859.

with agency—one that invades the body, occupies tissue, and corrupts. This was accompanied by an acute anxiety; this, alongside the pain, suffering, and abjection caused by the materiality of the tumour, helps to explain why patients requested extensive operations even when they knew these were not going to be curative. Thus, cancer was not only feared because it killed, but because it challenged fundamental notions of identity and bodily integrity.[123] Fear was clearly a crucial component of the patient's decision-making process. Simpson wrote:

> Every practitioner knows that, of all uterine diseases, cancer is the one which the female mind most constantly and most justly dreads. A patient scarcely ever suffers for a length of time under any severe affliction of the uterus, without her own anxieties and fears magnifying it into an instance of cancer, and investing it with all the horrors pertaining to this most fearful and loathsome malady.[124]

Both practitioner and patient were eager, therefore, to *get this thing out*, irrespective of whether this was the rational, effective, or curative thing to do. And, essential for the construction of surgical palliative care, even in the throes of death patients wanted their cancer gone. One surgeon commented on a female patient at the end of the nineteenth century, 'She will generally consent to anything to get rid of the haunting dread of that terror of her life—mammary cancer.'[125]

Surgery after Anaesthesia

Both James Young Simpson and Charles Bell did most of their work before the widespread adoption of chloroform. Anaesthesia was by no means unproblematic and anxiety over its safety was pervasive. In 1887, the *Liverpool Mercury* reported on the case of a woman 'who had died from the effects of chloroform administered for an operation. She suffered from cancer in the breast.'[126] Despite these concerns, anaesthetia's introduction transformed the experience of the cancer patient undergoing surgery and shifted the balance in assessments of risk and suffering. However, it had very little impact on cancer's definition as an incurable disease. For if anaesthesia, and later asepsis, made patients less likely to die on the

---

[123] Susan Sontag warned that the common, twentieth-century metaphor of cancer as a hostile enemy that had to be battled by all available means led to excessively aggressive, potentially harmful treatment. Susan Sontag, *Illness as Metaphor and AIDS and Its Metaphors* (London, 2013).

[124] Simpson, *Cases of Excision*, 15.

[125] Charles Creighton, 'Address in Pathology: On the Autonomous Life of the Specific Infections', *BMJ*, 2 (1883), 218–24, at 218.

[126] 'Special Telegrams &c.', *Liverpool Mercury*, 11 February 1887. For the history of anaesthesia see Snow, *Operations without Pain* and Pernick, *A Calculus of Suffering*.

operating table or from post-operative infection, neither could do much to prevent recurrence or substantially extend life.[127]

Of course, that does not mean that the surgery practised on cancer patients in the 1890s was identical to that performed on sufferers in the 1840s. Indeed, the late nineteenth century witnessed new operative techniques, particularly for breast cancer. While new practices—such as the radical mastectomy—were welcomed by medical men in the United States and across Europe, they were not without their critics. In 1896, Professor of Surgery at King's College London, W. Watson Cheyne, wrote, 'The last few years have seen marked alterations in the older methods of operating in these cases, and also the introduction of operations in regions and of an extent formerly not thought of.' Yet he recognized that these introductions had not been incorporated seamlessly into British theory and practice: 'Opinions differ very much at the present time as to the utility of many of these surgical procedures.'[128] Innovations in haptic skill prompted incremental and highly contested changes in cancer treatment and the latter half of the century was marked more by consistency than change. The precise terms of debate might have changed, but cancer's identity as a peculiarly lethal and intractable disease remained remarkably stable.

William Halsted's case notes are very similar to those from The Middlesex Hospital in the early nineteenth century, despite his reputation as responsible for a transformation in the curative abilities of surgery. His radical mastectomy was an operation in which the breast, underlying chest muscle, and lymph nodes of the axilla were removed.[129] Halsted noted in his 1894 essay in the *Annals of Surgery*, that 'Every one knows how dreadful the results were before the cleaning out of the axilla became recognized as an essential part of the operation. Most of us have heard our teachers in surgery admit that they have never cured a case of cancer of the breast.'[130] Halsted's mastectomy was supposed to be an advance in many ways, not least because it was 'literally an almost bloodless one'. This reputation relied on efforts in the mid-century to improve the safety of operations, and surgeons increasingly appreciated the value of conserving 'every drop of blood'.[131] Such labours seemed to prove fruitful as, 'not one death … resulted from the operation' out of seventy-six.[132] Crucially, however, the mastectomy was also supposed to

---

[127] For an account of the history of asepsis see Michael Worboys, *Spreading Germs: Disease Theories and Medical Practice in Britain, 1865–1900* (Cambridge, UK, 2000), 73–107.

[128] W. Watson Cheyne, 'Lettsomian Lectures on the Objects and Limits of Operations for Cancer', *BMJ*, 1 (1896), 385–90, at 385.

[129] Lerner, *The Breast Cancer Wars*, 4.

[130] William Halsted, 'The Results of Operations for the Cure of Cancer of the Breast Performed at the Johns Hopkins Hospital from June, 1889, to January, 1894', *Annals of Surgery*, 20 (1894), 497–555, at 504.

[131] Moscucci, *Gender and Cancer in England*, 62; J. Spence, 'An Address in Surgery, Delivered at the Forty-Third Annual Meeting of the British Medical Association', *BMJ*, 2 (1875), 189–98, at 193.

[132] Halsted, 'The Results of Operations', 512.

cure—with the extensive removal of tissue, muscle, and lymph nodes designed to eliminate as far as possible any residual cancerous flesh from the region.

Like Bell and Simpson, after Halsted operated he solicited testimonials from his patients, incorporated patient experience, and presented an interest in their well-being. Halsted's case notes included the patient's narrative—'In August 1909 patient struck right breast against bedstead. It caused severe temporary pain of 15–20 minutes'—and identified the initial cause as physical trauma.[133] Like his professional ancestors at the Middlesex, he described this patient's tumour as the 'size of a walnut' and it seeped a 'watery' and 'yellow' discharge.[134] He corresponded with those of his patients who had travelled to his clinic in Baltimore. One woman responded to him in 1914:

> Dear Sir, I receive your letter and was very glad to receive it. I have been in bed helpless ever since July 21, 1913. My arm is swollen now so I that I can't keep my self [sic]. I have had [a local doctor] attending me ever since and I have been in bed. But it seems that he don't know what to do. I am not able to sit up at all.[135]

Halsted replied with, 'I am very sorry to hear that you are not well. If you can meet me at the Johns Hopkins Hospital ... I shall be glad to make an examination.'[136] Many of the patients Halsted wrote to never replied. One man wrote in response to a query about his wife, 'I am very sorry to inform you that [she] ... died on the 12 Day of June 1913. Thank you very kindly for writing.'[137]

Alongside these narrative testimonials, Halsted also collected data on his surgical practices. Indeed, his 1894 essay also includes another form of 'curative' activity: the tabulation and visualization of results. Halsted standardized and 'smoothed' his surgical efforts by presenting his data in pages and pages of tables, graphs, and lists, transforming messy operations into the clean lines of lithograph. Between June 1889 and June 1902, Johns Hopkins admitted 343 cancer patients. Of them, 222 (72.8 per cent) were considered 'operable', whereas eighty-three (27.2 per cent) were considered 'inoperable'. Sixty-seven per cent of the 'inoperable' patients were in fact operated on, 'with the hope of alleviating pain or removing a disagreeable tumour'—or, in other words, to palliate suffering.[138] Just as earlier in the century, Halsted reflected that in most of the inoperable

---

[133] Johns Hopkins University Archive, Box No. 32, Folder No. 8, 12448, Case Note, Surgical No. 25282, 1910.

[134] Ibid.

[135] Johns Hopkins University Archive, Patient Correspondence from 'JHH Cases of Carcinoma of the Breast, 1895–1920', Letter to Dr Halsted, 18 June 1914.

[136] Ibid., 1 October 1914.   [137] Ibid., 7 July 1914.

[138] Johns Hopkins University Archive, Box No. 33, Folder No. 5, 12632, Statistical Study of Cases of Carcinoma of the Breast Admitted to the Johns Hopkins Hospital June 1889 to June 1902.

cases 'the tumour has been present a considerable time' and the inoperability was due 'to the delay in seeking surgical advice'.[139] Halsted then focused on just the 161 patients operated on between June 1889 and August 1899. Of those, sixty cases (37.2 per cent) were still alive in 1902. Seventy-four cases, of the original 161, lived longer than three years without evidence of recurrence.[140]

Despite these promising results, at the turn of the twentieth century, elite and prominent practitioners were still lamenting the limits of surgical intervention in ways that Charles Bell and James Young Simpson would have recognized. The *British Medical Journal* (*BMJ*) wrote in 1903:

> Surgery, working in the light of a more accurate pathology and with the help of asepsis, can indeed show better results than it did even a couple of decades ago; anything that can fairly be called a cure, however, is still the exception. Moreover, surgery is applicable only within a comparatively narrow range, and there are evident limitations to its possible developments.[141]

Moreover, Halsted's work received a mixed reception in Britain. Some, like Henry T. Butlin, Surgeon to St Bartholomew's Hospital, thought the operation had promising potential. In Butlin's 1888 tract on breast cancer he was ambivalent about the utility of surgery, but Halsted's 1894 essay prompted him to shift his position. In the 1890s Butlin championed a more radical surgical approach.[142] He wrote in 1898 that he hoped Halsted's radical mastectomy would 'do something to encourage both medical men and their patients to take a more hopeful view of the possibilities of operation against cancer of the breast'.[143] However, crucial to Halsted's assessments of his own practice—and to the uneasiness of most British doctors—was his 'three-year' watershed. The time period appeared again and again in his notes as a usable replacement for 'complete cure'. It relied on the work of the German surgeon Richard von Volkmann (1830–1889), who suggested that if patients were free from local recurrence for three years after operation then they were 'cured', because tumours that appeared after that time could equally be 'fresh outbreaks' and 'not a residue of the old infection'.[144]

British surgeons—while otherwise approving of Halsted's methods—were uncomfortable with this watershed and what it meant for the meaning of 'to cure'. In his Ingleby Lectures, published in the *BMJ* in 1897, Bennett May wrote of Volkmann's three-year limit:

---

[139] Ibid.   [140] Ibid.   [141] 'The Cure of Cancer', *BMJ*, 1 (1903), 1327–8, 1327.

[142] Henry T. Butlin, 'A Clinical Lecture on Halsted's Operation for Removal of Cancer of the Breast', *BMJ*, 2 (1898), 1665–8, at 1668.

[143] Ibid.

[144] A. Marmaduke Sheild, 'The "Cure" of Cancer by Operation', *The Lancet*, 147 (1896), 801–2, at 801.

I do not accept this, or indeed any other period as at all absolute owing to the way in which minute deposits may temporarily remain quiescent and latent. I have seen external recurrence after an interval of eleven years, and not infrequently a patient dies of the disease five, six, or more years after operation.[145]

Similarly, in 1904, W. L. Rodman wrote, 'The three-year limit of Volkmann is insufficient, and should be extended to at least five years. Recurrences may occur after ten or more years.'[146] Questioning the three-year watershed destabilized Halsted's definition of 'cured', at least for a community of elite British surgeons. That is not to say, however, that they rejected the time frame entirely; Rodman admitted, 'In this limited and provisional sense I accept it as a cure.'[147] He argued that a more flexible interpretation of 'cured' might, in this case, be appropriate: 'In some of them the disease was not "cured" in the sense of being wholly and permanently removed, but in several there is strong reason for thinking that this word "cure" may be justly used.'[148]

This tendency on behalf of some surgeons to redefine 'cured'—in part through the three-year limit—was recognized by A. Marmaduke Sheild. In a letter to *The Lancet* in 1896, he lambasted Cheyne's lectures, and suggested—wrongly—that he uncritically followed the teachings of Volkmann. He also mused on the definition of 'to cure':

Anyone taking up a dictionary may see that the uses of the word 'cure' are very numerous, and in relation to disease the term is so vague that qualifying phrases are often used, as a 'lasting cure', a 'perfect cure', a 'temporary cure', and the like... 'Cure' may, I think, justly be defined from the point of view of the public and the bulk of the profession as the removal or banishment of a disease which never returns and leaves the body and mind of the individual in a physical and mental condition equal or closely approximating to the perfection of normal health.[149]

However, this proposed definition was rarely deployed in the language of the late nineteenth-century medical periodical. Sheild diagnosed this tendency as an effort to evade the continuing challenges of cancer surgery: 'The results of operation for carcinoma of the breast in the past have been so bad that there is a natural and strong inclination to escape from a position not very creditable to surgery and to

---

[145] Bennett May, 'The Ingleby Lectures on the Operative Treatment of Cancer of the Breast', *BMJ*, 1 (1897), 1335–8, at 1335.
[146] W. L. Rodman, 'Carcinoma of the Mammary Gland: Early Diagnosis and Radical Operation Necessary for its Cure', *BMJ*, 2 (1904), 825–31, at 831.
[147] May, 'The Ingleby Lectures', 1335.   [148] Rodman, 'Carcinoma of the Mammary Gland, 831.
[149] Sheild, 'The "Cure" of Cancer by Operation', 801.

hastily assume that improvements in methods of operating can lead to results as favourable as the former modes were unsatisfactory.'[150]

However, unease over performing radical and disfiguring surgery for the sake of only a caveated 'cure' might have dissuaded practitioners in Britain from taking up Halsted's mastectomy in quite the numbers that his champions recommended. Rodman wrote in 1904: 'Though a decade has passed since Halsted's publication, nothing more radical has been or is likely to be offered, and many, I might justly say most, surgeons yet hesitate to go so far as he advised.'[151] If the radical mastectomy only gave cancer sufferers three years of life what, then, was the line between 'palliative' and 'curative'? Indeed, fin-de-siècle surgical discourse maintained a distinctly restrained and 'palliative' tone. Even in his enthusiastic support for Halsted's endeavours, Cheyne made clear the fundamental restraints on surgery: 'The primary object of operation in cancer is, of course, the prolongation of the patient's life and the alleviation of his local trouble.'[152] Indeed, the climate of late nineteenth-century medicine retained a pessimistic atmosphere. *The Lancet* reported on Edward Hamilton's address on the 'Progress of Surgery' in 1892, in which Hamilton insisted that, 'his hearers should not be exalted above measure by the great progress of surgery, he reminded them of the remaining opprobria, in the fact that cancer and tubercle were still incurable'.[153] Butlin reflected in 1898, 'The majority of medical men believe that "once cancer" means "always cancer".'[154]

Conclusion

This chapter has argued that the while the early nineteenth-century therapeutic landscape was diverse, and multiple treatments were available to the cancer sufferer, the first few decades after 1800 saw a subtle shift in understandings and priorities. Among elite practitioners, internal medicaments—popular in the eighteenth century and before—ceded ground to external treatments for the disease. The physical removal of the tumour was increasingly articulated as the only rational response to malignancy—although that removal could be performed by a range of techniques and tools. This shift reflects a matrix of theoretical and professional transformations in the early nineteenth-century medical landscape, but the hospital was key to the reification of surgery as the *ideal* method of treating cancer. Yet the institutionalization of cancer also destabilized surgery's position almost as soon as it had been secured. While the foundation of The Middlesex

---

[150] Ibid.   [151] Rodman, 'Carcinoma of the Mammary Gland, 825.
[152] Cheyne, 'Lettsomian Lectures', 385.
[153] Edward Hamilton, 'The Progress of Surgery', *The Lancet*, 140 (1892), 1284.
[154] Butlin, 'A Clinical Lecture', 1668.

Hospital's cancer ward was accompanied by optimism on behalf of surgical elites, this enthusiasm soon waned. The systematic study of large numbers of patients only confirmed cancer's incurability—no matter the skill and extent of the operation, the disease would soon return, rendering surgery impotent in the removal of cancer from body.

In response, practitioners reconstructed cancer surgery as palliative rather than curative. Thus, while they had failed to identify a new curative intervention, they had still done 'work' to resolve the cancer problem. In reconfiguring cancer surgery, they had manufactured a new category of medical practice and a new arena of medical knowledge. These elite practitioners were thus intimately involved in defining 'curative' and 'palliative', and in doing so had extended their reach and incorporated a greater number of sufferers into their remit as managers of corporeal disorder. We can see palliative surgery as both responding to the needs and demands of patients, and as an effort to intervene in cases otherwise beyond the reach of medical care. In drawing out these issues, this chapter contributes to our historical understanding of palliative care. Historians of palliative care tend to locate its emergence at the very end of the nineteenth century, with the development of dedicated hospices and professional specialisms.[155] While this chapter does not contest this structural or institutional history, it does suggest that there is a longer narrative of active intervention into the dying body that tells us much about how practitioners understood and justified their role in the early and mid-nineteenth century. Practitioners' efforts were in part about intervening for intervention's sake—about comprehending an intractable disease in a way that was better than doing nothing at all. Chapter 4 picks up on this thread of patient agency and explores the wider ramifications of conflict between professional expectation and lay demand in mid-nineteenth-century cancer therapeutics.

---

[155] See David Clark, *To Comfort Always: A History of Palliative Medicine since the Nineteenth Century* (Oxford, 2016).

4

Cancer Quackery

In 1860, Dr T. Spencer Wells compiled a compendium of treatments for and healers of malignancy. In *Cancer Cures and Cancer Curers* he described the experience of the 'wife of a distinguished admiral' who 'found a lump in her breast'.[1] This lump was soon diagnosed as cancerous and so she applied to a diverse set of practitioners and oscillated between different kinds of treatments. Relatively wealthy, she had access not only to a range of medical men but could travel the length and breadth of Britain in search of a cure. First, she visited Edinburgh, where a 'person named Beveredge' said he 'could rub it away'. He treated the lady with this dubious-sounding method for 'some weeks' but the tumour only grew. Disappointed, she returned to London and underwent caustic treatments for five weeks. She passed the time 'in misery' and suffered from the 'torture' of corrosive applications.[2] Finally, she sought the advice of a physician, Dr Birch. Open to both external treatments and internal medicaments, under his instruction she 'inhaled oxygen' three times a week, 'hoping that the effect of this gas on her blood might lead to healing of the open surface on her breast, and that then she would be "cured"'. None of these remedies worked and she died, 'breathing oxygen to the last'.[3]

This woman's experience of illness, interventions, and death reveals the crowded arena of cancer treatments in nineteenth-century Britain. Evidently, cancer sufferers took advantage of this therapeutic diversity. Thus far, I have focused on a close-knit circle of elite surgeons and physicians working in the metropolitan hospitals of London and Edinburgh. I have explored how these men insisted on the incurability of cancer and explained that they increasingly offered interventions designed only to ameliorate suffering rather than remove the disease from the body and produce a complete cure. This involved the provision of palliative rather than curative care—a distinction made rational by patient suffering and their desire to express a collective surgical identity predicated on compassion. However, while various patients demanded this sort of palliative intervention and implored surgeons to remove their cancers with the knife, there is also evidence to suggest that some of the people diagnosed with cancer—a disease that was not only known to be fatal, but was widely reported

---

[1] T. Spencer Wells, *Cancer Cures and Cancer Curers* (London, 1860), 63.   [2] Ibid.
[3] Ibid., 64.

The Cancer Problem: Malignancy in Nineteenth-Century Britain. Agnes Arnold-Forster, Oxford University Press (2021).
© Agnes Arnold-Forster. DOI: 10.1093/oso/9780198866145.003.0005

to cause a slow and agonizing death—were reluctant to resign themselves either to surgery or to a palliative course.

Charles Bell and James Young Simpson were only a fraction of the practitioners on offer. The nineteenth-century cancer sufferer—such as the admiral's wife—could choose from a diverse range of healers and remedies in their protracted efforts to rid their bodies of malignant disease. This chapter serves to nuance the story of nineteenth-century cancer therapeutics as set out in Chapters 1, 2, and 3 by bringing in patients and practitioners whose views on cancer diverged from those of the London and Edinburgh elites. Looking at sources beyond medical tracts, treatises, and journal articles, such as advertisements and obituaries, allows us to see how these individuals understood the available treatments and the disease itself. From these people's evidence and experiences, it is clear that the climate of pessimism surrounding cancer's intractability was not hegemonic and that various voices of dissent existed both within and without the 'regular' profession.

These dissenting voices offer a novel and important lens onto the processes whereby the identities of 'regular' and 'irregular' medicine, and the relationships between and within them, were redefined and reconstructed in this period. These processes have been subjected to much historical study. Scholars have tended to consider the eighteenth- and early nineteenth-century provision of health care as a 'medical marketplace', 'where physicians, surgeons, and apothecaries...melted into each other along a spectrum that included thousands who dispensed medicine full or part time'.[4] However, this spectrum was not undifferentiated and various historians have explored the mechanisms by which this differentiation took place.[5] Some scholars see these mechanisms in political terms, as products of debates occurring in the 1830s and 1840s which orbited around calls for medical reform. These debates were in line with contemporary political critiques and agitation, and medical radicals appealed for 'unity' and 'uniformity' among practitioners.[6] Other historians have seen professionalization as primarily cultural and emphasize modes of self-presentation as key to its development. They explore the linguistic means by which medical men came to view themselves in terms of a collective.[7] However, I want to argue that boundaries were also constructed

[4] Roy Porter, 'The Patient's View: Doing Medical History from Below', *Theory and Society*, 14 (1985), 175–98, at 188.

[5] Literature on nineteenth-century professionalization is plentiful. See Penelope J. Corfield, *Power and the Professions in Britain 1700–1850* (London, 1995); and Ivan Waddington, *The Medical Profession in the Industrial Revolution* (Dublin, 1984). For a review of the influence of the sociological notion of 'profession' on the history of medicine see John C. Burnham, *How the Idea of Profession Changed the Writing of Medical History* (London, 1998).

[6] M. J. D. Roberts, 'The Politics of Professionalization: MPs, Medical Men, and the 1858 Medical Act', *Medical History*, 53 (2009), 37–56.

[7] Michael Brown has looked at the role of language in efforts to form this mid-century 'medical collective' and in attempts to articulate a vision of the medical *profession* as a unitary and democratized body of practitioners connected by common ideals, knowledges, and practices. Michael Brown,

and deconstructed through cancer knowledge and practice—and particularly the disease's incurability and the notion of therapeutic efficacy. Moreover, attending to this aspect demonstrates the futility of trying to pigeonhole practitioners in terms of styles of self-presentation, which were extremely fluid.

Reconsidering the nineteenth-century medical marketplace with the aid of cancer exposes the fault lines within the 'medical collective' (between London elites and other 'regular' medical practitioners), as well as between the collective and other 'fringe', alternative, or 'irregular' practitioners.[8] Historians have suggested that elite practitioners constructed a version of the professional self predicated on the values of restraint, humility, and intellectual nuance. In contrast, quacks were marked out by their bombastic claims and promises of miraculous panaceas. However, this chapter suggests that styles of self-presentation could be adopted by almost anyone, depending on purpose, and that efforts to correlate specific groups of practitioner with specific performative styles are limited in the context of a complex mass of overlapping images and identities.[9] In looking at responses to a particular disease we can see how these conflicts and contestations between different practitioners took place in court cases, in the clinic, and in the pages of the periodical press. Not only does this allow us some access to the patient perspective, it recentres the importance of treatments in debates over medical identities. Indeed, after a decline in heroic therapies and the advent of medical scepticism and restraint later in the century, accusations of 'therapeutic nihilism' provoked patients to desert doctors for their 'quack' competitors.[10]

This chapter is divided into five sections. The first three sections, 'Lay Knowledge and Therapeutic Diversity', 'Removal without the Knife', and 'Curative Claims' will explore how the lay literate public came to know about and fear cancer, and how they learnt about different methods of treatment. In looking at who was offering those treatments, I will engage with the various categories of cancer practitioner, describe their place in the medical marketplace, and interrogate the types of remedies they were offering. I will show how healers capitalized on the construction of cancer as an incurable disease and advertised their interventions on the basis that they, unlike elite practitioners, would be able to provide a cure. The next section—'Incurability Contested'—will examine elite

---

'Medicine, Reform and the "End" of Charity in Early Nineteenth-Century England', *English Historical Review*, 124 (2009), 1353–88. See also Roy Porter, *Health for Sale: Quackery in England, 1660–1850* (Manchester, 1989); and Mark W. Weatherall, 'Making Medicine Scientific: Empiricism, Rationality, and Quackery in Mid-Victorian Britain', *Social History of Medicine*, 9 (1996), 175–94.

[8] I borrow the phrase 'medical collective' from Brown, 'Medicine, Reform and the "End" of Charity', 1378.

[9] Porter, *Health for Sale*, vii.

[10] Paul Starr, 'The Politics of Therapeutic Nihilism', *Hastings Center Report*, 6 (1976), 24–30; Charles E. Rosenberg, 'The Therapeutic Revolution: Medicine, Meaning and Social Change in Nineteenth-Century America', *Perspectives in Biology and Medicine*, 2 (1977), 485–502, esp. 502; Weatherall, 'Making Medicine Scientific', 177.

responses to these claims, and look at what exactly was at stake in debates over the incurability of cancer. It will argue that this aspect of the disease was used by elite surgeons and physicians to erect barriers among regular, irregular, and alternative practices and practitioners—and used by their opponents to challenge certain elements of the medical profession's dominance. In the final section, I use mesmerism as a case study to examine these issues in more detail.

I focus on the first three quarters of the nineteenth century in an effort to decentre the 1858 Medical Act, which gave statutory recognition for the first time to a distinct occupational category of 'legally qualified Medical Practitioner... entitled according to his Qualification to practise... in any Part of her Majesty's Dominions'. Indeed, recent scholarship on the Act has been lukewarm in its evaluation of its significance. This historiography replicates contemporary concerns that the legislation did not go far enough. Some reformers were bitterly disappointed, for example, that the Act did not criminalize quackery.[11] Having shown in Chapter 2 how the elite definition of cancer as incurable was constitutive with doctors' self-fashioning as humanitarian, enlightened, and emotional men, here I demonstrate how criticisms of that definition served to undermine such self-fashioning by challenging the image and identity of elites, offering alternative narratives, and indicating that others also possessed these characteristics.

Lay Knowledge and Therapeutic Diversity

In the nineteenth century, a vibrant print culture helped to construct a climate of fear around cancer. The Head of the Imperial Cancer Research Fund, E. F. Bashford, suggested, '"Cancer" as a scare headline possesses more power to arrest attention than any other in the vocabulary of medicine. In its two syllables, it spells something dreadful.'[12] Its incurability was well known, and newspaper articles and domestic medicine manuals layered a frank and diverse cancer discourse—making it near impossible for any member of the reading public to avoid knowledge of the disease and its likely prognosis. Obituaries provided vivid descriptions of the dying and their diseases. One published in 1797 recorded: 'The wife of a publican at Durham in Norfolk, on Thursday last died of a cancer; it originated in the mouth, but extended itself in the most shocking manner, until it eat [sic] away the entire of her face.'[13] The artist Thomas Gainsborough died from cancer in 1788 and an article on the death of 'one of the greatest geniuses that ever adorned any age or any nation', described the 'wen in the neck. Which

---

[11] See Roberts, 'The Politics of Professionalization', 53; and Weatherall, 'Making Medicine Scientific', 177.

[12] E. F. Bashford, 'Cancer, Credulity, and Quackery', *BMJ*, 1 (1911), 1222–30, at 1222.

[13] 'Editorial Article', *The Observer*, 18 June 1791, 2.

grew internally, and so large as to obstruct the passages.'[14] It devoted paragraphs to detailing the 'suppuration' and the tumour's 'protuberance'.[15] In 1823, a Methodist woman, Mrs Honor Rider, died from 'cancer in the throat, which at length entirely prevented the passage of food'.[16] In 1858, the Editor of the *Standard*, Dr Giffard, 'died of an excruciatingly painful disease—cancer'.[17] In contrast to the euphemistic language that makes up Susan Sontag's 'conspiracy of silence' in the mid-twentieth century, nineteenth-century obituaries were often candid about the cause of death.[18]

Domestic medicine manuals also emphasized cancer's special status among maladies: 'Cancer is one of the most fearful and justly one of the most dreaded diseases to which the human frame is viable.'[19] Publications of this kind went through multiple editions, would have been found in many a middle-class household, and entries on cancer followed immediately on from passages on candied fruits. Literate men and women with cancer were thus unlikely to be ignorant of their probable fate. In 1856, the spiritualist and artist, Emily Bowes Gosse, was diagnosed with breast cancer. In an account of his wife's treatment and subsequent death, Philip Henry Gosse wrote, 'Knowing, as we did, in what terrible agony cancer often ends, we looked forward with somewhat foreboding anxiety to the future.'[20] As shown in Chapter 3, the cancer diagnosis was accompanied by fear, anxiety, and dismay. James Young Simpson wrote, 'Every practitioner knows that, of all uterine diseases, cancer is the one which the female mind most constantly and most justly dreads.'[21]

As we have seen, the hospital and its associated elite practitioners could offer only limited hope to those experiencing this emotional distress and there is evidence to suggest that some patients were aware that elite practitioners would only provide palliative care. *The Observer* wrote in 1857: 'When a patient entered the ward of the hospital she did so with the settled conviction in her own mind that she would never again be restored to the society of her friends. It was to her

---

[14] David Henry and John Nichols (eds.), 'Deaths', *Gentleman's Magazine: and Historical Chronical*, August 1788, 753.

[15] Ibid.   [16] 'Recent Deaths', *Wesleyan-Methodist Magazine*, October 1823, 706.

[17] Leigh Hunt, Albany William Fonblanque, and John Forster (eds.), 'Obituary', *The Examiner*, 13 November 1858.

[18] Sontag argues that, 'conventions of treating cancer as no mere disease but a demonic enemy make [it] not just a lethal disease but a shameful one'. Susan Sontag, *Illness as Metaphor and AIDs and Its Metaphors* (London, 2013), 6. James T. Patterson provides additional evidence for this in nineteenth-century America in *The Dread Disease: Cancer and Modern American Culture* (Cambridge, MA, 1989). Barbara Clow has disputed Sontag's 'conspiracy of silence' with evidence from early twentieth-century Canada. Barbara Clow, *Negotiating Disease: Power and Cancer Care, 1900–1950* (Montreal, 2001); and 'Who's Afraid of Susan Sontag? Or, the Myths and Metaphors of Cancer Reconsidered', *Social History of Medicine*, 14 (2001), 293–12.

[19] Spencer Thomson, *A Dictionary of Domestic Medicine and Household Surgery* (London, 1859), 80.

[20] Philip Henry Gosse, *A Memorial of the Last Days on Earth of Emily Gosse* (London, 1857), 60.

[21] James Young Simpson, *Cases of Excision of the Cervix Uteri for Carcinomatous Disease* (Dublin, 1846), 15.

"the Valley of the Shadow of Death".[22] One woman had reportedly entered 'so deeply imbued with the idea that she should never leave the hospital, that she had disposed of all her clothing, and nearly the whole of her property'.[23] For some of those diagnosed with cancer in the nineteenth century, death was seen as an inevitable consequence of the disease and they found solace in the palliative care of friends, family, or local practitioners.

However, we can also speculate that some of the people diagnosed with a disease that was not only known to be fatal, but was widely reported to cause a slow, agonizing, and distressing death, were reluctant to resign themselves to death and palliative care alone. In 1839, Physician to the Royal Berkshire Hospital, Charles Cowan, reflected, 'The love of life is deeply entwined in the human heart, and the desire to retain or recover health, and to avoid pain, are powerful and absorbing incentives.'[24] Elite, hospital-based practitioners might have been convinced by the incurability of cancer—and found the definition productive in one way or another—but for some patients, the prognosis brought nothing but despair. Indeed, while some of Charles Bell and James Young Simpson's patients expressed gratitude for their palliative care, one woman treated at the Middlesex was, 'grieved beyond measure at the ill-success of the treatment'.[25] She had clearly expected something more than palliation and was devastated at the outcome. This suggests that there was a fundamental disconnect between what the surgical elites surveyed in Chapter 3 offered, and what some of the cancer-suffering public expected or demanded from their clinical interactions.

Nineteenth-century cancer sufferers chose from a busy medical marketplace and could seek a range of treatments both in tandem and consecutively. Drawn from a variety of social and professional backgrounds, these healers ranged from 'regular' university-educated physicians, hospital-based surgeons, and village doctors, to 'irregular' quacks and purveyors of patent medicines. While, in the early years of the century, successful completion of an apprenticeship was all that was needed for entry into 'regular' medical practice, there were qualifications for those who wanted them and could pay. Within 'regular' practice, there was a rigid—at least in terms of formal affiliation—distinction between physicians, surgeons, and apothecaries, in declining degrees of authority and prestige. The Royal College of Physicians drew its Fellows from the graduates of Oxford and Cambridge—trained in the writings of Galen and Hippocrates. The Royal College of Surgeons in London

[22] 'The Cancer Ward of Middlesex Hospital', *The Observer*, 13 April 1857, 5.   [23] Ibid.
[24] Charles Cowan, *The Danger, Irrationality, and Evils of Medical Quackery; Also, The Causes of its Success; The Nature of its Machinery; The Amount of Government Profits; With Reasons Why It Should be Suppressed: And an Appendix Containing the Composition of Many Popular Quack Medicines: Addressed to all Classes* (London, 1839), 9.
[25] Alexander Shaw, Charles H. Moore, Campbell de Morgan, and Mitchell Henry, *Report of the Surgical Staff of the Middlesex Hospital, to the Weekly Board and Governors, Upon the Treatment of Cancerous Diseases in the Hospital, on the Plan Introduced by Dr Fell* (London, 1857), 94.

was granted a Royal Charter in 1800 and surgeons were trained by apprenticeship. There were also private medical schools like the Great Windmill Street School of Anatomy, where Charles Bell taught from 1812 to 1824.[26] Few patients, however, would encounter these university-educated physicians or the hospital-based surgeons. Even if we assume that people with cancer *wanted* to be treated by men who could only promise palliative care, these elite practitioners were often prohibitively expensive in private practice, and the institutions to which they volunteered their time were usually only accessible to those who lived nearby. While London had its cancer hospitals, other cities and towns did not. An article in *The Lancet* lamented the uneven spread of medical provision across Britain and the resultant proliferation of irregular practice in the provinces, 'You know not what we miserable provincials have to contend with ... [w]ith you a general practitioner in London has not perhaps much surgery; the hospitals are near, and access is easy to several well-known, operating surgeons ... [b]ut remember London is not Great Britain.'[27]

Instead, most cancer patients were likely to be treated by healers who had completed an apprenticeship but were not 'elite' surgeons or physicians (practitioners educated at Oxbridge, members of learned societies, and/or affiliated to a royal or voluntary hospital). These 'regular' practitioners might not have been educated at Oxford or Cambridge, but would still have undergone some form of training. This category included the village doctor, or, in places where physicians were scarce, the local surgeon-apothecary. Membership of the Society of Apothecaries was acquired by examination by those wishing to dispense in London, and with the 1815 Apothecaries Act the organization became the main examining body for entry into general medical practice.[28] This category included men like Mr Blaker, a medical attendant in Brighton who cared for the wife of a fishmonger, Mrs Gardener, who had suffered from cancer of the breast for six months.[29] Or Dr Scott, from Leeds, who unsuccessfully urged his patient to undergo an operation to remove two cancerous tumours from her body.[30] These practitioners might have already been known to their patients—members of the community who had formerly treated them for other maladies. Or they could have been introduced through friends and acquaintances. When Emily Bowes Gosse was treated for breast cancer in the 1850s, she showed her tumour to her friend, 'who immediately accompanied her to Dr Laseron'.[31]

---

[26] Susanne C. Lawrence, 'Private Enterprise and Public Interests: Medical Education and the Apothecaries' Act, 1780–1825', in R. French and A. Wear (eds.), *British Medicine in an Age of Reform* (London, 1991).

[27] Joseph Ashbury Smith, 'On the State of the Medical Profession in England, and on Quackery in the Manufacturing Districts', *The Lancet*, 63 (1854), 402–3, at 403.

[28] Lawrence, 'Private Enterprise and Public Interests'.

[29] 'Living Dissection', *Satirist, And the Censor of the Time*, September 1835, 295.

[30] 'Strange Charge of Manslaughter at Leeds', *Bradford Observer*, 11 March 1869, 8.

[31] Gosse, *A Memorial of the Last Days*, 5.

These regular practitioners shared space in the medical marketplace with a varied selection of alternative or 'fringe' practitioners and irregular 'quacks'. According to Porter, 'fringe' medicine was an ideological movement whose opposition to regular medicine had 'designs on men's minds more than their pockets'.[32] They were ideological rather than just commercial rivals to conventional medicine.[33] Increasingly popular and powerful as the century progressed, 'fringe' medicine included homeopathy, hydropathy, and mesmerism—'medical heresies arising within the regular ranks'.[34] Those who practised fringe medicine usually had some form of regular training, institutional affiliation, or elite associations. Irregular 'quacks', on the other hand, tended to lack such credentials. Porter defines 'quacks' as those who 'drummed up custom largely through self-orchestrated publicity; who operated as individual entrepreneurs rather than as cogs in the machine of the medical community'.[35] By the 1850s, contemporary observers estimated there were 5,000 to 6,000 providers of medical services practising with inadequate or fraudulent qualifications.[36]

Removal without the Knife

While their freedom to decide between different practitioners was constrained by their financial means, geographical location, and ability to travel, cancer sufferers used a range of mechanisms to choose between healers and their remedies. These mechanisms included the type of treatment; the practitioner's exotic, oriental, or noble associations; and perhaps most importantly, the remedy's promised capacity to *cure* cancer. We know that these aspects were important to patients because they feature again and again in the writings of those selling or providing treatments. Irregular practitioners differentiated themselves from regular surgeons, physicians, and apothecaries by advertising in newspapers. By the 1760s, most provincial centres had at least one weekly newspaper, with many towns supporting two or three.[37] The 'advertisements and notices' pages of these papers and periodicals invariably offered pills, potions, and people, all offering treatments for cancer.[38]

---

[32] Porter, *Health for Sale*, 232–4.
[33] Or as P. S. Brown put it, 'demarcation of the "fringe" is therefore a matter both of medical theory and of social boundaries'. P. S. Brown, 'Social Context and Medical Theory in the Demarcation of Nineteenth-Century Boundaries', in W. F. Bynum and Roy Porter, *Medical Fringe and Medical Orthodoxy 1750–1850* (London, 1987), 230.
[34] Ibid., 216.   [35] Porter, *Health for Sale*, 6.
[36] Roberts, 'The Politics of Professionalization', 42.
[37] Hannah Barker, 'Medical Advertising and Trust in Late Georgian England', *Urban History*, 36 (2009), 379–98, esp. 379. See also, Hannah Barker, 'Catering for Provisional Tastes: Newspapers, Readership and Profit in Late Eighteenth-Century England', *Historical Research*, 69 (1996), 42–61.
[38] This proliferation of print was made possible by late eighteenth-century economic development and population growth, accompanied by an expansion in the manufacture and consumption of consumer goods. Barker, 'Catering for Provisional Tastes', 42.

These advertisements capitalized on public fears of surgery and promised to treat cancer without recourse to the knife.[39] Articles published in the periodical press publicized the horrors of surgery and reported on cases of 'medical torture'.[40] In 1844, the *Leeds Mercury* reported that Elizabeth Crowther was cured from cancer 'without cutting'.[41] Similarly, in 1838 'Dr Drummond & Co.' placed an advertisement in the *Manchester Guardian*, promising to cure cancer 'without the use of the knife'.[42] Opportunities for the cancer curer were plentiful and Britain attracted medical men offering effective treatments from across the Atlantic. Dr J. Weldon Fell was an American surgeon who arrived in London in the 1850s claiming to possess a new cure for cancer.[43] His entrance onto the British medical stage was greeted with sycophantic fanfare in the periodical press, with Mrs Valentine Bartholomew writing in the *Ladies' Cabinet* in 1856, 'His heart seems filled with sympathy to overflowing for the sufferers of his race.'[44] Another article advertised his peculiar talent to cure cancer 'without the aid of the knife'. It was partly this ability that persuaded his patient Emily Bowes Gosse, the wife of the naturalist Philip Henry Gosse. While her regular doctor had advised 'instant excision', Emily was drawn to Fell who had supposedly invented a 'new process, without the need of an operation'.[45]

Indeed, while there was much cross-over in the type of treatment used by different sorts of practitioners, the use of the knife worked to differentiate between irregular and regular healers. Adverts that appeared on the same or subsequent pages of a single paper all offered to treat 'without cutting' and there were considerable therapeutic similarities between the various irregular practitioners. They had, therefore, to draw on a range of strategies to distinguish themselves from the competition. Patients were drawn in by a variety of means, including rhetorical tricks that were deployed in the sale of a whole range of medicaments for a wide variety of maladies. Advertisements used persuasive methods that were not specific to cancer remedies, but were also used in missives that promised effective treatment for fevers, dropsies, aches, and pains of all sorts.

Many advertisers claimed a specific intellectual or social trait or aptitude that set them apart from others. For example, female healers often claimed a peculiar understanding of female complaints. In his published advertisements, Dr Cavania offered a 'lady doctor' to give advice to women suffering from cancer, enabling

---

[39] This continued throughout the nineteenth century. Bashford referenced 'the natural dread of the knife' in 1911. Bashford, 'Cancer, Credulity, and Quackery', 1224.

[40] 'Living Dissection', 295.

[41] 'Advertisements & Notices', *Leeds Mercury*, 24 February 1844.

[42] 'Classified Advertisement', *Manchester Guardian*, 18 August 1838, 1.

[43] The USA was a repeatedly cited as a source of quackery because Americans were, according to the *BMJ* in 1907, full of 'proverbial cuteness' and 'a credulous people'. 'A Prophet of Quackery', *BMJ*, 1 (1907), 644–5, at 644.

[44] Valentine Bartholomew, 'Dr Fell versus Cancer', *Ladies' Cabinet*, 1 November 1856, 268.

[45] Gosse, *A Memorial of the Last Days*, 6.

them 'to Consult one of their own sex'.[46] This was relevant to cancer, as the disease frequently affected sexual and reproductive organs, and thus shame, modesty, and discretion played a role in a practitioner's appeal and the prospective patient's decision-making. Advertisements often presented their pills, potions, and tonics as panaceas that could cure any disease under the sun. In 1799, *The Observer* ran an advertisement for a medicine that promised 'the most efficacious Remedy' for 'Cancers, Leprosy, Scrophula, Scurvy, Itch, Ulcers...sore Nipples, Pimples and Blotches in the Face, and all other Eruptions, Scorbutic and Cutaneous Diseases, the Intermittent Fevers, Ague, Worms, the Bit of venomous Insects in the East and West Indies'.[47] This practice formed part of the nineteenth-century patent medicine convention, offering value for money alongside extravagant claims. Others used jargon, 'Oriental', and exotic references to sell remedies. In the 1850s, 'The Black Doctor' attained a degree of fame and then notoriety for his promises to cure cancer by means of 'foreign medicines' imported from his home country of Suriname.[48] However, these efforts were not confined to the irregular practitioner. The crucial ingredient of Fell's application was the *Sanguinaria* root, which he described as 'a root used by the North American Indians on the shores of Lake Superior, which the Indian traders told me was used by them with success in these affections'.[49] In deriving legitimacy from the natural knowledge of the Native Americans, Fell was turning the vice of his American citizenship into an exotic virtue and drawing on persuasive techniques used by healers or stereotypical 'quacks' in the pages of the periodical press.

Irregular 'cancer curers' also invoked home-grown prestige, publicized royal and cosmopolitan associations, provided quoted testimonials, and promised long lists of successful cases.[50] A classified advertisement, published in *Lloyd's Evening Post*, asserted that the Countess Dowager of Chatham had authenticated the 'remarkable Cure of William Betty, who had a malignant CANCER, of Eight Years duration, which had nearly consumed his Mouth, Nose, Eyes, and a great Part of his Face'.[51] An advertisement for a cancer cure published in the *Manchester Guardian* in 1821 promised 'several hundred' published testimonies and 'many thousands unpublished'.[52] Another, published in 1844, said that 'references may be had, and persons seen under treatment [to provide] amply sufficient proofs of the pre-eminence of his modes of cure'.[53]

[46] 'Advertisements & Notices', *Hull Packet and East Riding Times*, 5 April 1867.
[47] 'Classified Ad 5', *The Observer*, 21 April 1799, 1.
[48] 'The Black Doctor', *The Observer*, 8 January 1860.
[49] J. Weldon Fell, *A Treatise on Cancer, and its Treatment* (London, 1857), 56.
[50] Moreover, social class could protect men who practised medicine without qualifications from professional vitriol. Irvine Loudon, 'The Vile Race of Quacks with which this Country is Infested', in Bynum and Porter, *Medical Fringe*, 107.
[51] 'Classified Ads', *Lloyd's Evening Post*, 20 January 1792.
[52] 'Classified Ad 5', *Manchester Guardian*, 29 September 1821, 1.
[53] 'Classified Ad 7', *Manchester Guardian*, 4 May 1844, 4.

None of this suggests, however, that procedures to remove cancerous tumours without the knife were the sole preserve of irregular healers. As argued in Chapter 3, 'regular' practitioners were partial to caustic treatments in appropriate cases.[54] Throughout the nineteenth century, The Middlesex Hospital's cancer ward—'ever alive to the importance of doing all in its power to advance the treatment of this intractable complaint'—adopted the unusual policy of system-atically trialling treatments on the patients held within.[55] In 1856, they tested Fell's treatment. The hospital minutes contain a detailed description of the remedy. Nitric acid was applied 'by the means of a small bit of sponge tied to the end of a stick' to the whole surface of the affected breast, 'the object of this application was to remove the skin'.[56] On the following day, the surgeon sliced a series of parallel scratches on the surface of the now exposed flesh. These cuts were about half an inch apart, reaching from top to bottom. Then, he spread a purple mucilaginous paste made from flour, chloride of zinc, and other ingredients over the incisions. The next day, the scratches were deepened and the purple substance was reapplied.

After a few days of this repeated exercise narrow strips of linen rag, soaked in the purple paste, were inserted into the long parallel scores. Every day the strips of rag were renewed and the scratches were deepened. This process killed the cancerous flesh, transforming it into 'a woody hardness, and a deep black colour'. Once the incisions had reached the bottom of the tumour, the surgeon applied a 'girdle' around the line where the growth met living, healthy flesh. Gradually, the tumour would detach and eventually drop out of its cavity; likened by Philip Henry Gosse to a hard, penny bun.[57] For reasons left unexplained, none of this was conducted under chloroform. Following a trial of several weeks on over fifty patients, The Middlesex Hospital's surgical staff decided that Dr Fell's method was 'in entire accordance with known principles of surgery', 'ingenious', 'safe', and 'easy of application by well-instructed surgeons'.[58] Thus, and as shown in Chapter 3, caustics were regularly used by orthodox and elite surgeons, and it would be anachronistic to equate 'surgery' with 'the knife' alone.

Even contemporary practitioners observed that this therapeutic fluidity blurred boundaries between regular and irregular doctors. In 1844, The Lancet reported on the case of Edwin James Port, a forty-nine-year-old chemist, who was indicted for manslaughter for causing the death of Mary Harris.[59] Port had no medical training and no institutional affiliation, however, as The Lancet wryly noted, while

---

[54] See 'Internal or External Treatments', Chapter 3.
[55] Shaw et al., Report of the Surgical Staff, 8.   [56] Ibid.
[57] Gosse, A Memorial of the Last Days, 33.   [58] Shaw et al., Report of the Surgical Staff, 8.
[59] 'Chester Assizes: Accusation of Manslaughter against One of "Graham's Own". Quack Plasters for Cancer. Trial at Chester, before Mr. Baron Gurney', The Lancet, 44 (1844), 382–3.

he was 'neither a licensed physician nor surgeon ... that made no difference in the case'. Port had treated Mary Harris for breast cancer, with a 'plaister' containing arsenic. Dr Zachariah Barnes Vaughan—a physician, surgeon, and expert witness—was called to provide evidence.[60] He reflected on the challenges involved in assessing effective or even rational remedies for the disease: 'The treatment of cancer is one of the most difficult subjects to the profession. There are great doubts as to the best mode of treatment.'[61] But he observed that even orthodox practitioners used arsenic in their treatments. Vaughan told the court that 'Cooper's *Surgical Dictionary*' (referenced in Chapter 3) 'is an authority in the profession' and 'arsenic is one of the substances used in open cancer'. Nonetheless, he insisted that it 'require[d] the greatest caution'.[62] The use of caustics evidently traversed the boundaries between regular and irregular conduct. Vaughan reflected on the imprecise border between different types of treatment: 'Some medicines, once deemed quackeries, are now used in the profession.'[63] This practitioner could not advocate charging this man with culpable negligence and felony because Port had acted in accordance with his own practice.

It is also worth noting that it was not only irregular practitioners who advertised in the press, and it was not only 'quacks' who used testimonies and extravagant claims in their self-presentation.[64] Occasionally, regular practitioners advertised in the pages of the periodical press and P. S. Brown has observed that poverty compelled some medical men to sell patent medicines.[65] While it was common for irregular practitioners to provide or promise enthusiastic testimonials, regular practitioners could also use extravagant insistence, bombastic certainty, and testimonials from happy and satisfied patients to convince their readership of the value of their therapies. For example, in 1824, Thomas J. Graham, a member of the Royal College of Surgeons of England, railed against conventional opinion in his text *Practical Observations on the Cure of Cancer*, and championed the 'value of the remedies employed'. He provided a series of cases in which his 'mild method' effected a complete cure, and insisted, 'I could easily have related many other cases of cancer (amounting at least to the number of forty) which were cured by the same means.'[66]

---

[60] As Ian Burney has demonstrated, the authority of medical knowledge, inside and outside the courtroom, was a prominent contemporary issue, for it was at this time that medical reformers like Wakley were campaigning for the medicalization of the coroner's inquest. Ian Burney, *Bodies of Evidence: Medicine and the Politics of the English Inquest, 1830–1926* (Baltimore, MD, 1999).

[61] 'Chester Assizes', 382.   [62] Ibid.   [63] Ibid.

[64] Irvine Loudon refers (politically incorrectly) to those medical practitioners who adopted the manners and appearances of the quack as 'medical transvestites'. Loudon, 'The Vile Race of Quacks', 107.

[65] Brown, 'Social Context and Medical Theory', 216.

[66] Thomas J. Graham, *Practical Observations on the Cure of Cancer, Illustrated by Numerous Cases of Cancer in the Breast, Lip, and Face; which Have Been Cured by a Mild Method of Treatment, that Immediately Alleviates the Most Agonizing Pain* (London, 1824), 4.

Curative Claims

Perhaps of most importance to the patient was the remedy's promised capacity to *cure* cancer. Thus, practitioners marketing their wares in the pages of the press traded in a persuasive language tailored to cancer and its peculiar challenges. They engaged with the question of curability and targeted elite practitioners' inability or unwillingness to provide curative rather than palliative interventions. Thus, advertisements promised a cure, even—or especially—when conventional practitioners had given patients up as hopeless. It is no surprise, therefore, that advertised remedies directed themselves, explicitly, towards the 'class of those who suffer from cancer—a *class* hitherto almost universally abandoned'—those for whom orthodoxy could only palliate.[67] Note the pejorative 'abandoned'—regular surgeons and physicians were negligent, whereas these other practitioners were indiscriminate in their compassion. Crucially, therefore, these advertisements not only offered alternative treatments—claiming greater skill, insight, or good fortune than their elite counterparts—they also offered a challenge to cancer's incurability. If surgeons affiliated to a voluntary hospital or with elite credentials tended to be convinced of the malady's intractability, then other practitioners promised 'complete cures' for the 'dread disease'.

This narrative of elite and institutional failure was repeated in almost every advert for cancer treatment. The 1792 successful cure by Mr Roop was, for William Betty, one of last resort: for the 'Surgeons of Exeter Hospital (as well as an eminent Practitioner at Bath, under whose Care he had been placed, at her Ladyship's Expense, three Times) could render him no relief'.[68] Betty had sought treatment elsewhere, but it had failed. Not content with palliative care, he had submitted to Roop's 'cure' and been rewarded for his efforts. In 1867, the *Hull Packet and East Riding Times* advertised the treatments of Dr Cavania. It boasted, 'Many [cancerous] limbs have been shown to their medical advisers who had turned them out of Hospitals as being incurable, because they refused amputation.' These 'miraculous cures' drew patients from across the country.[69] Such offerings often contrasted the ability of labourers and skilled craftsmen who worked as irregular healers with the inability of trained doctors. The *Leeds Mercury* reported in 1844 that Elizabeth Crowther was cured by John Whitely, a stonemason, 'without cutting, after being given up incurable by several Surgeons and Physicians'.[70] A stonemason had succeeded where regular medical practitioners had failed.

However, just as some advertised, several regular surgeons and physicians also offered curative interventions, revealing further overlap between these two groups.

---

[67] Shaw et al., *Report of the Surgical Staff*.   [68] *Lloyd's Evening Post*, 20 January 1792.
[69] 'Advertisements & Notices', *Hull Packet and East Riding Times*, 5 April 1867.
[70] 'Advertisements & Notices', *Leeds Mercury*, 24 February 1844.

In Chapter 3, I referred to the case of Bedford surgeon Samuel Young. In 1810, he suggested a system of compression to remove cancer from the bodily economy. Young published a collection of cases in which his remedy had proven successful and assured his readers that 'the cure cannot fail of being effected'.[71] Supported initially by prominent lay and professional figures like Thomas Denman, Sir Benjamin Brodie, and Samuel Whitbread, the method was soon judged ineffective. Both Samuel Young and the testimonial-providing Thomas J. Graham were hospital-based practitioners and members of learned societies. They were both supported by powerful lay and medical individuals, but nonetheless questioned cancer's incurability and drew on rhetorical tricks—like those that appeared in advertisements—to convince their opponents of the efficacy of the treatment.

Thus, cancer sufferers took advantage of a crowded medical marketplace and were eclectic in the treatments they sought. While they were restricted by their location and social status, they also had many remedies and practitioners from which to choose. They were desperate, but they still needed to be enticed. A diverse range of healers used different offerings, promises, and persuasive techniques to lure paying patients. These various providers of medical care, advice, and interventions drew on overlapping and flexible modes of self-presentation that blurred the boundaries between 'regular' and 'irregular' practitioners. However, key to both the decision-making process of the patient and the advertising strategies of the practitioner, was the promise to cure an incurable disease. It was 28this that set some apart from the elite surgeons or physicians, and it was this that appealed to cancer patients.

Incurability Contested

Remedies that promised to be able to cure, rather than just palliate, posed a real threat to those who had built their identity around the construction of cancer as an incurable disease. As shown in Chapter 2, the first half of the nineteenth century was a time of intense flux within the medical community. Moreover, for many regular practitioners in early and mid-nineteenth-century England, the spectre of irregular practice loomed large. *The Lancet* wrote in 1835, 'Never have quacks, quackish doctrines, and quack medicines, exercised a greater influence over the minds and bodies of the people of this country, than they exert in the present epoch.'[72] *The Lancet* had actively pursued medical reform from its foundation in 1823, seeking a meaningful, legislative way to differentiate between regular and

---

[71] Samuel Young, *An Inquiry into the Nature and Action of Cancer; with a View to the Establishment of a Regular Mode of Curing that Disease by Natural Separation* (London, 1805), 97.

[72] 'Means of Checking the Operations of Quacks', *The Lancet*, 1 (1835–6), 948.

irregular practitioners and pursuing the criminalization of quackery. After sixteen unsuccessful attempts, it partially succeeded with the passage of the 1858 Medical Act, which did not, however, outlaw irregular practice.[73]

Thus, while the vibrant medical marketplace offered a range of healers and remedies (appealing to patients because it provided a sense of agency and choice), it threatened the primacy and intellectual claims of the elites, particularly when it undermined their 'ideology' of cancer. Historian Mark W. Weatherall argues that while debate within the 'boundary' of orthodoxy was 'safe, even fertile and necessary', in contrast, the 'intrusion of rejected medical knowledge' was felt keenly by those invested in making medicine 'scientific' in the mid-century.[74] It was less the presence of these remedies that threatened the elite medical or surgical practitioner, but rather that these treatments represented and traded on an alternative interpretation of cancer: that it was, or could be, cured.[75] In their defence, these surgeons and physicians attached the label of 'quackery' to those who promised to be able to cure the disease. 'Cancer curer' came to be synonymous with 'cancer quack'. Chair of Surgery at University College, John Eric Erichsen, referred to 'the cancer-curing quacks' or 'the "cancer-curer" as he calls himself'.[76] To be a quack was to offer a cure. Crucially, too, the question of cancer's curability was also used to make more subtle distinctions *within* the supposedly orthodox medical community. After all, the medical marketplace did not just include patent medicines and their inventors—the caricatures of the mercenary charlatan—but also orthodox practitioners running private practices or operating out of hospitals. Thus, this mechanism of differentiation—whether practitioners promised to be able 'to cure' cancer—could be deployed in multiple settings and to multiple ends.

However, these accusations by regular practitioners did not go unchallenged. Not only did some of those labelled 'quack', or heterodox in some other way or another, defend themselves against the charge—claiming authority and ability—but many of them argued that the 'orthodox' practitioners were wrong to insist on cancer's incurability, and that their commitment to this fatalistic outlook reflected broader ills in the medical faculty like self-interest, dogmatism, and pecuniary preoccupations. Thus, debates over cancer's curability took place across indistinct boundary lines. As one physician observed, 'Unfortunately, quackery exists in the

---

[73]   Roberts, 'The Politics of Professionalization', 37.

[74]   Weatherall, 'Making Medicine Scientific', 178.

[75]   P. S. Brown and Michael Brown have both argued that James Morison, purveyor of the popular (and much-derided) 'Morison's Pills', was 'frankly and aggressively anti-medical' and that he constructed an alternative system of health, the body, and therapeutics. Brown, 'Social Context and Medical Theory'; Michael Brown, 'Medicine, Quackery and the Free Market: The "War" against Morison's Pills and the Construction of the Medical Profession, c.1830–c.1850', in Mark S. R. Jenner and Patrick Wallis (eds.), *Medicine and the Market in England and Its Colonies* (Basingstoke, 2007).

[76]   John Eric Erichsen, 'Clinical Lectures Delivered at University College Hospital', *BMJ*, 1 (1860), 239–40, at 239.

profession as well as out of it: where there is a demand there will be a supply.'[77] Crucially, too, these permeable borders were drawn between practitioners irrespective of institutional status, association, or training—and medical men of every conceivable background and persuasion drew on competing and overlapping rhetorical modes of performance and image construction. For example, both regular and irregular practitioners made use of testimonials and newspaper advertisements. This complicates our picture of nineteenth-century medical professionalization by suggesting that 'quacks' could not be identified by their self-aggrandizement alone.

As part of their defence against so-called quackery, regular practitioners levied accusations of dishonesty, cruelty, and a fundamental misunderstanding of cancer's character at those who advertised their 'cures' in periodicals and the press. A *British Medical Journal* (*BMJ*) article, published in 1860, stated: 'The amount of misery and suffering entailed upon human beings by them is quite indescribable. The probability in cases of cancer is, that the disease was incurable; but that is no reason why the friends of the patients should be tortured with false hopes.'[78] In cases of malignancy, and according to elite discourse, 'cancer curers' increased rather than lessened the distress of those 'who suffer under this awful malady'.[79] Towards the end of the century, a 'cancer curer' named Thomas McGrath was sued by a patient because 'his negligent and improper treatment aggravated the disease to such an extent that the arm of the plaintiff had to be amputated at a later date'.[80] According to this critique, the suffering inflicted by 'cancer curers' was emotional as well as physical. Not only did their treatments often cause pain, their offers of curative treatments only heightened the emotional agony of cancer because they misled their patients, fooling them into believing they had more life left than they did. 'Cancer curers' capitalized on desperation, profiting while people died.

The spectre of 'false hopes' was called on time and time again by elite practitioners in their diatribes against the 'cancer curer':

> Where legitimate medicine fails, the patient, tortured, probably, by the misery of deferred hope, with the dread of death perhaps before him, is easily induced to throw himself into the arms of the charlatan, who is ready to indulge him in unbounded expectations.[81]

The cruel and misleading promises of the 'cancer curer' were contrasted with regular practitioner's kind honesty. Cambridge surgeon A. Marmaduke Sheild

---

[77] Robert M. Glover, *On the Philosophy of Medicine, on Quackery, &c. Being the Last of a Course of Lectures Delivered in the School of Medicine, Newcastle-upon-Tyne* (London, 1851), 5.

[78] 'Quacks Abroad and At Home', *BMJ*, 1 (1860), 52–3, at 52.

[79] 'Cancer Cures', *BMJ*, 1 (1873), 650–1, at 650.   [80] 'A "Cancer Curer"', *BMJ*, 1 (1895), 158.

[81] Glover, *On the Philosophy of Medicine*, 3.

argued that it was the medical profession's 'duty' to 'speak with absolute truth regarding such matters, and especially not to use terms likely to mislead either the public of the bulk of the profession, who largely take their views of treatment and prognosis from the centres of medical teaching'.[82] In a lecture given in Newcastle in 1856, surgeon and physician Robert M. Glover wrote, 'How great a contrast does this candour present to the vain glorious boastings of the quacks!'[83]

Accusations of deliberate and fraudulent misdiagnosis were key to accusations of quackery. Surgeon Joseph Ashbury Smith recounted an anecdote in *The Lancet*:

> Some years ago, a relative of mine suffered from a slight ulceration on the inside of the cheek, caused by a broken tooth. The tooth had been removed by a surgeon at Chesterfield, but the diseased part not readily healing the patient become alarmed; somebody told him it was 'a cancer', and he came to consult the old charlatan at Manchester. He was told, of course, that it *was* 'cancer', and ordered into lodgings. Every morning he attended at the surgery, and every morning for *six months* paid him. At length, when perhaps both were weary, or money enough had been extracted, the process...was suspended, the sore allowed to heal, and the patient went home, *believing to this hour that he had been cured of a* CANCER.[84]

The use of 'charlatan' in this quotation and Ashbury's emphasis on the lengthy period of pay imply deceit. However, Glover's 'quacks' were not just transgressing morally and ethically, but intellectually, too. As shown in Chapter 3, elite practitioners diagnosed cancer retrospectively—they identified the disease only once, and only because, it had killed the patient, revealing the inextricable and practical connection between cancer and incurability. If they were not deliberately deceiving their patients, 'cancer curers' instead erred in their diagnosis of the disease. The *BMJ* stated: 'with unqualified persons, any external lump or tumour, however benign, is instantly diagnosed as cancer and promptly plastered'.[85] Elsewhere, medical and surgical elites often acknowledged the difficulties inherent in diagnosing cancer—even for the most 'qualified' practitioner (see Chapters 2 and 6). In this instance, the *BMJ* set up an inaccurate dichotomy between 'qualified' certainty and 'unqualified' error or deliberate misdiagnosis.[86] Irrespective of whether the practitioner was guilty of fraudulently or mistakenly misdiagnosing

---

[82]   A. Marmaduke Sheild, 'The "Cure" of Cancer by Operation', *The Lancet*, 147 (1896), 801–2, at 802.

[83]   Glover, *On the Philosophy of Medicine*, 3.

[84]   Ashbury Smith, 'On the State of the Medical Profession', 403.

[85]   'Clerical Errors', *BMJ*, 2 (1900), 1733.

[86]   As Charles E. Rosenberg has noted, there is 'social power' in the naming and diagnosis of disease. This is a power that early nineteenth-century practitioners had to fall back on in absence of therapeutic success. Charles E. Rosenberg, 'The Tyranny of Diagnosis: Specific Entities and Individual Experience', *Milbank Quarterly*, 80 (2002), 237–60.

a benign ulcer as malignant, in doing so he or she misrepresented cancer as a curable disease.

Critics of this misdiagnosis argued that the misrepresentation through incorrect diagnosis of cancer as a curable disease not only misled the patient, but damaged public faith in the orthodox medical community. Sheild wrote:

> In dealing with maladies like cancer or phthisis any new modes or results of treatment are closely criticised and watched by an observant section of the public. Nothing shakes their confidence in medical men so much as statements regarding the cure of what they regard as incurable disease which afterwards when applied in individual instances or in important personages are found false or misleading.[87]

Adhering to the codes of the profession served the community and doing otherwise threatened it with collapse. Misleading cancer patients about the curative efficacy of treatments might damage the fragile contract of trust between the medical faculty and the laity. Erichsen argued that while the stakes were high for the 'regular practitioner', if the 'cancer-curing quacks' failed to effect a cure then they suffered little damage to their professional reputation. Instead, 'quacks' capitalized on the famed incurability of cancer, arguing that the occasional failure when treating such a challenging disease was only to be expected; they benefited from orthodoxy's insistence that they could only offer palliative care. If, on the other hand, the quack used his caustics and destroyed a tumour, 'which, being non-malignant, though erroneously believed to be a cancer, does not return', then the patient and 'her friends' would assume the quacks had succeeded where conventional medicine had failed.[88] The 'cancer curer' could, therefore, only gain.

Indeed, failure to cure cancer only rarely made the irregular practitioner vulnerable to attack. Throughout the nineteenth century, court cases that attempted to find cancer quacks guilty for fraudulence or malignant intent did so without the help and umbrage of the dead patient's family. Instead, friends and loved ones usually expressed gratitude to the practitioner, even when the latter's efforts had been in vain. In Bradford in 1869, Richard Atkinson, a 'gentleman', was charged with the manslaughter of Mary Scott. She had suffered 'for about two years from an ulcerated breast', and Atkinson had offered to 'apply a plaster' because he had 'previously cured a woman of a similar disease'. However, Scott died three weeks after the first treatment. Despite their loss, the inquest had not taken place at the request of the family, 'who were fully satisfied with what the accused had done'. Indeed, her relatives were 'opposed to any such inquiry taking place' and believed that Atkinson 'had done the best he could'.[89]

---

[87] Sheild, 'The "Cure" of Cancer by Operation', 801.   [88] Erichsen, 'Clinical Lectures', 239.
[89] 'Multiple News Items', *Bradford Observer*, 11 March 1869, 8.

As argued, regular surgeons and physicians could also promise curative treatment and their orthodoxy did not protect them from criticism or accusations of impropriety. Fell's location within The Middlesex Hospital might have afforded him protection from accusations of quackery. The surgical staff of the Middlesex were convinced of the utility of Fell's application. They incorporated it into the institution's therapeutic arsenal and it appeared as a treatment in case notes well into the late nineteenth century. However, they insisted that it could only *ameliorate* suffering and was useful as a palliative rather than curative treatment. The staff concluded in their assessment of the trial that even under Fell's treatment, 'Cancer retains its notoriously malignant character'.[90] Fell, however, was marketing himself and his application as explicitly curative—*not* palliative. Fell's commitment to the curative value of his treatment (and, by implication, the *curable* nature of cancer) resulted in a radical change in his fortunes and reception. While initially rapturous, Fell's coverage in the British press rapidly turned sour. *The Lancet* had, in January 1857, reported positively on the trial, writing that 'This experiment reflects great credit on the medical officers of the Middlesex Hospital.'[91]

By April, however, the publication's opinion of Fell and his practices had altered dramatically. *The Lancet* denigrated his supposed coupling of 'Medicine and Mystery', and compared his experimentation to shamanic craft:

> Somewhere in that respectable institution there is a secret chamber where things are done that mortal eye must not look upon. The high priests—those initiated into the mysteries of the inner shine—only are permitted to know the fearsome secrets of that awful place... Perhaps the scene of operations is hung with sable draperies; the atmosphere is loaded with sulphurous vapours; blue lights burn dimly, and cast a lurid glare over the objects of the scene... Perhaps after all there is nothing to conceal. When we say *nothing* to conceal, we mean that supposing the veil of mystery to be drawn aside, we should see *nothing* worth seeing.[92]

In arguing that Fell's treatment was '*nothing* worth seeing', the writer was suggesting that it was ineffective and that his remedy could not produce a complete cure. *The Lancet*'s particular gripe was with Fell's tendency towards concealment—a tendency Fell himself admitted: 'My first impulse was to make it public at once... but circumstances, added to reflection and the advice of some medical friends, induced me to depart from this course.'[93] Those who worked for *The Lancet* were appalled, reflected on their previous praise and turned their ire

---

[90] Shaw et al., *Report of the Surgical Staff*, 35.
[91] 'The Middlesex Hospital and Treatment of Cancer', *The Lancet*, 69 (1857), 128.
[92] 'Secret Surgery, and the "Mystery Men" of the Middlesex', *The Lancet*, 69 (1957), 358.
[93] Fell, *A Treatise on Cancer*, v.

towards the hospital itself: 'When we applauded the authorities of the Middlesex for taking the reputed "cancer cure" up, we were not prepared for such "hole and corner" work as is going on there now.'[94]

Similar scenes played out in a scathing article published in the *BMJ* that assessed the propriety and efficacy of the Cancer Hospital (later the Royal Marsden). This example demonstrates how claims of curability and accusations of quackery could take place within institutions usually considered 'elite'. In its published registers and mortality rates, the hospital reported that 796 inpatients and outpatients had come under observation in the previous year, and that fifty-four of the inpatients were discharged 'cured, or the disease arrested', eighty-nine were successfully operated on, and thirty-eight were 'discharged cured without operation'.[95] The *BMJ*'s critique of the report was sarcastic:

> In it we find this, to us, novel statement. We give it for the benefit of those who may be as ignorant as ourselves: 'The possibility of arresting cancer for a great number of years, and, in some instances, curing it, by a combination of local and constitutional remedies, we believe to be fully established, and that with far less suffering and annoyance to the patient than was formerly the case.'

The *BMJ* dismissed the hospital's claims, 'We should regard it as a miracle that fifty or sixty patients a year are cured of cancer, but that out of the walls of the institution in which the cures have been effected there is not a single competent member of the profession who knows anything of the matter.'[96] They regarded the cure of cancer on such a scale as a 'miracle'—they relegated it to the fantastical, and in doing so associated the Cancer Hospital with mysticism and quackery.[97] This case demonstrates the limits to fertile, necessary debate within the boundaries of 'regular' medicine—the idea that cancer might be curable moved beyond healthy, intellectual debate and into the realm of the absurd.[98]

In contrast to the Cancer Hospital's confidence, regular practitioners frequently reflected on the therapeutic futility of mid-century medicine. One wrote, 'Assuredly the uncertain and most unsatisfactory art that we call "medical science" is no science at all, but a mere jumble of inconsistent opinions, of conclusions hastily and often incorrectly drawn, of acts misunderstood or perverted, of comparisons without analogy, of hypothesis without reason, and of theories not

---

[94] 'Secret Surgery', 358.   [95] 'Cancer Cures', 650.   [96] Ibid.

[97] This was a common rhetorical strategy used to denigrate 'cancer curers'. In 1908, the *BMJ* published an article peppered with 'cured' and 'curers' encased in meaningful inverted commas, and concluded with a flourish, 'In my opinion, the "cure" is worse than a farce, and one may ask how is suffering humanity to be saved from the tragedy of self-destruction by faith in these direful "miracles".' J. Lynn Thomas, 'A Note upon a Case of Cancer in the Right Breast "Cured" by the Cardigan "Cancer Curers": The Aftermath: A Danger-Signal to the Public', *BMJ*, 2 (1908), 1676–8, at 1678.

[98] Weatherall, 'Making Medicine Scientific', 178.

only *useless*, but *dangerous*.'[99] Thus, there was widespread ambivalence regarding the curative powers of the medical profession across the social spectrum.[100] This malaise was particularly relevant to malignancy. As Dr Zachariah Barnes Vaughan noted in 1844, cancer was 'one of the most difficult subjects to the profession... I have not always been successful in my treatment of diseases. Medicines that I have prescribed may have been injurious.'[101]

Mesmerism: A Case Study

The subtle role of cancer's curability in identity formation and boundary-making can be seen most clearly in the language of practitioners who occupied that liminal space between regular and irregular practitioners—and specifically, those alternative doctors who practised mesmerism. In 1848, John Elliotson (1791–1868), presented a case in which a woman's 'true cancer' was cured with mesmerism. Mesmerism—or 'animal magnetism'—was the idea that all living and animate beings possessed an invisible natural force that could be invoked to send people into trances, heal wounds, and anaesthetize pain.[102] Mesmerism's status was highly contested—practised and championed by orthodox surgeons and physicians, but also subject to accusations of quackery and impropriety. Historian Alison Winter has argued that it played a central role in everything from physics and 'social consensus', to, most relevant here, controversies over medical authority.[103]

Elliotson bore many of the marks of medical orthodoxy. He was made Professor of the Principles and Practice of Medicine at University College London in 1832, and Senior Physician to University College Hospital in 1834. However, in August 1838, the inveterate editor of *The Lancet*, Thomas Wakley, conducted a series of mesmerism experiments in front of several witnesses. Wakley denounced mesmerists as frauds and proclaimed their practice a fiction.[104] Elliotson was forced to resign. This complicated relationship with elite practice and traditional institutions was born out in his 1848 essay, published after his fall from grace. Elliotson was a keen advocate of mesmerism. He began his text with various nods towards what he recognized as the orthodox consensus on cancer before going on to challenge that interpretation. Initially he conformed to conventions of cancer's

---

[99] Samuel Dickson, *The 'Destructive Art of Healing': A Sequel to the 'Fallacies of the Faculty'* (London, 1856), 4.

[100] The *Saturday Review* remarked in 1858, 'The great augmentation in the number of people who get cured not according to received rule makes itself felt even in the House of Commons.' *Saturday Review*, 10 July 1858, 30.

[101] 'Chester Assizes', 382.

[102] John Elliotson, *Cure of a True Cancer of the Female Breast with Mesmerism* (London, 1848).

[103] Alison Winter, *Mesmerized: Powers of Mind in Victorian Britain* (Chicago, 1998).

[104] 'Dr Elliotson's Experiments in "Mesmerism" at the House of Mr. Wakley with Two Girls Deceiving', *The Lancet*, 36 (1838), 805–14.

incurability. His original purpose was to 'render [the patient] insensible to the pain of the surgical removal of the breast', because he saw 'no other chance for her; and this indeed was a poor chance, for cancer invariably returns in the same or some part if the patient survives long enough'.[105] He also made use of a common critique levied at unorthodox practitioners: 'When a disease termed cancer has not returned, I have no doubt that it had not been cancer; and such a terrible thing as the removal of breasts not cancerous has always been but too frequent among surgeon.'[106] Elliotson was unsurprisingly familiar with the terms of the debate and the subtle codes of cancer and professionalism in use in the mid-nineteenth century.

However, his text soon departed from the received consensus. He reported how he mesmerized the woman daily. During her 'sleep-waking', Elliotson, her mother, and her niece made 'contact passes upon her breast over the linen'. Anxious about accusations of impropriety, Elliotson was careful to clarify that he did so 'over her dress'.[107] To his surprise, 'the mass began to diminish', and during 1847 the disease 'steadily gave way'. By September 1848, the tumour had 'completely dissipated', the breast was 'perfectly flat, and all the skin thick and firmer than before the disease existed. Not the smallest lump is to be found.'[108] Thus, Elliotson could not only promise 'considerable relief' from cancer, but, 'in many cases a positive cure'.[109]

Elliotson and his supporters used this case not only to contest cancer's incur-ability, but also as a tool to critique the metropolitan medical elites who had excluded him from their community. As shown in Chapters 1 and 2, the elite definition of cancer as incurable was crucial to these practitioners' self-fashioning as humanitarian, enlightened, and emotional men. Thus, criticisms of that defin-ition served to undermine such efforts by challenging the image and identity of elites, offering viable alternatives, and demonstrating that others also possessed these characteristics. Elliotson accused elite, regular practitioners of 'holding fast to their physiological notions with determined obstinacy' and with a sense of 'duty'.[110] Instead, their 'real duty' was—according to Elliotson's co-editor, William Collins Engledue (1813–1858)—'following out, by persevering inquiry, the diffi-culties of all physiological problems; and after this, in honest recognition and avowal of what they have satisfactorily ascertained'.[111]

---

[105] Elliotson, *Cure of a True Cancer*, 11.   [106] Ibid.

[107] Ibid., 15. Yet Elliotson was well aware that such activities drew the ire of observers. He quoted a Harveian Oration at the London College of Physicians, 'Among quacks, the imposters, called mesmer-ists, are in my opinion the especial favourites of those, both male and female, in whom the sexual passions burn strongly, either in secret or notoriously. Decency forbids me to be more explicit.'

[108] Elliotson, *Cure of a True Cancer*, 15.

[109] William Collins Engledue, 'Introductory Remarks', in Elliotson, *Cure of a True Cancer*, iv.

[110] Ibid., vi.

[111] Ibid. Engledue was an English physician, surgeon, apothecary, mesmerist, and phrenologist; he co-edited, with Elliotson, *The Zoist: A Journal of Cerebral Physiology & Mesmerism, and their*

He pleaded for flexibility and humility from the community, 'the views of the teachers of an imperfect science should not be received as dicta from which there is to be no swerving; but rather as the probable interpretation of facts'.[112] Accusations of 'dogma' or adherence to 'dicta' played a crucial role in the construction of medical boundaries and identities in the nineteenth century. However, the insult could be slung across both sides of the divide, and mutate according to intent. As historians like John Harley Warner and Mark W. Weatherall have pointed out, however, interpretations of this rhetoric are plural. Terms like 'empirical' and 'rational' were fluid.[113] 'Rational' medicine could be logical and reasoned, or it could be simplistic and dictatorial. Similarly, 'empirical' medicine could be free from prejudice, or negatively associated with 'trial and error' and a lack of educated theory.[114]

Just as mesmerism and other 'fringe' practices like homeopathy were characterized as 'dogmas' by regular practitioners, accusations of elite stagnancy and an unwillingness to accommodate change were also common in nineteenth-century cancer discourse. Elite commitment to the incurability of cancer made these practitioners vulnerable to charges of 'obstinacy'. This obstinacy caused suffering to patients because, as the accusations went, sufferers were denied access to curative treatment only because their doctors might lose face and have their 'doctrine' of incurable cancer disproven. Graham argued that despite the 'indolent scepticism of some professional men', it was an 'unquestionable fact' that cancer 'has often been cured by art'.[115] Medical tracts and treatises frequently described cancerous tumours as 'indolent', and the word's use here suggests that the medical elites' inaction was pathological in both spirit and consequence.

This contradicted elites' own insistence as to their kindness and care. As suggested in Chapter 3, they implied that their commitment to an incurable disease marked them out as benevolent practitioners and their efforts to provide palliative care were framed in compassionate terms. These elevated practitioners insisted that their acknowledgement of cancer's incurability was a kindness because it prevented the cultivation of 'false hopes'. Moreover, it is worth noting that this consternation over the supposed inflexibility of orthodox practitioners did not reflect how these elites chose to present themselves, and self-effacement as well as intellectual nuance and restraint were central to the identity of the scientific gentleman. Even Walter Hayle Walshe—who was otherwise committed to cancer's incurability—cautiously warned against inflexible and a priori assumptions

Applications to Human Welfare, an influential British journal, devoted to the promotion of the theories and practices of mesmerism and phrenology.

[112] Engledue, 'Introductory Remarks', vi.

[113] John Harley Warner, *The Therapeutic Perspective: Medical Practice, Knowledge, and Identity in America, 1820–1885* (Cambridge, MA, 1986), 41–5. Weatherall, 'Making Medicine Scientific', 178.

[114] Weatherall, 'Making Medicine Scientific', 178   [115] Graham, *Practical Observations*, 7–8.

on behalf of practitioners. While there might be 'delusion in the extravagant estimates' of some surgeons who claimed high rates of success, 'there is still more serious error in the dictum of those surgeons who...having witnessed a considerable number of unsuccessful operations, generalise these results and shut their eyes to every fact of opposite tendency'.[116] Hayle Walshe recognized the value of modesty and humility. This was simultaneously a critique of the supposed dogmatism of those who insisted on cancer's incurability, the flamboyant pronouncements of 'cancer curers', and an indication that the elites did not see themselves as inflexible and were instead keen to present as intellectually liberal.

Conclusion

For many 'regular' practitioners in mid-nineteenth-century England, the spectre of unlicensed practice loomed large. In 1858, after decades of attempted reform, the British parliament passed the Medical Act, which gave statutory recognition for the first time to a distinct occupational category of 'legally qualified Medical Practitioner'. While this is a tempting turning point in the history of professionalization, recent scholarship has been lukewarm in its evaluation of the Act's significance. This literature replicates contemporary concerns that the legislation did not go far enough and highlights those reformers who were bitterly disappointed that the Act did not criminalize quackery. Cancer provides insight as to why such campaigns had proven unsuccessful. There was widespread anxiety over the limited practical utility of orthodox medicine. The increasing public commitment to 'science' and to the benevolence of the medical profession was not matched by belief in the latter's therapeutic superiority. As suggested earlier in this chapter, doctors even levied this critique at themselves.

This ambivalence over the curative powers of the medical profession spread across the social spectrum and both the popular and periodical press contributed to public anxiety regarding cancer's unusual threat and incurability. The *Saturday Review* remarked in 1858, 'The great augmentation in the number of people who get cured not according to received rule makes itself felt even in the House of Commons.'[117] The laity not only knew of the suffering inflicted by the disease, but were aware that elite practitioners could offer little more than palliation. Thus, patients exerted agency in their choice of healer and remedy and, despite financial and geographical constraints, selected from a vibrant medical marketplace. Key to this decision-making process—and essential to the advertising strategies of a whole range of practitioners—was the promise to cure an incurable disease

---

[116] Walter Hayle Walshe, *The Anatomy, Physiology, Pathology, and Treatment of Cancer* (Boston, MA, 1844), 149.

[117] *Saturday Review*, 10 July 1858, 30. Cited in Roberts, 'The Politics of Professionalization', 47.

without the knife.[118] Non-elite purveyors of cancer treatments made use of what Javier Moscoso calls the 'moral economy of hope', and positioned their offerings in contrast to the palliative efforts of their elite counterparts.[119] Re-examining the medical marketplace through the lens of therapeutic efficacy reveals that debates over the curative abilities of one treatment or another constructed and deconstructed boundaries between regular and irregular practitioners. Moreover, the discourse of incurability also exposed fault lines *within* regular medical practice, as well as between orthodox and alternative or irregular healers. Crucially, too, criticisms of the definition of cancer as incurable served to undermine elite self-presentation. After all, and as demonstrated in Chapters 1, 2, and 3, that definition was critical in their image of themselves as humanitarian, enlightened, and emotional men. Those who questioned the incurability of cancer challenged that image, offered alternative and less flattering portrayals in its place, and demonstrated that others also possessed the positive characteristics usually attributed to elite practitioners (humanity, compassion, benevolence).

Debates over restraint, dogmatism, and inflexibility set the scene for the construction of 'scientific medicine' in mid- to late Victorian Britain.[120] Widespread commitment to cancer's incurability can also be seen as a precursor to the 'therapeutic nihilism' that infiltrated elite medical discourse after the 1850s. Critics of orthodox medical men emphasized the limited practical utility of orthodox medicine. As shown, doctors even levied this negative assessment at themselves. The conflict over the curability of cancer continued into the second half of the nineteenth century, as did anxieties over the therapeutic limitations of regular medicine.

Throughout the century, cancer continued to be constructed by elite elements of the medical community as incurable. Moreover, this incurability continued to be levied as a differentiating factor between groups of practitioners, and continued to form part of the self-expression and maintenance of regular medical authority. However, as historian M. J. D. Roberts has observed, authority is a relational category—it rests on more than assertion and insistence and requires some measure of cultural acceptance.[121] Just as elite surgeons and physicians continued

---

[118]   Bashford argued that the 'cancer curers' 'knowingly and deliberately trade upon the anxieties and credulity of the public in all that pertains to the etiology and treatment of cancer'. Bashford, 'Cancer, Credulity, and Quackery', 1222.

[119]   Javier Moscoso, 'Exquisite and Lingering Pains: Facing Cancer in Early Modern Europe', in Rob Boddice (ed.), *Pain and Emotion in Modern History* (Basingstoke, 2014); Javier Moscoso, *Pain: A Cultural History* (Basingstoke, 2012).

[120]   See John Harley Warner, 'Science in Medicine', *Osiris*, 1 (1985), 37–58; John Harley Warner, 'Ideals of Science and Discontents in Late Nineteenth-Century American Medicine', *Isis*, 82 (1991), 454–78; John Harley Warner, 'The Rise and Fall of Professional Mystery: Epistemology, Authority and the Emergence of Laboratory Medicine in Nineteenth-Century America', in Andrew Cunningham and Perry Williams (eds.), *The Laboratory Revolution in Medicine* (Cambridge, UK, 1992); W. F. Bynum, *Science and the Practice of Medicine in the Nineteenth Century* (Cambridge, UK, 1994).

[121]   Roberts, 'The Politics of Professionalization', 51.

to insist on cancer's incurability, swathes of the suffering public refused to accept the definition and continued to seek medical attention from those who promised a complete cure. While Roberts argues that the Medical Act of 1886 revealed a distinct shift since 1858 'in the quality of lay respect for professional authority', and various scholars have suggested that the diversity of the medical marketplace dwindled as the nineteenth century moved on, cancer paints a different picture.[122] Advertisements for remedies for the disease continued apace into the early twentieth century. Key surgical, scientific, and public health 'successes' that had helped to shore up medical authority in the second half of the nineteenth century (anaesthetic, asepsis, control of cholera, and the identification of various disease-causing microbes) had little effect on the intractability of malignancy.

Thus, an article published in the *Woman's Herald* in 1891 spoke with the same disaffection the *Saturday Review* had expressed forty years earlier. It described a particularly popular alternative therapy, 'The Mattei Cancer Cure'. Count Mattei, 'the hermit of La Rochetta', used 'electro-homeopathic' remedies to treat and resolve malignant diseases. The author of the article reflected on the appeal of the remedies in light of the horrors of cancer: 'The world knows no greater scourge than cancer. Other diseases may be as fatal, but few are as agonizing, and of these all are speedier in their effect than this painful and insidious malady.'[123] The article critiqued, therefore, the medical faculty's unwillingness, 'to give credit to those searchers for truth who are not members of its bodies'. The author finished his rhetoric with, 'Who is there amongst us who would not rather be cured of cancer by a quack than left to die according to the rules and regulations of the College of Physicians?'[124] Just as practitioners of different sorts critiqued each other for dogmatism and a priori assumptions about cancer's incurability, the laity fired similar shots at the profession. This author was suggesting that, for patients, it was only the outcome that mattered—they had no commitment to medical science, only to the healing arts. Thus, for lay observers, and throughout the nineteenth century, irregular practitioners offered just as good a solution to the 'cancer problem' as their regular alternatives. This challenge frustrated attempts not only to clarify cancer as an incurable disease, but also to construct and affirm conventional medical authority.

For medical men who encountered cancer in the nineteenth-century clinic, the disease's incurability was not just an obstacle to overthrow but a galvanizing and intellectually provocative idea that had shifted medicine and professional identity in profound and lasting ways. As delineated in Chapters 1, 2, and 3, it enabled the construction of professional credentials and community values; made hospitals into places for treating 'terminal' illness; made possible the invention of new forms and rationales of intervention; and carved boundaries between orthodox and

[122] Ibid., 53.   [123] 'The Mattei Cancer Cure', *Woman's Herald*, 17 January 1891, 199.
[124] Ibid., 198.

unorthodox practitioners. However, and as Part II of this book will show, it also brought into being certain modes of investigating the disease, such as mapping, the microscope, and discourses of progress and decline. For scientists and social commentators—as well as surgeons—cancer's incurability was an invaluable opportunity to demonstrate the power and promise of their respective investigative techniques.

PART II
CAUSES

5

Counting and Mapping Cancer

In the nineteenth century, cancer was made into an incurable disease. By about 1850, this persistent intractability coincided with a new interest in the vital statistics of the nation, and the systematic collection of data pertaining to birth, marriages, and causes of death, to produce fresh anxiety. This data suggested that not only was cancer incurable, but that it appeared to be increasing in incidence. In response, some medical practitioners sought strategies beyond the clinic to elucidate the evasive malady. The continued therapeutic futility with respect to cancer provoked a diversification of investigative efforts, and elements of the medical community refocused on the disease's aetiology, prevention, transmission, and potential communication. Indeed, this new interest in the vital statistics of the nation was itself an effort to rationalize, comprehend, and even control cancer—characteristics associated with 'modern medicine' in nineteenth-century Britain.

The mid-nineteenth century saw the British populace increasingly quantified on a local, regional, and national scale.[1] This practice derived in part from the development of statistical methods and epidemiology and grew alongside a quantitative study of people and their activities more generally. These intellectual movements were increasingly institutionalized and professionalized, and by the 1860s the government was systematically undertaking a large quantity of official numerical enquiries into the health of the nation.[2] The main source of disease statistics was the *Annual Report of the Registrar-General on Births, Deaths and Marriages in England*, first presented to parliament in 1838.[3] In 1839, the statistician William Farr joined the General Register Office (GRO) and proceeded to

---

[1] See, J. Eyler, *Victorian Social Medicine: The Ideas and Methods of William Farr* (Baltimore, MD, 1979); Ruth G. Hodgkinson, 'Social Medicine and the Growth of Statistical Information', in F. N. L. Poynter (ed.), *Medicine and Science in the 1860s: Proceedings of the Sixth British Congress on the History of Medicine* (London, 1968); Kathrin Levitan, *A Cultural History of the British Census: Envisioning the Multitude in the Nineteenth Century* (Basingstoke, 2011); Donald A. Mackenzie, *Statistics in Britain 1865–1930: The Social Construction of Scientific Knowledge* (Edinburgh, 1981); Graham Mooney, 'Professionalization in Public Health and the Measurement of Sanitary Progress in Nineteenth-Century England and Wales', *Social History of Medicine*, 10 (1997), 53–78; and Simon Szreter, 'The GRO and the Public Health Movement in Britain, 1837–1914', *Social History of Medicine*, 4 (1991), 435–63.

[2] Hodgkinson, 'Social Medicine', 184.

[3] Edward Higgs, 'Registrar General's Reports for England and Wales, 1838–1858', Online Historical Population Reports, http://histpop.org/ohpr/servlet/AssociatedView?path=Browse&active=yes&mno=2052&assoctitle=Registration%20(Amendment)%20Act,%201858&assocpagelabel, accessed 13 October 2016.

The Cancer Problem: Malignancy in Nineteenth-Century Britain. Agnes Arnold-Forster, Oxford University Press (2021).
© Agnes Arnold-Forster. DOI: 10.1093/oso/9780198866145.003.0006

tabulate regional and national vital statistics—births, marriages, and deaths—for each of the country's divisions. The GRO also calculated the annual mortality by each cause and the proportion of deaths in 100,000 affected by each class of disease in each region. Parallel reports were later produced for Scotland, Wales, and Ireland. Farr developed various tools to ameliorate the process of gathering and interpreting national data, including a standard nosology, standardized death rates, and mathematical models from complex epidemiological phenomena such as the curve of an epidemic and the relationship between population density and mortality.[4] Narrative prefaces to each annual report situated individual investigations within a broad chronology and enabled doctors and public health professionals to comment on yearly shifts in the disease profile of the nation.[5]

Cancer was integrated into this practice from the outset. From the *Fourth Annual Report* causes of death were recorded, alongside the person's sex, age, and profession. The causes were divided into 'Epidemic, Endemic, and Contagious Diseases', 'Sporadic Disease of Uncertain or Variable Seat', 'Sporadic Diseases of Special Systems and Organs', and 'External Causes: Poisoning, Asphyxia, Injuries'. Cancer was categorized within 'Sporadic Disease of Uncertain or Variable Seat'.[6] The Medical Officer of Health (MOH) reports, first produced in 1848, ran parallel to the GRO's output.[7] These reports were the first time the health of the metropolis had been both systematically recorded and published for anyone to see. They also required the development of a new kind of health professional—the Medical Officer of Health—whose main role was the numerical investigation of disease.[8] They, too, provided vital data on birth and death rates, infant mortality, incidence of infectious and other diseases, and a general statement on the condition of the population. The MOHs tabulated causes of death according to disease and stratified by age. From 1856, the reports included cancer in their nosology (see Figure 5.1).

As the quantity of data on cancer and its incidence accumulated, observers began drawing conclusions about the disease's relative rates in different years. Cancer appeared to be increasing. The *Forty-Second Annual Report*, published by the GRO in 1879, recorded that among men of all ages cancer was the case of 4,121

[4] J. Eyler, 'The Conceptual Origins of William Farr's Epidemiology: Numerical Methods and Social Thought in the 1830s', in Abraham M. Lilienfeld (ed.), *Times, Places, and Persons* (Baltimore, MD, 1980), 1.

[5] Edward Higgs, 'The Annual Report of the Registrar-General, 1839–1920: A Textual History', in Eileen Magnello and Anne Hardy (eds.), *The Road to Medical Statistics* (Amsterdam, 2002), 55.

[6] George Graham, 'Statistical Nosology', in *Fourth Annual Report of the Registrar-General* (London, 1840–1), 93–105.

[7] The Wellcome Library have digitized the Medical Officer of Health reports for London from 1848 to 1972: https://wellcomelibrary.org/moh/, accessed 14 April 2020.

[8] For more on the MOHs and their role within preventive medicine see Anne Hardy, *The Epidemic Streets: Infectious Disease and the Rise of Preventive Medicine, 1856–1900* (Oxford, 1993); and John Welshman, 'The Medical Officer of Health in England and Wales, 1900–1974: Watchdog or Lapdog?' *Journal of Public Health*, 19 (1997), 443–50.

16

QUARTERLY RETURN OF DEATHS

IN THE

PARISH OF ST. MARTIN-IN-THE-FIELDS,

For the Months of April, May, June, 1856.

		Death at all ages.	Under 3 years.	At 5 and under 20.	At 20 and under 40.	At 40 and under 60.	At 60 and under 80.	80 and upwards.
1.—Zymotic Class	Small Pox	1	1	—	—	—	—	—
	Measles	3	3	—	—	—	—	—
	Scarlatina	3	3	—	—	—	—	—
	Hooping Cough	4	4	—	—	—	—	—
	Diarrhœa	5	5	—	—	—	—	—
	Typhus	5	—	1	1	1	2	—
	Rheumatic Fever	1	—	—	—	1	—	—
	Erysipelas	3	—	—	1	2	—	—
2.—Dropsy, Cancer, &c.	Hæmorrhage	1	—	—	..	1	—	—
	Dropsy	5	1	—	—	1	3	—
	Cancer	1	—	—	—	—	—	1
3.—Tubercular Class	Scrofula	2	1	1	—	—	—	—
	Tabes Mesenterica	8	7	1	—	—	—	—
	Phthisis	15	1	1	5	8	—	—
	Hydrocephalus	4	4	—	—	—	—	—
4.—Dis. of Brain, Nerves, &c.	Cephalitis	2	2	—	—	—	—	—
	Apoplexy	3	—	—	2	1	—	—
	Paralysis	7	—	—	3	2	2	—
	Convulsions	2	2	—	—	—	—	—
	Dis. of Brain	2	—	—	—	2	—	—
5.—Dis. of Heart, &c.	Dis. of Heart	5	—	—	—	4	1	—
6.—Dis. of Lungs, &c.	Laryngitis	2	2	—	—	—	—	—
	Bronchitis	6	1	—	—	3	2	—
	Pneumonia	3	2	1	—	—	—	—
	Asthma	2	—	—	—	1	1	—
7.—Dis. of Digestive Organs.	Teething	3	3	—	—	—	—	—
	Ascites	2	—	—	—	2	—	—
	Enteritis	1	—	—	1	—	—	—
	Peritonitis	1	—	—	—	1	—	—
	Dis. of Pancreas	1	—	—	—	1	—	—
	Dis. of Liver	3	—	—	—	2	1	—
	Fistula	1	—	—	1	—	—	—
8.—Dis. of Kidneys	Dis. of Kidneys	2	—	—	—	2	—	—
9.—Dis. of Uterus, &c.	Child birth	1	—	—	1	—	—	—
10.—Dis. of Joints, Bones, &c.	Dis. of Bones	1	1	—	—	—	—	—
11.—Dis. of Skin, &c.	Carbuncle	2	—	—	1	1	—	—
17.—Violence, Privation, &c., &c.	Debility from Birth	4	4	—	—	—	—	—
	Debility from Age	8	—	—	—	—	6	2
		125	47	5	16	35	19	3

Figure 5.1 'Quarterly Return of Deaths in the Parish of St. Martin-in-the-Fields'

Source: From *Medical Officer for Health Report for St Martin-in-the-Fields* (London, 1856), 16. Wellcome Collection.

deaths, on par with diseases like diarrhoea (5,712), whooping cough (5,804), scarlet fever (9,148), and measles (4,678). It also caused many more deaths than cholera, the quintessential Victorian malady (122).[9] However, cholera was, of course, an epidemic disease and 1879 was not an epidemic year. Among women the figures were even more dramatic, with cancer causing 8,508 deaths, more than any other disease. The narrative preface elaborated on these high numbers, and expressed concern over the increased mortality from cancer, which had 'maintained the increase to which it has been gradually mounting for many years'.[10]

Responses to this supposed increase became increasingly fretful. In 1883 the *British Medical Journal (BMJ)* published an article entitled 'An Inquiry into the Causes of the Increase in Cancer', in which the author lamented, 'A cursory examination only is sufficient to divulge that the fell disease [cancer] claims year by year a higher ratio of victims.'[11] Meditations on the 'gradually mounting' rates of cancer predominated in intellectual discourse on the disease.[12] The language was also invariably melodramatic: 'We have, then, confessedly, to face the fact that cancer is increasing in our midst at a rate which bids fair to become more and more serious with the advance of time.'[13] Commenters made use of an emotive vocabulary to express their concern: 'Unhappily...a strict examination of the facts and figures bearing upon it, must lead to the painful and disquieting conviction that cancerous disease is, year by year, becoming more fatal in this country.'[14] This bleak prognosis—both for individuals afflicted and for the population as a whole—filtered through multiple strata of later nineteenth-century society. Concern over the new 'cancer epidemic' appeared most frequently in medical periodicals, particularly the *BMJ* and *The Lancet*. However, it was not confined to medical discourse. Instead, evidence for, and debates about, the increase in cancer appeared in a variety of publications. 'The rapid increase of cases of death by that dread disease cancer', stated the *New York Times* in 1902, 'is exciting attention in Europe as it has here.'[15] Vital statistics, however, not only offered a challenge to the medical community—drawing their attention to a painful 'reality'—they also presented an opportunity. They offered up other avenues of investigation, which were particularly welcome in the present climate of perceived therapeutic inadequacy, and promoted a series of different 'approaches' to the 'cancer problem'. One such 'approach' was mapping.[16]

[9] Brydges P. Henniker, 'Deaths from Several Zymotic and Other Causes, and Inquest Cases, in the Divisions, Counties, and Districts of England', in *Forty-Second Annual Report of the Registrar-General* (London, 1881).

[10] 'Introduction', in *Forty-Second Annual Report*, xxx.

[11] Hugh P. Dunn, 'An Inquiry into the Causes of the Increase of Cancer', *BMJ*, 1 (1883), 708–10, at 708.

[12] Ibid.   [13] Ibid.   [14] Ibid.

[15] 'Malaria a Cure for Cancer', *New York Times*, 7 April 1902.

[16] In its investigation of Victorian notions of space, environment, and region, this chapter dialogues with the recent 'spatial turn' in historical research in writing. Beat Kümin and Cornelie Usborne, 'At Home and in the Workplace: A Historical Introduction to the "Spatial Turn"', *History and Theory*, 52 (2013), 305–18.

In the 1870s, Dr Alfred Haviland plotted the distribution of cancer on vividly coloured maps of Britain.[17] From these diagrams he concluded that cancer's incidence was determined by geographical location and drew connections between the landscape and the causation of the disease. This interpretation not only depended on an eighteenth-century tradition of medical geography, but was indebted to contemporary developments in epidemiology and sanitary science.[18] Haviland's maps were reliant on the vital statistics published by the GRO and he was devoted to numerical methods as a way of advancing scientific knowledge and as a technology to inform medical practice. His maps were both an investigative tool—designed to elucidate an obscure and incurable disease—and a rhetorical device—intended to convince others of his model of cancer causation. Haviland's maps have been subjected to very limited scholarly study and yet they reveal an early integration of cancer and public health in Victorian Britain, the respective historiographies of which have rarely intersected.[19] Literature on nineteenth-century sanitary reform, medical statistics, and mapping is plentiful. However, this research has tended to focus on urban geographies. As a result, and despite Haviland's obvious dependence on these public health practices and causative theories, because he focused on the countryside his mapping of cancer differed in crucial ways from the sanitary maps of other epidemiologists. Haviland looked at pastoral environments and laced the rural landscape—rivers, soil, and trees—with pathological potential. Moreover, he was not alone in doing so, and this chapter will locate Haviland within a community of map-making and 'map-thinking' peers. It will also explore the continuation of spatial interpretations of malignancy in the fin de siècle and look at the cancer mapping done after his death in 1903.[20]

This chapter's first section, 'Mapping and Medicine' will begin by setting the sanitary science scene and provide context about mapping and public health in the first half of the nineteenth century. The second, third, and fourth sections—'Dr Alfred Haviland', 'Cancer and the Countryside', and 'Haviland's Contemporaries'— will look at Haviland, his maps, and his fellow cancer map-makers. The final section, 'New Concepts of Cancer Mapping', will argue that environmental understandings of cancer's causation, as well as mapping as a technology, continued to be prominent in cancer investigation well into the twentieth century, and have proven themselves

---

[17] Alfred Haviland, *The Geographical Distribution of Heart Diseases and Dropsy, Cancer in Females and Phthisis in Females, in England and Wales* (London, 1875).

[18] Gregg Mitman and Ronald L. Numbers, 'From Miasma to Asthma: The Changing Fortunes of Medical Geography in America', *History and Philosophy of the Life Sciences*, 25 (2003), 391–412, esp. 399.

[19] Historical geographer Tom Koch is one of the few scholars to direct substantial attention to Haviland. Tom Koch, *Cartographies of Disease: Maps, Mapping and Medicine* (Redlands, CA, 2005). However, Haviland also appears in Ornella Moscucci's account of gender and cancer from 1860 to 1948. Ornella Moscucci, *Gender and Cancer in England, 1860–1948* (London, 2016), 26–30. See also: Agnes Arnold-Forster, 'Mapmaking and Mapthinking: Cancer as a Problem of Place in Nineteenth-Century England', *Social History of Medicine*, 33 (2020), 463–488.

[20] 'Alfred Haviland, M.R.C.S.', *BMJ*, 1 (1903), 1522.

highly adaptable and compatible with a range of conceptualizations of disease causation. I demonstrate this point by showing how, at the very end of the nineteenth century, discussion over so-called 'cancer houses' reflected an ongoing interest in cancer mapping which continued to draw inspiration from Haviland while also making use of new germ theories of disease.

Mapping and Medicine

In the context of a succession of disease epidemics, mapping was an increasingly prevalent public health practice in nineteenth-century Britain. It was used to investigate and illustrate the course and concentration of disease incidence and deployed to make arguments about appropriate and inappropriate interventions. For example, in the aftermath of the cholera epidemic that struck Leeds in 1832, a map that indicated the areas of the city where cases clustered was included in the *Report to the Leeds Board of Health*, and its author used the map to claim an environmentalist aetiology for the disease and argue for improved civic order and cleanliness. The minutes of the board meeting on 16 January 1833 read as follows:

> We are of the opinion that the streets in which malignant cholera prevailed most severely, were those in which the drainage was most imperfect; and that the state of the general health of the inhabitants would be greatly improved, and the probability of a future visitation from such malignant epidemics diminished, by a general and efficient system of drainage, sewerage and paving, and the enforcement of better regulations as to the cleanliness of the streets.[21]

This quotation reveals the complex interplay of reasons and rationales for disease mapping in the nineteenth century. They were investigative, persuasive, and justifications for intervention and reform. The map in this *Report* revealed where 'malignant cholera prevailed most severely', persuaded readers that this proved a causal relationship between place and disease, and justified increased urban regulation.

The findings of the *Report* were also included in Edwin Chadwick's *Report on the Sanitary Conditions of the Labouring Population of Great Britain*, published in 1842.[22] Chadwick is credited with bringing medical mapping into the British mainstream. Born in Manchester in 1800 to a middle-class family with limited financial means, he expertly climbed the social and professional ladder. Following a stint working for Jeremy Bentham he was asked to serve on a Royal Commission

---

[21] *Report of the Leeds Board of Health, MDCCCXXXIII* (Leeds, 1833).
[22] Edwin Chadwick, *Report on the Sanitary Conditions of the Labouring Population of Great Britain: A Supplementary Report on the Results of a Special Inquiry into the Practice of Internment in Towns* (London, 1843).

to investigate the effectiveness of the Poor Laws. Inculcated into the realm of reform, and following a series of mass epidemics—cholera in 1832, influenza in 1837, and typhoid in 1838—he shifted his professional gaze to the problems of sanitation and disease.[23] While his work was reliant on an eighteenth-century tradition of medical geography—the idea that disease could be dictated by the place a person lived—his mapping of particularly pathological areas and his use of diagrams to justify the sanitary reform of usually urban space signalled a turning point in the science of epidemiology and public health.

Chadwick and his fellow map-makers used maps as key mechanisms by which large amounts of evidence could be collected (they delineated spaces that information gatherers could focus their attentions on), analysed, and then represented.[24] The practical benefits of mapping are obvious—it takes the many and varied intricacies of human existence, eliminates extraneous information, and reduces complex, obscure spaces to clearly understandable lines and symbols.[25] The original London underground map, for example, was only comprehensible because the creator untangled the overlapping multitude of train lines and eradicated unnecessary details. The text that supported the various sanitary maps was replete with visual metaphors—they 'elucidate', 'display', and 'reveal'.[26] Surgeon and medical historian, D'Arcy Power used comparable language, contrasting the relative opacity of numbers and tables with the easily consumable medium of maps: 'Although the actual numbers are not very imposing in this series of cases, a *glance* at the maps will show the remarkable manner in which the disease is distributed.'[27] Mapping was, therefore, a way to make the complexity of disease more easily accessible to the professional gaze. It made the correlation between disease incidences and different pathological places visible to the naked eye— uncovering the complex and dynamic relationship between geography, the built environment, human activity, and disease.[28]

The process by which this correlation was transformed into causation reveals the persuasive, rhetorical function of medical mapping. In the nineteenth century, maps were increasingly part of material and consumer culture. They featured in schoolrooms, decorated middle-class homes, and appeared in the pages of newspapers and periodicals. As a result, a wider audience was inculcated into

[23] Christopher Hamlin, *Public Health and Social Justice in the Age of Chadwick: Britain, 1800–1854* (Cambridge, UK, 2008), 84–120.

[24] Tom Koch, 'Social Epidemiology as Medical Geography: Back to the Future', *GeoJournal*, 72 (2009), 99–106, esp. 102.

[25] Pamela K. Gilbert, *Mapping the Victorian Social Body* (Albany, NY, 2004), 7.

[26] Pamela K. Gilbert, 'The Victorian Social Body and Urban Cartography', in Pamela K. Gilbert (ed.), *Imagined Londons* (Albany, NY, 2007), 15.

[27] Quoted in Tom Koch, *Disease Maps: Epidemics on the Ground* (Chicago, 2011), 250; emphasis added.

[28] Gilbert, 'The Victorian Social Body and Urban Cartography', 14.

the 'language' of cartography.[29] Various practitioners, therefore, used maps to present different frameworks of disease causation. For example, Chadwick used maps to make a claim for a miasmatic aetiology of cholera. He argued—along with many others—that the evolving industrial city contained within it specific conditions that predisposed inhabitants to ill health. In this anti-contagionist schema, disease was intimately tied to pathological urban spaces—the slum, factory, and workhouse. Chadwick and his co-theorists suggested that the environment could both act as a carrier for disease agents ('ferments' that could arise *de novo* given favourable conditions) and weaken the body, making it vulnerable to infection.[30] The 1849 cholera map of Bethnal Green is labelled as 'Shewing [sic] the Cholera Mist', and the shading is evocative of a spreading atmospheric density (see Figure 5.2). 'A Cholera Map of the Metropolis' from the same year similarly uses intensity of colour to call to mind the extension of disease miasma (Figure 5.3). Later in the century, John Snow famously used his diagram of cholera deaths in Soho, London, to argue that the disease was transmitted by drinking water.[31]

Mapping was also used to justify intervention into, and the alteration of, Victorian urban environments. Both Chadwick and the Leeds Board of Health used their maps to make the case for the transformation of the city and its slums in aid of epidemic control. Chadwick's efforts and agitation contributed to the 1848 Public Health Act and the creation of local boards of health.[32] These were local authorities in urban areas of England and Wales with powers to control sewers, clean the streets, regulate environmental health risks, including slaughterhouses, and ensure the proper supply of water to their districts. Chadwick inspired a proliferation of sanitary maps, largely depicting industrial spaces, that were deployed in the investigation of disease in the nineteenth century.[33]

Dr Alfred Haviland

While the mapping of cancer in the mid- to late century cannot be understood without this context of urban sanitary mapping—they too were investigative,

---

[29] J. B. Harley, *The New Nature of Maps: Essays in the History of Cartography* (Baltimore, MD, 2006), 7.

[30] Michael Worboys, *Spreading Germs: Disease Theories and Medical Practice in Britain, 1865-1900* (Cambridge, UK, 2000), 23. For a full analysis of Chadwick's understanding of disease aetiology see Hamlin, *Public Health and Social Justice*; and 'Providence and Putrefaction: Victorian Sanitarians and the Natural Theology of Health and Disease', *Victorian Studies*, 28 (1985), 381-11.

[31] John Snow, *On the Mode of Communication of Cholera*, 2nd edn (London, 1855). See also: http://www.ph.ucla.edu/epi/snow/mapmyth/mapmyth.html, accessed 14 April 2020.

[32] Hamlin, *Public Health and Social Justice*, 254-74.

[33] Maps of the metropolis and its boroughs were a regular feature of public health print media throughout the nineteenth century, and in the 1890s Charles Booth applied mapping to the problems of poverty and health in the capital. Koch, *Cartographies of Disease*, 62-3.

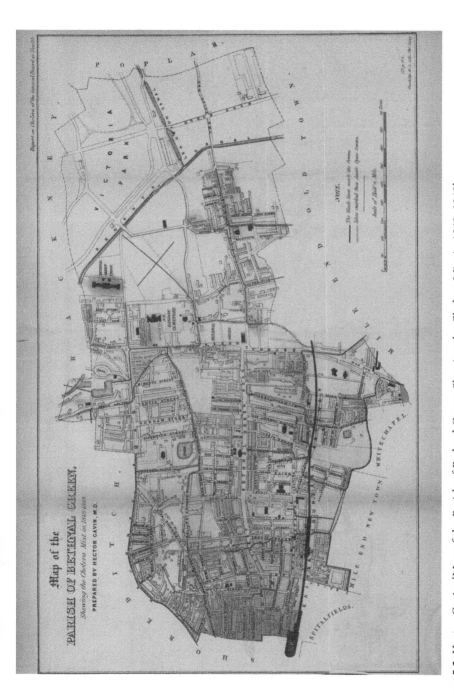

Figure 5.2 Hector Gavin, 'Map of the Parish of Bethnal Green, Shewing the Cholera Mist in 1848–1849'

Source: Wellcome Images.

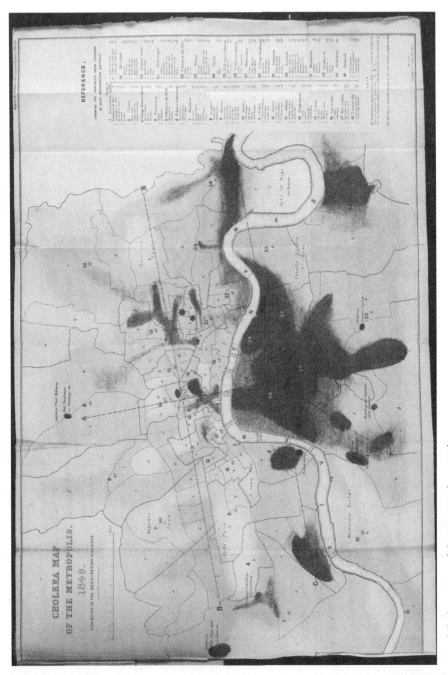

Figure 5.3 'Cholera Map of the Metropolis, 1849'
Source: Wellcome Images.

persuasive, and interventionist—diagrams of malignancy departed from these principals and practice in crucial ways. Most scholarship on nineteenth-century disease mapping has looked at the depiction of infectious diseases. However, some public health practitioners created maps of chronic and constitutional maladies, like dropsy, heart disease, and rickets. One such practitioner was Dr Alfred Haviland, who, in 1874, plotted cancer incidence on maps of England. Haviland was born in Somerset, educated in London, and trained as a doctor at St Thomas' Hospital.[34] He was a prolific writer and his publications reveal a deep commitment to the climatological, topographical, and geographical determinants of health and disease, further evidenced by his lecture course on the 'Geographical Distribution of Diseases', given at St Thomas'.[35] In his 1855 book *Climate, Weather and Disease*, Haviland wrote, 'It will be the endeavour of the author in the following pages to present to the student some of the more remarkable facts, that prove the dependence of many diseases, for their origin and continence, on certain meteoric phenomena.'[36] He waxed lyrical on the value of investigating climate:

> In studying Climate we study man; for in tracing its effects in all their variety on the human frame and mind, we make ourselves acquainted with his laws, customs, psychical and physical capabilities, vices, virtues, and all that appertains to that protean animal.[37]

This tendency towards environmental explanations for disease was typical for the time and intimately tied to an Enlightenment tradition of medical geography.[38]

Haviland was also fully embedded within the nineteenth-century community of public health practitioners and invested in sanitary reform as a mechanism to improve the well-being of the population. He wrote books that dealt with sanitation (*The Sanitary Regulations of Ancient Rome*) and public health (*Scarborough as a Health Resort*—the preface was written by J. W. Taylor, the local MOH), and Haviland was MOH for the combined sanitary authority of Northampton, Leicester, Rutland, and Buckinghamshire.[39] In the second edition of his most successful work, *The Geographical Distribution of Diseases in Great Britain*

---

[34] Frank A. Barrett, 'Alfred Haviland's Nineteenth-Century Map Analysis of the Geographical Distribution of Diseases in England and Wales', *Social Science and Medicine*, 46 (1998), 767–81.

[35] In 1855, he wrote two tracts, *The Sanitary Regulations of Ancient Rome* (London, 1855), and *Climate, Weather, and Disease: Being a Sketch of the Opinions of the Most Celebrated Ancient and Modern Writers* (London, 1855). In 1874, he published his most celebrated work, *The Geographic Distribution of Disease in Great Britain* (London, with a second edition in 1892); this was followed by *Geology in Relation to Sanitary Science* (London, 1879), and *Scarborough as a Health Resort: Its Physical Geography, Geology, Climate and Vital Statistics* (London, 1883).

[36] Haviland, *Climate, Weather and Disease*, vii.   [37] Ibid., 5.

[38] German physician L.L. Finke produced a world map of disease in 1792; F. A. Barrett, 'Ginke's 1792 Map of Human Diseases: The First World Disease Map?', *Social History of Medicine*, 50 (2000), 915–21.

[39] Haviland, *Scarborough as a Health Resort*.

(published in 1892), Haviland reflected on his professional autobiography and the genesis of his interest in geographical and climatic origins of disease, noting the relationship between his experience of public health practice and environmental determinants of ill health. In 1849, he had 'medical charge of [his] native town, in the West of England, at the time of the direful visitation of Asiatic Cholera epidemic of that year'.[40] Throughout the pestilence—and desperate for an explanation of cholera's aetiology—he was 'constantly taking meteorological observations', and he noted the 'relationship between cholera and the wind'.[41]

Haviland's professional, intellectual, and ideological relationship with the public health community also provided him with an investigative tool: mapping. For the *Geographical Distribution*, he produced six small and three very large coloured maps (they fold out of the book, covering a desk), showing heart disease, cancer, and tuberculosis mortality for England and Wales. He also printed three maps of London showing the distribution of each disease. In the second edition, he created geological and contour maps of the Lake District, overlaying the regional distribution of cancer. *Scarborough as a Health Resort* began with a large-scale (again, fold-out) map of the town, with all its climatological and topographical features carefully engraved.

Maps were useful and Haviland deployed the technology with enthusiasm throughout his long career. However, his ability to make maps and think geographically was dependent on the collection and tabulation of vital statistics by the GRO. He was explicit about the debt mapping owed to the quantification of the social body. He was devoted to the GRO's *Annual Reports*, referred to them as 'That valuable epitome of knowledge', and dedicated his 1855 tract *Climate, Weather and Disease* to the current MOH, George Graham.[42] The GRO data allowed those interested to assess the distribution of health and ill health across the country and analyse region by region. Haviland wrote that the GRO reports 'rendered the geographical distribution of disease in England and Wales a possibility'.[43] However, spatial approaches to disease pre-date the GRO. The gathering of data required the division of the nation into political jurisdictions within which health and population information could be adequately collected. Haviland called that process of division 'mapping', and in doing so recognized that the quantifying of the British population was inherently geographical: 'The *mapping* of England and Wales into 11 divisions, 53 counties, and 625 union districts, affords the means of analysing the distribution of heart-disease or any other cause of death.'[44] The relationship between the numerical method and geography was not one of cause and effect. Rather, the two shared a spatial

---

[40] Haviland, *The Geographical Distribution of Diseases in Great Britain*, 2nd edn, 5.   [41] Ibid.
[42] Haviland, *Climate, Weather and Disease*, 5.
[43] Haviland, *The Geographical Distribution of Diseases in Great Britain*, 2nd edn, 8.
[44] Alfred Haviland, 'Abstracts of Lectures on the Geographical Distribution of Disease in England and Wales: One', *BMJ* 2 (1871), 453–4, at 453; emphasis added.

conceptualization of disease and the population. Public health was, from the outset, geographically configured.

Haviland's commitment to an environmental framework of disease causation, as well as his use of mapping as a critical analytic, was dependent on his professional participation in public health in the early nineteenth century. However, his involvement in social statistics at a time when cancer was perceived as a growing epidemic threat also explains his new focus on malignancy after c.1860. Haviland's main aim was to uncover the aetiology of cancer and decode the enigma of its increase. As shown in the previous four chapters, nineteenth-century tracts and treatises on the disease were replete with lamentations over cancer's mysterious status. In line with commentaries published earlier in the century, Haviland called cancer 'A disease, which hitherto has baffled all the skill of generation after generation of our professional brethren.'[45] It was 'a most painful and loathsome disease', one that 'kills by inches, and seldom admits of any cure except by the knife, and even that remedy does not always succeed'.[46] Even at the advent of the twentieth century it was persistently enigmatic.

Haviland outlined his general methodology for understanding the cause of cancer in an 'Abstract of Lectures on the Geographical Distribution of Diseases in England and Wales', delivered at St Thomas' Hospital, London, and published in the *BMJ* in 1870:

> In the first place, we see what proportion the death-rate from a cause of death bears to the population in each of the eleven divisions; we colour blue or red those divisions which are above or below the average, and then study this gross distribution carefully. The next process is to colour the counties in the same way, and observe where the distribution at all coincides with that of the divisions; and the third process is to discover whether the proportional mortality of each county is influenced by the mortality in the districts. Having done this, we again review our work, and calculate the effect of each of the many causes surrounding us in the production of the distribution, which our coloured map reveals.[47]

Here, Haviland claimed the distribution of disease—arranged visually—allowed the observer to explain any variations in incidence: the 'coloured map reveals'. He suggested that 'to ascertain the geographical distribution of a disease is the first step towards a knowledge of its natural history'.[48] He used mapping 'to discover where diseases prevail, and were they do not thrive',[49] and 'to search for, in those

---

[45] Alfred Haviland, 'Abstracts of Lectures on the Geographical Distribution of Disease in England and Wales: Two', *BMJ* 2 (1871), 573–5, at 574.

[46] William Buchan, *Domestic Medicine; or A Treatise on The Prevention and Cure of Diseases, by Regimen and Simple Medicines* (London, 187?), 320.

[47] Haviland, 'Abstracts of Lectures: Two', 574.

[48] Haviland, *The Geographical Distribution of Diseases in Great Britain*, 2nd edn, 10.   [49] Ibid.

localities, the causes of prevalence, or absences, or scarcity, whether they reside in their local airs of waters, or are due to general or local climates, geological structure, physical configuration, or social surroundings'.[50] He went on to lament: 'That part of the study of the Natural History of Disease, which treats of its geographically distribution, has been much neglected; hence a powerful aid in the preventive treatment of many of the grand causes of death has been allowed to remain unused.'[51]

In his tract *The Geographical Distribution of Diseases in Great Britain*, he attended to the distribution of three maladies: cancer, phthisis, and heart disease, which, 'in certain well-defined areas throughout England and Wales...consecutively caused high death rates, whilst in other equally well-defined areas they had failed to exceed their average death rate in the country'.[52] He framed his investigation as a search for 'the causes of this unequal but apparently fixed distribution', and argued that their spread was dependent on 'the soil and the atmosphere'—the precise details of which he was endeavouring to uncover.[53] To do so, he used GRO data for the decade 1851–60 to map out female cancer incidence in England and Wales in beautiful simplicity (Figures 5.6 and 5.7). Havilland's use of colour is interesting. Choropleth (coloured) mapping was first used in France in 1826 and geographers have examined the nineteenth-century transformation of colour from a decorative feature into a crucial and explanatory element of design, 'indispensable to the cartographic objective'.[54] Haviland explained his colour coding:

> I selected red and blue with the view of aiding the medical memory, the first being typical of red, life-giving arterial blood, the symbol of health and low mortality as indicated by death-rates below the average, while the second represents the colour of effete and used-up venous blood, the emblem of disease and high death-rates, or a mortality above the average...The lowest mortality is indicated by the darkest red and the highest by the darkest blue.[55]

Here Haviland draws metaphorical comparison between the individual body and the body politic. Just as cancer marks itself on the landscape of the flesh—black masses devoid of a health—it marks itself on the national landscape. In his maps of 'The Geographical Distribution of Cancer Females, 1851–1860' (Figures 5.6 and 5.7), the relatively cancer-free arterial blood drains from west to east, with London a blue dot.

---

[50] Ibid., 11.   [51] Haviland, *Scarborough as a Health Resort*, 7.

[52] Haviland, *The Geographical Distribution of Diseases in Great Britain*, 2nd edn, viii.   [53] Ibid.

[54] Karen S. Pearson, 'The Nineteenth-Century Colour Revolution: Maps in Geographical Journals', *Imago Mundi*, 32 (1980), 9–20, at 9.

[55] Haviland, 'Abstracts of Lectures: Two', 573.

However, Haviland also went further. He understood cancer to operate on multiple different 'scales'—from the body all the way through to the nation—and he repeatedly inscribed the relationship between the individual and social body. Recently, social geographers have scrutinized the production of scale as a political-economic process. Rather than taking the scales of social and cultural activity for granted (such as the nation state), these scholars are gesturing towards ways in which scale was contested and constructed.[56] Thus, while Haviland's maps fixed the scale of cancer at the national or regional levels, he was also seeking to reveal what was happening at the scale of the human body. For Haviland, therefore, the body (and its scale) can only be understood through reference to the scale of the region or nation. He required environmental representations to make sense of cancer (and chose a rural environment to do so), thus demonstrating that scales are relational and not natural or inherently fixed.

Mapping also made visible, in a different way, an often undetectable disease. As argued in Chapter 1, medical men were well aware that malignancy could navigate its way through the internal textures of the body without necessarily manifesting external signs. The medical philosopher Elisha Bartlett spoke at length on the obscurity of cancer, making use of a variety of visual metaphors:

Almost all diseases are occasionally so impressed and modified, by inappreciable or unknown influences, that their usual diagnostic signs are wanting, or very much obscured,—the diseases being *latent*, as it is called. Cancerous disorgan-isation of the stomach, in some instances, gives no indication of its existence, insufficiently distinct to render its detection possible, during life, even by the most competent and careful observers.[57]

Mapping could therefore help to reveal, or at least visualize, the 'obscured' cancer, organize the 'cancerous disorganization', and detect what clinical observation had thus far failed to observe. Putting cancer on the macro level of maps gave it a different kind of visibility to that of the micro level of individual examination.

The inability to identify and treat latent cancers was connected intrinsically to the 'disorganization' noted. This not only suggests a metaphorical relationship between the practices of public health mapping and the practicalities of detecting cancer in the individual, but also a more fundamental way of thinking. Just as the organization of public health knowledge into existence could constitute a 'treat-ment' for the social body, the lessons of public health seemed relevant, and even useful, for practitioners confronting cancer in the individual body. Similarly, Haviland wrote in 1875, 'Perchance *some light might be thrown upon* the aetiology

[56] 'Scale', in Linda McDowell and Joanne P. Sharp (eds.), *A Feminist Glossary of Human Geography* (London, 1999), 242.
[57] Elisha Bartlett, *An Essay on the Philosophy of Medical Science* (Philadelphia, PA, 1844), 140.

of that fatal class of malignant diseases, registered as causes of death under the term cancer, if the available statistics, as published by Dr William Farr, C.B., were to be treated on the same geographic principles as had been demonstrated in the cases of phthisis and heart disease.'[58] In this way, mapping was a 'solution' to the problem of cancer's incurability. While clinical intervention might have limited success, illustrating the spatial distribution of cancer was a productive and pragmatic response to the intractability of the disease.

The map of the 'Divisions' (Figure 5.4) provided insufficient detail and so Haviland zoomed in on the 'Counties' (Figure 5.5). If the former suggested an east–west contrast in cancer incidence, the latter painted a more complex picture. Haviland's maps of heart disease had been clear in their implications—the malady was 'more fatal in the unventilated valley-system of England and Wales than in the open areas freely-exposed to the prevailing winds and sunshine'.[59] This relationship aligned neatly with commonly held nineteenth-century assumptions—which manifested in multiple ways and in multiple people—that sunshine and free-flowing, dry air had therapeutic (or preventative) health benefits. Cancer, while no doubt associated with the landscape, was harder to elucidate. Haviland, therefore, focused on the Lake District—a bright-red area of low cancer mortality—and plotted four maps: a geological map of the theoretical rocks and soil distribution and a contours map (Figure 5.6), a map of cancer at all ages, and a map of cancer at over thirty-six years of age (Figure 5.7). He then correlated areas of high mortality and areas of low mortality with the geological substrata and the topographical features: 'I studied the registration district-map of England side by side with an early impression of Greenough's splendid physical and geological map of England and Wales.'[60]

For Haviland, 'the high mortality groups' could be 'seen to skirt the lower courses of fully-formed rivers that seasonally flood the riparian districts'. Indeed, the intense blue of London could be explained by its straddling of the Thames: 'The Thames Basin has long been known as one of the great cancer fields of England and Wales.' Haviland concluded that cancer was more fatal among women in 'clayey flooded areas than on elevated calcerous soil'.[61] He had a low opinion of clay:

> In the history of diseases clays are connected with the most deadly scourges to which the human race has been subjected, such as those that have arisen in our

[58]   Haviland, 'Abstracts of Lectures: Two', 573; emphasis added.
[59]   Haviland, *The Geographical Distribution of Diseases in Great Britain*, 2nd edn, viii.
[60]   Alfred Haviland, *A Paper on the Influence of Clays and Limestones on Medical Geography; Illustrated by the Geographical Distribution of Cancer among Females, in England and Wales* (London, 1891), 3.
[61]   Haviland, *The Geographical Distribution of Diseases in Great Britain*, 2nd edn, viii.

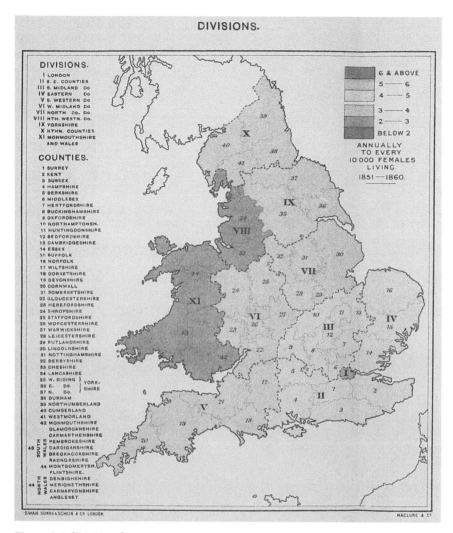

Figure 5.4 'Divisions'

Source: From Alfred Haviland, *The Geographical Distribution of Diseases in Great Britain*, 2nd edn (London, 1892), 36–7. Wellcome Collection.

own times from vegetable decomposition after floods—as in the intense of cholera from the alluvial clays forming the delta of the Ganges,[62] and in the long list of malarial fevers all over the world which have had their origin in the deltas of rivers and inland marshes, characterised by alluvial clays saturated with

---

[62] It is worth noting that map-making (and concerns over sanitation and public health) were also crucial for interrogating cancer in the British colonies; see Chapter 7.

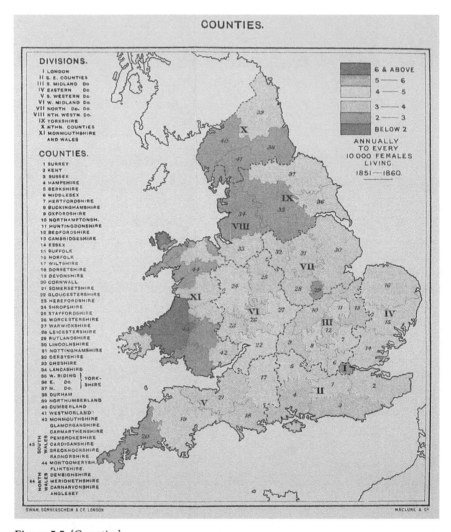

Figure 5.5 'Counties'

Source: From Alfred Haviland, *The Geographical Distribution of Diseases in Great Britain*, 2nd edn (London, 1892), 36–7. Wellcome Collection.

the products of the decomposed and decomposing vegetation, that had first been flooded, then killed, and lastly, left to rot in the sun.[63]

In contrast, his praise of limestone was unequivocally positive: 'Limestones have no such an appalling record. We know of no epidemic sweeping over the world, either air-borne or man-borne, that could be traced to a limestone nidus; on the

[63] Haviland, *A Paper on the Influence of Clays*, 8.

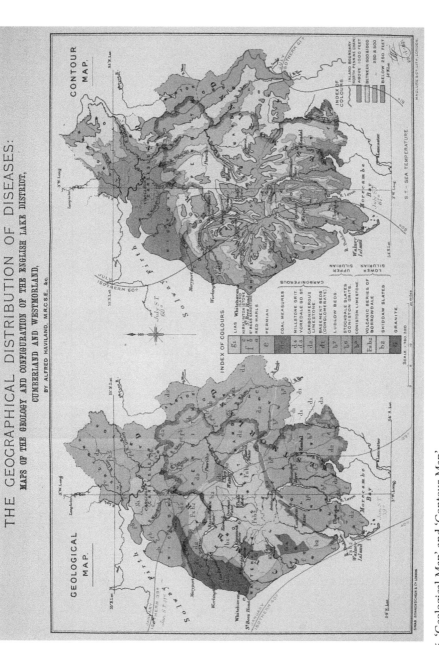

Figure 5.6 'Geological Map' and 'Contour Map'

Source: From Alfred Haviland, *The Geographical Distribution of Diseases in Great Britain*, 2nd edn (London, 1892). Wellcome Collection.

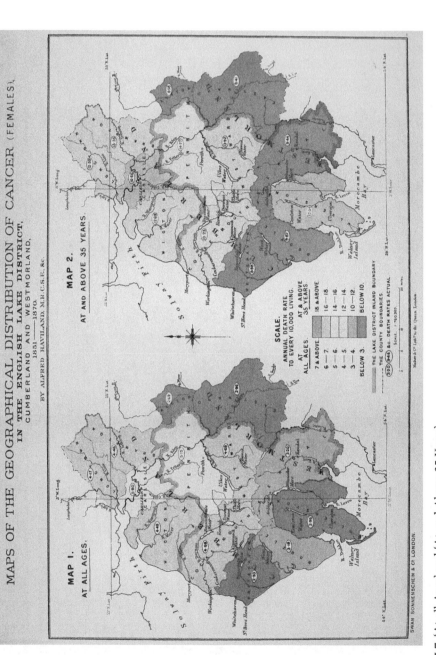

Figure 5.7 'At all Ages' and 'At and Above 35 Years'

Source: From Alfred Haviland, *The Geographical Distribution of Diseases in Great Britain* (London, 1892). Wellcome Collection.

contrary...they are associated with the earliest dawn of life.'[64] Rivers, flowing over clay soil, were in his opinion the cause of cancer: 'In the counties having a high mortality from cancer we find that the tributaries of the large rivers flow from soft marly or other easily disintegrated rocks into sheltered valleys, through which the main rivers flow.'[65] His conceptualization of cancer was thereafter referred to by others as the 'riverine thesis'.[66]

Cancer and the Countryside

Thus, rather than conceptualizing cancer as disease of towns and cities, Haviland framed it as a disease of rural environs. *The Fifth Annual Report of the Registrar-General* recorded that 'more deaths were referred to scrofula and cancer in the country than in the town districts'.[67] Haviland wrote about the cancer-causing properties of the Avon, the Severn, and the Wye rivers, he traces the Trent and the 'great Yorkshire rivers', and locates pathological potential in the 'high ridges of the Northumbrian and Cumbrian hills'.[68] Haviland mapped the agrarian Lake District. While the Thames Valley was coloured deep blue—indicative of high cancer mortality—the metropolis was not considered to be the cause of elevated incidence. Instead, it was the water, soil, rock—the 'natural' environment. While cholera and cancer both might be dependent on their environments, they were produced by very different spaces. Unlike the public health practitioners surveyed, Haviland did not argue that the uneven distribution of cancer incidence was an artefact of people living longer, healthier lives in the countryside. This not only shows us that public health in the nineteenth century was concerned with non-urban spaces, but that cancer was perceived as fundamentally different to the epidemic diseases of poverty. Mapping was, therefore, not simply an expression of Victorian anxieties about the new industrial town, but could equally be applied to

---

[64] Ibid., 9.   [65] Haviland, 'Abstracts of Lectures: Two', 574.

[66] While Haviland did not cite Max von Pettenkofer (1818–1901), Professor of Hygiene in Germany, his work shares much with the latter's concept of *Bodentheorie* (soil theory). In the 1860s von Pettenkofer claimed that soil pollution was the principal cause of epidemics, and in particular cholera. This connection between soil and disease was widespread, and reflected the persistence of localist-miasmatic aetiologies into the late nineteenth century. Men such as Charles Murchison and Alfred Smee, as well as von Pettenkofer, argued that disease-causing germs had to undergo a period of incubation in the soil to become infective. It was thus consistent to think of cancer as causally related to soil quality and Haviland was well situated within his intellectual context. However, Haviland was surprisingly vague about the precise relationship among rocks, soil, rivers, and cancer. While he referenced the possibility of a cancer 'germ', he stopped short of setting out of any clear aetiological model. Jacob Steere-Williams, 'Performing State Medicine during its "Frustrating" Years: Epidemiology and Bacteriology at the Local Government Board, 1870–1900', *Social History of Medicine*, 28 (2014), 82–107.

[67] *The Fifth Annual Report of the Registrar-General of Births, Deaths, and Marriages* (London, 1843), 408.

[68] Haviland, 'Abstracts of Lectures: Two', 575.

districts representative of health and well-being. While it may have originated because of those urban concerns, it was subsequently applied to other settings.

In Victorian literary tropes, the Lake District and the Thames Valley were usually associated with health, affluence, images of bucolic England, and British national identity. Keir Waddington argues that this association of rurality with health was 'reinforced by the environmental determinism central to Chadwickian conceptions of public health ... and gained power in the late nineteenth century in response to growing fears of urban degeneration'.[69] An 1883 *Spectator* article on a defeated plan for a new railway that would cut across the region waxed lyrical on the rural beauty of the Lakes: 'We turn and pass down the vale, by the side of Ennerdale Water ... One thing strikes us at once. The singular loveliness of the wild strip of land between lake and mountain-wall.'[70] The article goes on to suggest that the Lakes were distinctly healthful and beneficial to England's 'true wealth':

> Parliament has been wise in remembering that England's true wealth lies not in her mineral supply, so much as in her supply of healthy souls in healthy bodies. Parliament does not forget that the work of the world demands that there shall be rest-spaces for the weary workers.

The Lakes provided an essential reprieve from the traumas of industrial labour. They were a favourite destination for tourists and visiting dignitaries alike in the nineteenth century, with the King of Saxony including them in his tour of northern English attractions in 1844.[71] In reconceptualizing them as diseased spaces—lacing the Lake District with pathological potential—Haviland marked himself out as distinct from contemporary commentary and implied remapping of our understanding of the Victorian landscape.

These various spatial configurations of cancer also tell us something more diffuse about how the disease's aetiology was conceptualized in the nineteenth century. Haviland and others all understood cancer as produced by rural places. However, there was a paradox in this correlation between countryside and cancer. If the bucolic was also disease-causing, then how did that sit with contemporary conceptualizations of the city as marked by industrial overcrowding and attendant

---

[69] Keir Waddington, '"In a Country Every Way by Nature Favourable to Health": Landscape and Public Health in Victorian Rural Wales', *Canadian Bulletin of Medical History*, 32 (2014), 183–204, 187. More generally, W. J. T. Mitchell suggests that landscapes are cultural products and can be read as 'symbols in religious, psychological, or political allegories; characteristic structures and forms ... can be linked with generic and narrative typologies such as the pastoral, the georgic, the exotic, the sublime, and the picturesque'. W. J. T. Mitchell, 'Introduction', in W. J. T. Mitchell (ed.), *Landscape and Power* (Chicago, 2002), 1. See also Jeremy Burchardt, *Paradise Lost: Rural Idyll and Social Change in England since 1800* (London, 2002), 25–34, 67–76; and Simon Schama, *Landscape and Memory* (London, 1995).

[70] 'The Defeated Ennerdale Railway', *The Spectator*, 21 July 1883, 929.

[71] 'Court and Fashionable', *John Bull*, 20 July 1844, 456.

poverty and poor health?[72] Much of late eighteenth- and nineteenth-century rhetoric was devoted to pathologizing the city, as Noah Webster wrote, 'Why should cities be erected if they are only to be the tombs of men?'[73] Nonetheless, connections between cancer and rural idylls fit with broader understandings of cancer that existed in the second half of the nineteenth century. Global geographies of the disease plotted populations on a gradient—from immune to cancer riddled—at one end sub-Saharan African colonies, at the other Anglo-Saxon or Teutonic races: 'Observation has shown that cancer has a certain geographical distribution. It prevails extensively in some parts of the globe, and is scarcely known in others.'[74] This mapping was marshalled as evidence for cancer as a 'disease of civilization' (see Chapter 7).[75] Not only was the disease on the increase, the epidemic was confined to nations that were understood as biologically, and in every other way, superior. By extension, in the domestic context cancer was flourishing in the English countryside.[76]

Haviland's mapping of cancer in rural environs reveals something subtle in his understanding of mapping and its role in public health. His maps—in so many ways familiar to the standard narrative of maps as the insidious and modernist tools of state control over deviant *populations*—here seem to veer off in a different direction, used to interrogate and even control *nature*. Chadwick and his allies were explicit in their understanding of the urban environment as pathological; however, historians have tended to read against the grain and interpret sanitary reform and the map-making that accompanied it as an attempt to organize *people* as well as, or instead of, *spaces*. Haviland's interest in rural spaces might be understood as a way to organize the landscape into submission, but at heart he was more interested in the management of the relationship between people and places and an implicit return to Hippocratic ideas. In 1891 he would argue that

---

[72] These conceptualizations had foundation in demographic reality. In 1801, rural inhabitants enjoyed an approximately eleven-year advantage in life expectancy at birth compared to their urban counterparts. By 1911, this difference was much reduced, but countryside dwellers still retained an advantage. R. I. Woods, 'The Effect of Population Redistribution on the Level of Mortality in Nineteenth-Century England and Wales', *Journal of Economic History*, 45 (1985), 645–51. For more on this 'urban penalty' see G. Kearns, 'The Urban Penalty and the Population History of England', in A. Brandstrom and L. G. Tedebrand (eds.), *Society and Healthy during the Demographic Transition* (Stockholm, 1988).

[73] Koch, 'Social Epidemiology as Medical Geography', 101.

[74] Hugh P. Dunn, 'English Experience with Cancer', *Popular Science Monthly*, 36 (1885), 689.

[75] Nascent in this is the now-prevalent idea that cancer is a pathology of progress. See Charles E. Rosenberg, 'Pathologies of Progress: The Idea of Civilization as Risk', *Bulletin of the History of Medicine*, 72 (1998), 714–30.

[76] In many ways, this construction of the English countryside as a bucolic idyll was misaligned with its current economic state—rural England was in the middle of an agricultural depression and various places were targeted by public health practitioners for their own version of sanitary reform. See Edward Hunt and S. J. Pam, 'Responding to Agricultural Depression, 1873–96: Managerial Success, Entrepreneurial Failure?', *Agricultural History Review*, 50 (2002), 225–52; Waddington, '"In a Country Every Way by Nature Favourable to Health', 191.

One of the functions of the medical geographer is to ascertain where certain diseases prevail, and to indicate those areas on his maps as guides ... to the busy medical practitioner who requires to know *at once*, for the sake of the patients who consult him as to where they ought not to reside if they would avoid the diseases they dread, and where are to be found the localities in which there is the greatest chance of escaping them.[77]

Haviland thought of his map-making as usefully preventative, suggesting a way for humankind to 'manage', through mapping, their relationship with nature and change this into something healthy. The disease-causing properties of certain spaces might not be alterable—mountains, rivers, and streams cannot be moved— but they could at least be avoided.

Prevention and avoidance were crucial for a man who, like most of peers, believed cancer to be incurable. In 1875, he wrote,

It is a fact which we cannot disguise, that up to the present date we know of no cure for Cancer, and more than this, with all our deep and unwearied study of its physical and pathological nature, we have not even got a clue to one; in fact, so far as treatment or a remedy is concerned, we are now simply waiting for some such lucky chance.[78]

However, he was not despondent and believed he, as a map-maker and MOH, could still be of use in efforts to solve the 'cancer problem'. He rejected the 'vulgar adage' 'what can't be cured must be endured', and insisted that his objects were 'based upon higher and worthier principles'.[79] He argued that his perseverance had 'already led to such grand results in ... investigation of causes' and suggested that these efforts—his mapping—contributed to 'the knowledge how to prevent many unnecessary diseases and a great amount of premature death'.[80] While a cure for cancer might be the goal, prevention was a useful temporary substitute.

Haviland's Contemporaries

While Haviland was the most prolific cancer map-maker, he was not alone in conceptualizing the disease as a problem of geography or climate. Environmental understandings of cancer appeared before Haviland's map-making and persisted well into the twentieth century. Just over ten years prior to the publication of *The Geographical Distribution*, Surgeon to The Middlesex Hospital's Cancer Ward,

[77] Haviland, *A Paper on the Influence of Clays*, 5.
[78] Haviland, *The Geographical Distribution of Heart Diseases and Dropsy*, 91.   [79] Ibid.
[80] Ibid.

Charles H. Moore, published a book full of spatial thinking. Working to uncover the cause of cancer he suggested, 'Somewhere, among the personal, social, industrial, traumatic, or geographical conditions of the patient, in the *debris* of foregoing disease, or in his ancestral entail, the case of Cancer surely lies within reach of an adequate search.'[81] He devoted one chapter of his work to the 'geographical conditions' and posited that 'if a disease common to all the human race is yet unequally distributed, some cause influencing its prevalence or its rarity might be disclosed by an examination of the circumstances'.[82] He suggested that there must be something meaningful about the uneven scattering of cancer incidence in Britain: 'Can we find in the distribution of Cancer among large masses of people, any rule which would connect its rarity or frequency with the general conditions of their life?'[83] He connected cancer to broader understandings of disease and locale: 'It is notorious, that very different states of general healthiness exist in large divisions of the community.'[84] He, like Haviland, relied on governmental statistics and laid out his rationale for taking the death rate as a reliable stand-in for incidence: 'In the instance of a malady so fatal as Cancer, the death-rate only too accurately represents its numerical prevalence among the people, the Government returns are suitable for the inquiry before us.'[85] From that data he concluded: 'If the country be divided by a line from Bristol to Peterborough...the mortality from Cancer in the five southern divisions is considerably in excess of that on the north of the line. Its greatest prevalence, according to the records, is in London and the counties south of it.'[86] Moore makes limited effort to explain this unequal distribution, but in setting out his justification for the utility of geographical investigations into cancer he laid the groundwork for subsequent efforts to turn such thinking into map-making.

Nor did Haviland have the last word on cancer mapping. Studies into the spatial distribution of the disease proliferated in the decades surrounding 1900, and many were regional in focus. In 1884, the Medical Congress appointed an 'International Committee' for the 'prosecution of Collective Inquiries'.[87] It put forward a plan for the investigation of the aetiology of various as-yet-unexplained diseases, including rickets, rheumatism, and cancer. The goal was to distribute enquiries to all medical practitioners within a country and use the responses to map the geographical distribution of the disease under scrutiny. While they had little success in central Europe as 'little interest could be aroused in collective work', in Denmark, Sweden, and Norway 'the investigation was taken up with more zeal'. Reports from these countries, together with one from the American Medical Association, were presented to Medical Congress held in Washington in

---

[81] Charles H. Moore, *The Antecedents of Cancer* (London, 1865), iv.   [82] Ibid., 36.
[83] Ibid., 37.   [84] Ibid., 40.   [85] Ibid., 38.   [86] Ibid., 43.
[87] Isambard Owen, 'Reports of the Collective Investigation Committee of the British Medical Association: Geographical Distribution of Rickets, Acute and Subacute Rheumatism, Chorea, Cancer, and Urinary Calculus in the British Islands', *BMJ*, 1 (1899), 113–16, at 113.

1888. Britain's efforts were coordinated by the Collective Investigation Committee of the British Medical Association, under the direction of Isambard Owen, Secretary to the Committee. The Collective Investigation Committee circulated an 'inquiry paper' to every registered medical practitioner in the United Kingdom, which asked, 'Are the following diseases, or any of them, common in your district; that is, would a medical man in average practice in it be likely to meet with, on the average, a case a year?' The data derived was used to create a map of the distribution of cancer across the British Isles, which was published in 1889.[88]

The committee enquired about rickets, acute rheumatism, chorea, urinary calculus, and cancer. As in Haviland's maps, places in which the disease was 'common' were coloured blue, and those where it was 'uncommon' were marked with red. More than 3,000 completed papers were returned and eight maps were produced from the information contained: England and Wales, Scotland, Ireland, the Orkney and Shetlands Islands, the Channel Islands, and one each of Manchester, Edinburgh, and Greater London. The disease appeared to be evenly distributed, and any clustering in the major cities was explained by the accompanying report in the *BMJ* as resulting from the density of medical institutions in these urban places.[89] Cancer seemed to be particularly common in the Orkney and Shetlands Islands and in the Channel Islands. In London, the report noted how cancer, 'tended to collect in the flat lands adjacent to the river', and they referenced Haviland's riverine thesis.[90]

In 1899, the Committee...to Investigate the Influence of Locality on the Prevalence of Malignant Disease in the Counties of Warwick, Stafford, Salop, and Worcester published their interim report. This committee consisted of various local doctors, including Dr R. M. Sion, Dr T. Law Webb, Dr Thomas Wilson, Dr Douglas Stanley, and Dr E. N. Nason, who were appointed at a meeting of the Birmingham and Midland Counties Branch of the British Medical Association. The committee had, by this point, met four times and collected a 'large amount' of evidence from the counties of Warwick, Stafford, Salop, and Worcester. They echoed Haviland's concern over rivers and clay, concluding that 'The districts in which malignant disease occurs with the greatest frequency are usually ill drained, low-lying or flat, or border on streams.'[91] Reflecting on another investigation, conducted by a Dr W. H. Symons and published in *Public Health*, the committee wrote, 'The town [Bath] is built partly on a sand bed, partly on a clay bed of varying thickness overlying a bed of limestone. This clay has in many cases been

---

[88] For an analysis of Collective Investigation Committee more broadly, see Harry Marks, ' "Until the Sun of Science...the True Apollo of Medicine Has Risen": Collective Investigation in Britain and America, 1880–1910', *Medical History*, 50 (2006), 147–66.

[89] Owen, 'Reports of the Collective Investigation Committee', 114.   [90] Ibid.

[91] 'The Influence of Locality on the Prevalence of Cancer', *BMJ*, 1 (1899), 812–13, at 812.

thrown out into mounds to get at the limestone; houses have been built upon these clay banks and, speaking generally, these are the houses where cancer occurs.'[92]

Haviland proved a point of reference for many of these analyses (which generally faded into obscurity) and for subsequent general reflections on the geographical distribution of cancer. For example, in 1898 the *BMJ* referred to the 'well-known views of Mr. Haviland'.[93] Similarly, in 1899 Cambridge doctor E. Lloyd Jones published an article entitled, 'The Topographical Distribution of Cancer', in which he 'sought to determine in what manner cancer is distributed in the borough of Cambridge and in the surrounding county'.[94] He referenced Haviland repeatedly, claiming that 'most observers agree with Haviland that limestone and chalky districts are comparatively free from cancer'.[95] Haviland also appeared in a 1903 *BMJ* article on cancer mortality: 'The connexion of the disease with geological formation as shown by Haviland in his cancer map of England and Wales.'[96] In 1904, Alexander Urquhart wrote in the *BMJ*, 'The south-eastern division of England has long been regarded as showing a high death-rate from cancer, and the Thames valley in particular has had this unenviable reputation.'[97] He referenced Haviland and applied new statistics to an old problem which seemed to 'justify the conclusion that the Thames valley is still associated with a relatively high mortality from cancer'.[98] Haviland's theories and data were being talked about in the medical and public health press well into the 1960s.[99] His name also appeared beyond the national borders of Great Britain and was referenced favourably in a French medical thesis from 1897.[100] He was given a long obituary in the *BMJ* and his work was reviewed rapturously in various periodicals. The *Medical Times and Gazette* wrote about *The Geographic Distribution of Disease*: 'It is a national work, and hence the author has a right to expect to find upon the list of his subscribers at least every sanitary board, not only in England and Wales, but wherever the English language is read.'[101] The *British and Foreign Medico-Chirurgical Review* added: 'The undertaking is novel, an honour to British Medicine, and calculated to promote the pursuit of a department of pathology hitherto greatly neglected.'[102] Thus, Haviland's ideas about the pathological potential of Britain's natural environment had purchase. He was influential on conceptualizations of cancer's causes, shaping the landscape of research in direct and diffuse ways.

---

[92] Ibid.   [93] 'Cancer in Relation to the Dwelling', *BMJ*, 2 (1898), 1571–2, at 1571.

[94] E. Lloyd Jones, 'The Topographical Distribution of Cancer', *BMJ*, 1 (1899), 813–15, at 814.

[95] Ibid.   [96] James Braithwaite, 'Cancer Mortality', *BMJ*, 1 (1903), 1289.

[97] Alexander Urquhart, 'Notes on Recent Cancer Mortality in the Thames Valley', *BMJ*, 1 (1904), 825–6, at 825.

[98] Ibid.   [99] 'Soil and Stomach Cancer', *BMJ*, 1 (1965), 1–2, esp. 1.

[100] Henri Jouve, *Thèse pour Le Doctorat en Médecine sur La Topographie et La Contagion du Cancer* (Paris, 1897), 13.

[101] Quoted in Haviland, *The Geographical Distribution of Diseases in Great Britain*.   [102] Ibid.

New Concepts of Cancer Mapping

One way in which Haviland's geographical framing of cancer proved particularly influential was in the popularity of, and preoccupation with, so-called 'cancer houses', 'cancer streets', and 'cancer villages'. These were dwellings, roads, and settlements which seemed to manifest an unusual frequency of cancer incidence. In the 1890s, surgeon and medical historian D'Arcy Power devoted considerable time and energy to investigating these places. He was not alone, and the question of 'cancer houses' drew attention from a range of medical practitioners as well as from the lay press. These places served as sites of theoretical contestation and coexistence, and discussions of their existence and distribution required the making and circulation of cancer maps. However, unlike Haviland's maps, these more geographically circumscribed diagrams were often used to argue for a range of aetiological mechanisms. Not only did they suggest that cancer was transmitted from the surrounding environment, they also claimed that malignancy might be carried by an as-yet-undiscovered microbe or through family bloodlines. Power mapped cancer occurrence for the years 1872–88 in a British village of 1,036 persons and demonstrated the uneven incidence of cases to identify the location of 'cancer streets' and 'cancer houses'.[103] In keeping with Haviland's focus on the countryside, people preoccupied with cancer houses mostly looked at smaller enclaves, like villages and hamlets, not the metropolis or its industrial co-cities. While Power had originally thought that 'the question [of cancer] might be solved in the laboratory', he subsequently focused his attention on the spatial distribution of the disease. He described one 'cancer house' in detail:

> Mr. Wynter Blyth narrates the case of three successive tenants of a house in Buckland Brewer, who died of cancer. Mrs. V. frequently visited the last of the tenants, to whom she was not related, and she subsequently became affected with cancer of the breast and lung. Her niece, a girl of 14, slept with her and nursed her. This girl developed cancer of the breast, and was operated upon.[104]

The successive occupants had been 'in perfect health' before entering the house, which suggested to Power that there was something pathological about the building itself. Precisely what this 'something' was, was open to debate.

Like Power, Dr E. Lloyd Jones surveyed 5,685 houses and produced maps of the locales in question (Figure 5.8).[105] In 1899, he made a record of all the cases of cancer occurring in Cambridgeshire over the previous nineteen years. The method he adopted 'consisted in copying out . . . the death-certificates, dividing the names

---

[103] D'Arcy Power, 'Cancer Houses and their Victims', *BMJ*, 1 (1894), 1240.   [104] Ibid., 1240.
[105] Lloyd Jones, 'The Topographical Distribution of Cancer', 814.

XL.14.2.2.									
L.1.	R.1. Unaffected Houses 62, 1 to 62, Cancer 1.								
L.2.	R.2 Unaffected Houses 13, Cancer 0.								

XLVII.2.2.		XLVII.2.3.		XLVII.2.4.		XLVII.2.5.		XLVII.3.7.	
L.1. Unaffected Houses 27, 1 to 13, Cancer 2.	R.1. Unaffected Houses 125, 1 to 17.8, Cancer 7.	L.1. Unaffected Houses 49, 1 to 8.1, Cancer 6	R.1. Only about 2 Residences.	L.1. No houses.	R.1. (Common land.)	L.1. Few houses.	R.1.	L.1. Unaffected Houses 62, 1 to 31, Cancer 2.	R.1. Unaffected Houses 30, 1 to 10, Cancer 3.
L.2.	R.2. Unaffected Houses 61, 1 to 7.6, Cancer 8.	L.2. Unaffected Houses 83, 1 to 9.2, Cancer 9.	R.2. Unaffected Houses 45, 1 to 11.2, Cancer 4.	L.2. Unaffected Houses 31, 1 to 5.1, Cancer 6.	R.2. Unaffected Houses 80, 1 to 6.1, Cancer 13.	L.1. Unaffected Houses 121, 1 to 30.2, Cancer 4.	R.2. Unaffected Houses 128, 1 to 16, Cancer 8.	L.2. Unaffected Houses 13, 1 to 2.1, Cancer 6.	R.2.

Figure 5.8 Cancer Houses

Source: E. Lloyd Jones, 'The Topographical Distribution of Cancer', *BMJ*, 1 (1899), 815.

into classes'. These 'classes' ranged from 'persons who died in their own house' to 'persons who died in the workhouse'. From this data, he compiled a list of all the houses in which people had been taken ill with cancer. He then visited all the houses and marked each on an ordnance survey map—'scale of 10 feet to a mile'— showing the affected and non-affected houses in red or black. Much like Haviland, he concluded that 'damp situations are more apt as a rule to harbour cancer than dry ones' and that dwellings built on chalky soil tended to be cancer free.[106] In 1912, Karl Pearson, the influential statistician and proponent of eugenics, published an exhaustive article in Francis Galton's journal *Biometrika* on the statistics germane to the 'cancer house' hypothesis. Pearson closed his analysis with the claim: 'I think these data certainly justify a fuller inquiry into the whole question. They provide some evidence, of more than mere impression, that the hypothesis of "cancer houses" is worthy of a fuller consideration.'[107] Some suggested a geographical explanation for the prevalence of cancer houses:

> These cancer districts seem more especially to lie about the beds of rivers which are liable to overflow their banks, and the nature of the soil into which the overflow takes place appears to have a very marked influence in the production of cancer; it is the stiffer clay soils which hold the water for a considerable time, which seem to be particularly noxious.[108]

[106] Ibid.

[107] Karl Pearson, 'On "Cancer Houses" from the Data of the Late Th. Law Webb, M.D.', *Biometrika*, 8 (1912), 430–5, at 435.

[108] Arthur Jackson, 'An Address on the Incidence of Cancer', *BMJ*, 2 (1899), 1465–7, at 1465.

There is also plenty of evidence to suggest that cancer mapping entered public discourse and was deployed persuasively in an expanding range of contexts. 'Cancer houses' in particular were a popular topic of debate in the turn-of-the-century press. *The Observer* published an article in 1907 entitled 'Cancer Houses: Does the Disease Infect our Dwellings?' which asked whether 'rooms inhabited by cancer patients liable to convey the disease years after the patient is dead?'[109] The *Times of India* published a similar editorial on 'Cancer Houses: Infection or Coincidence?' It was subtitled 'Disease-Haunted Buildings', and in it they reported on D'Arcy Power's investigations and claimed: 'The disease appeared to haunt certain buildings, quite irrespective of their size, age, or condition.'[110] As late as 1933, the *BMJ* reported on the 'stigma' of 'cancer house', and how it 'must often inflict serious pecuniary losses on the owners of the house in question'.[111]

In 1909, the doctor and medical writer, Charles E. Green, published the first edition of his book *The Cancer Problem: A Statistical Study*. It was printed again and again until the 1930s, going into over fifteen editions. In it, he 'mapped out' his geographical-germ theory of cancer causation.[112] Cast in the Haviland mould—he referenced both him and Charles H. Moore—Green was committed to an environmentalist investigation of cancer and dependent on the statistics of the GRO.[113] In the 1912 edition he insisted that the data proved 'that cancer is much more prevalent in some districts than in others',[114] and that 'there are most striking topographical variations in the incidence of the disease.[115] Clearly, not only had environmentalist understandings of cancer persisted through the 'bacteriological revolution', Green had continued to be profoundly influenced by such conclusions and methodologies. He referred to 'the very generally accepted idea' that 'the proximity of tall trees has some connection with cancer'.[116] While he discounts this as a credible theory, he does so using mapping: 'It will be seen that the rural districts of Orkney have a mortality above the average, amounting to 5.32, and as there is only one tree of any size in Orkney, which is looked upon as a curiosity and is situated in the centre of Kirkwell, it is obvious that the tree theory falls to the ground.'[117]

Green wrote about how he 'motored over practically the whole of Scotland in the endeavour to find any clue to these pronounced differences [in cancer incidence]'.[118] He was studying cancer in situ—seeing it in the place it manifested. Much like Haviland, he focused on the countryside and investigated Nairn, 'a beautiful rural county' in Scotland. He concluded: 'those where the death-rate was

---

[109] 'Cancer Houses: Does the Disease Infect our Dwellings?', *The Observer*, 8 September 1907, 3.
[110] 'Cancer Houses: Infection or Coincidence? Disease-Haunted Buildings', *The Times of India*, 1 October 1907, 9.
[111] 'France', *BMJ*, 1 (1933), 716–17, at 717.
[112] Charles E. Green, *The Cancer Problem: A Statistical Study*, 2nd edn (London, 1912).
[113] Ibid., 2.   [114] Ibid., 2.   [115] Ibid., 42.   [116] Ibid., 45.   [117] Ibid.
[118] Ibid., 45–6.

low were comparatively flat, or at most had low, swelling, undulating hills, with houses built on their sides, whereas those where the mortality was high were intersected with gulleys and valleys, with the houses as a rule situated in the hollows'.[119] On the other hand, 'Towns lying in a cup have by far the highest cancer mortalities, while those on a level site with level surroundings show the lowest percentage. Those on hilly sites are slightly higher than those on sloping sites.'[120] How could this distribution be explained? For Green, it spoke to contemporaneous debates over cancer's origin, 'the Cell Theory, and the Parasitic... In other words, is it of intrinsic or extrinsic origin?'[121] His statistics 'prove that *it must be some element in the environment of the sufferer which brings on the disease*, and if we admit this, we must admit an extrinsic origin'.[122] In line with the aforementioned compatibility of various cancer theories, he suggested a mechanical, chemical, parasitic cause—'or a subtle combination of the three'.[123] The extrinsic origin of cancer is dealt with in more detail in Chapter 6—where I discuss how medical men reached a similar conclusion to Green, but through the microscope rather than with the help of mapping.

What, then, did Green think was the element in the environment that made certain areas cancerous? Alongside his mapping, he made use of occupational cancer statistics and discovered 'that the chimney-sweep has by far the highest mortality figure of all trades'.[124] He concluded that soot was the active agent in producing malignant disease, 'as is shown by the appalling mortality among chimney-sweeps and by other indications'.[125] Green also made use of existing cancer maps in his interrogations. He included in his book a copy of a plan of a village, which the original maker had used to suggest that cancer was infectious (Figure 5.9).[126] Green, however, drew a different conclusion:

> This plan is worth of most careful study, as the author has indicated the slope of the ground by arrows. If these arrows are followed, they will be found in a most remarkable way almost to point to the houses in which cases have occurred... If, then, the lie of the ground seems to have a mysterious influence on the local incidence of cancer, how can this be explained?[127]

He also deployed two further diagrams that intended to demonstrate how the topography of the land as well as the built environment could collude to make certain houses and areas more or less vulnerable to chimney soot and its cancer-causing properties (Figures 5.10 and 5.11). Again, he borrowed these images from another book—one designed to explain the dangerous nature of chimneys, but with no reference to cancer. Maps might have been made to express one

---

[119] Ibid., 46.   [120] Ibid., 51.   [121] Ibid., 3.   [122] Ibid.   [123] Ibid., 20.
[124] Ibid., 27.   [125] Ibid., 31.   [126] Ibid., 56.   [127] Ibid.

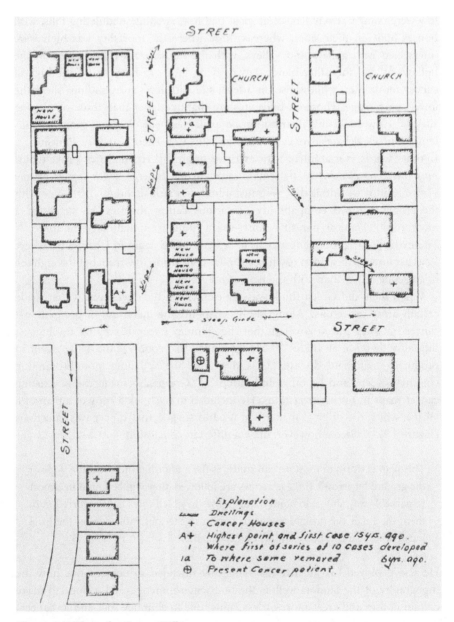

Figure 5.9 Map of a Cancer Village

Source: Charles E. Green, *The Cancer Problem: A Statistical Study*, 2nd edn (London, 1912), 57.
Wellcome Collection.

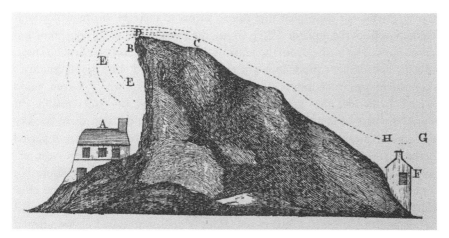

Figure 5.10 Topography of the Land
Source: Charles E. Green, *The Cancer Problem: A Statistical Study*, 2nd edn (London, 1912), 60.
Wellcome Collection.

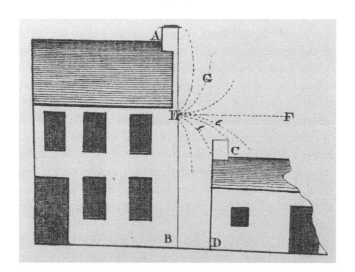

Figure 5.11 Proximity to Chimneys
Source: Charles E. Green, *The Cancer Problem: A Statistical Study*, 2nd edn (London, 1912), 61.
Wellcome Collection.

aetiological framework, but used by someone else to suggest an alternative or competing schema.

Green then moved from a local scale to a global one. He referenced the cancer surgeon W. Roger Williams's 1908 book on *The Natural History of Cancer*, which dedicated a chapter to the international geographical distribution of the disease.[128] William concluded that cancer seems to increase 'in frequency with remoteness from the Equator'.[129] To Green, the explanation for this phenomenon was obvious: 'The further from the Equator the greater necessity for artificial heat, with the concomitant productions of combustion ... [and] In tropical countries where there are no chimneys the disease is almost unknown.'[130] Green was a convert to the idea that cancer was produced by a parasite—'after reading an enormous mass of literature on the subject, I am convinced that there is every indication that cancer may be of parasitic origin'[131]—but believed the soot played a crucial role in making bodily cells susceptible to infection. Green's cancer-causing disease agent was a 'minute fungi' that grew best in any 'medium *not too fully oxidised*'.[132] Chimney smoke supposedly restricted oxygen to the cells, which rendered them 'liable to the attacks of the minute fungi'.[133] Green's explanation of the cancer-causing properties of soot synthesized environmental and germ theories of disease.

Many others also suggested that an infectious disease agent was responsible for cancer houses, lying latent in the drapes and furnishings of domestic dwellings. For example, an article published in the *BMJ* in 1906 drew comparison between 'infected cages' as the 'source of spontaneous cancer developing among small caged animals' and 'cancer houses'.[134] Similarly, one commentator wrote in 1909, 'Just as among human beings there are cancer districts, streets, and houses, so among mice there are strains and cages in which the same phenomenon occurs.'[135] Cancer houses were places where environmental and germ theories of cancer coalesced. In 1909, Dr Robert J. Simons reported on a noteworthy case: 'A short time ago a man came into my consulting room one evening. He had tuberculous glands in his neck, and in trying to elicit a family history he gave me the following remarkable and interesting account.' The man's family lived on a farm in Glamorganshire, in an old house that had at one time been rather large. At some later date the house had been divided into two smaller houses by a partition wall, and a family of farmers occupied each section. Within these two houses (or rather, one house) there had been five fatal cases of cancer in a period of twenty-one years.[136] Simons claimed:

> It seems there is something more than coincidence here, and that probably there are predisposing, if not determining, factors to be found in the house and its surroundings. The house is built on the side of a stream that courses down the

---

[128] W. Roger Williams, *The Natural History of Cancer: With Special Reference to its Causation and Prevention* (London, 1908).

[129] Ibid., 22.   [130] Green, *The Cancer Problem*, 61.   [131] Ibid., 20.   [132] Ibid., 72.

[133] Ibid.

[134] H. G. Gaylord, 'Evidences that Infected Cages are the Source of Spontaneous Cancer Developing among Small Caged Animals', *BMJ*, 2 (1906), 1555–8, at 1555.

[135] Etienne Burnet, *The Campaign against Microbes*, trans. E. E. Austen (London, 1909), 10.

[136] Robert J. Simons, 'A Cancer House', *BMJ*, 1 (1909), 275–6, at 275.

valley. The stream, which is often swollen with floods, is not sluggish, but the subsoil is always saturated with moisture. The valley is thickly wooded, and many trees are affected with arboreal tumours, one tree, an ash, close to the house, being much disfigured by these bosses.[137]

He suggested a 'connexion between the prevalence of cancer and the prevalence of arboreal tumours'.[138] The cancer-causing agent living within these tree tumours was passed on to the inhabitants of the house via a vector. This theory was likely informed by recent developments in the aetiology of malaria.

Debates over cancer houses at the very end of the nineteenth century suggest that while geographical conceptualizations of malignancy and the plotting of its incidence persisted into the fin de siècle and beyond, mapping was a highly adaptable medium and increasingly presented a range of different aetiological models of disease. As discussed further in Chapter 6, germ theories of disease proliferated in this period and the idea that cancer might be communicated by a microbe became more and more attractive to some medical and scientific practitioners. Reflecting on the shifting scientific landscape in the second edition of *The Geographical Distribution of Diseases* (1892), Haviland wrote:

> Since 1868 . . . the powerful aid of the microscope has been invoked, and in some specific, forms of diseases has detected *flagrante delicto* some of these long hidden *vera causae* at their deadly work . . . True, the hidden cause of cancer still baffles the most expert microscopist; so did the cause of Tuberculosis and many other pathogen in times gone by.[139]

For Haviland, germ theory was entirely consistent with mapping and could be integrated with environmentalist understandings of disease.

In 1914, *The Spectator* stated: 'The attempt to solve the mysteries of cancer is made along two main lines; there are the researches of the pathologists and bacteriologists; and there is the tabulation of statistics which show the incidence of the disease.'[140] While these were framed as two separate methodologies, they could—and often did—produce equivalent theories. Maps could reveal an environmental cause of cancer, just as they could be used to demonstrate a germ theory of the disease.[141] The persistence of medical geography was entirely consistent with contemporary germ theories that frequently suggested that the environment

---

[137] Ibid., 275–6.   [138] Ibid., 276.

[139] Haviland, *The Geographical Distribution of Diseases in Great Britain*, 2nd edn, viii.

[140] 'Logic and Disease', *The Spectator*, 11 April 1914, 600.

[141] Some historians have argued that the environmentalist credo of the public health movements declined in influence as the nineteenth century progressed and eugenic theories and bacteriology emerged. Mitman and Numbers, 'From Miasma to Asthma', 391; Simon Szreter, 'Introduction: The GRO and the Historians', *Social History of Medicine*, 4 (1991), 404–14.

might predispose the body and make it susceptible to infection.[142] Moreover, evolutionary understandings of micro-organisms were concerned with the effects of climate on the living germs.[143] In other words, as the century moved on, cancer map-making was less and less tied to a particular understanding of disease causation and more associated with a particular methodology. Place remained their critical analytic, but multiple theories of disease causation and transmission could coexist within that arena.

Conclusion

The mapping of cancer reveals the extent to which the disease was integrated into the medical landscape of the nineteenth century. Between c.1860 and 1914, and correlating with a new preoccupation with statistics and epidemiology, cancer was constructed as a disease of place. In the process, it transitioned from a disease of individual tragedy to a public health problem. Tables and maps allowed practitioners to 'see' cancer in new ways. Much like its movement through the corporeal body, cancer's presence in the *body politic* was diffuse. The disease travelled along tributaries (along lymphatic channels or systems of rivers and streams), and infected distant parts. In this period, therefore, cancer came to be reconceptualized as a malady that affected the entire population—people in aggregate—rather than primarily a disease of the individual clinical interaction. This was only possible after cancer had been—quite literally—placed on the national map and integrated with the collection of population statistics. In other words, mapping made cancer comprehensible within the framework of a nationally oriented public health.

Moreover, while I may have argued for an integration of cancer into the history of Victorian public health, I contend that this integration will not be easy or simplistic. Haviland's chosen scales and foci reveal something not just about cancer itself, but about the larger context of mapping and modern life. Unlike sanitary mappers, he was not preoccupied by the threat of urban 'civilization' and industrial overcrowding. Instead, cancer maps overwhelmingly represented rural places: unlike 'other' epidemic diseases, cancer featured on maps of the whole country, rather than just cities or towns. Cancer was seen not only to affect (rural) parts of the population largely otherwise neglected by public health practitioners and historians alike, but it was understood as a disease of relevance to the entire nation state. This fact perhaps allows us to move beyond interpreting map-making solely through the lens of power and the social control of problematic populations. If the cartography of cholera, for example, has been interpreted by historians as a way of rationalizing irrational urban environments and their occupants, what does

---

[142] Worboys, *Spreading Germs*, 23.
[143] Mitman and Numbers, 'From Miasma to Asthma', 399.

the mapping of cancer on a rural and national scale reveal about the particularities of malignancy and the generalities of public health in the nineteenth century? In some ways, the curious case of Haviland aligns with what we already know about the rationales for public health in the nineteenth century. He can be read as committed to sanitary reform and statistical methodologies, and as working to make visible an obscure and threatening disease. However, his choice of place cuts across our expectations and his motivations are left unclear. Haviland was not interested in controlling or organizing the landscape, but instead concerned by the management of the relationship between people and space. Haviland thought of his map-making as usefully preventative, suggesting a way for humankind to organize, through mapping, their relationship with nature into something healthy. The disease-causing properties of certain spaces might not be alterable—mountains, rivers, and streams cannot be moved—but they could at least be avoided.

In this chapter, I have looked at the text and images made by men who searched for malignancy's origin in the landscape—those who 'paid attention to the subject of cancer from the point of view of . . . locality'. However, mapping was only one of the many tools deployed in the decoding of the 'cancer problem' in the latter half of the nineteenth century. Running parallel to the activities of Alfred Haviland, Charles H. Moore, and Charles E. Green, bacteriologists, parasitologists, pathologists, and histologists took up new tools and turned their attention to world invisible to the naked eye. Chapter 6, 'Cancer under the Microscope', interrogates the world and work of these practitioners and examines their relationship with cancer in both the laboratory and the clinic.

6

Cancer under the Microscope

In Chapter 5, I looked at the text and images made by men who searched for malignancy's origin in the landscape. Those who 'paid attention to the subject of cancer from the point of view of . . . locality'.[1] However, mapping was only one of the many tools deployed in the decoding of the 'cancer problem'.[2] Running parallel to the activities of Alfred Haviland, Charles H. Moore, and Charles E. Green, bacteriologists, parasitologists, pathologists, and histologists took up the microscope and turned their attention to a world invisible to the naked eye. Like their map-making peers, these new professionals were frustrated by medicine's therapeutic limits, concerned by the disease's persistent incurability, and anxious over cancer's increasing incidence. Like mapping, the microscope was one of a range of medical 'interventions' that proliferated after c.1860 and aimed to make sense of the nature, emergence, potential spread, and prevention of cancer.[3]

This new intervention took place in a new setting and was part of a new project or 'way of knowing'.[4] If 'hospital medicine' was 'one aspect of a project of medical "analysis"', then 'laboratory medicine'—often the home of the microscope— broadly correlated to experimentalism and was increasingly common in the second half of the nineteenth century.[5] From the 1830s onwards, new microscopic instruments became available—free from the optical defects of spherical and chromatic aberrations that had afflicted earlier models. Thus, in the first half of the nineteenth century, investigators took advantage of these achromatic lenses to launch numerous and sustained enquiries into the minute structure of the living body and its surroundings.[6] The microscope became a symbol of medical and scientific progress and its use promised theoretical and therapeutic transformation.

---

[1] 'The Causation of Cancer', BMJ, 1 (1901), 1281–2, at 1281.

[2] The phrase 'the cancer problem' was used frequently in turn-of-the-century medical journal articles on the topic. John T. MacLachlan and E. Wardman-Wilbourne, 'The Cancer Problem', BMJ, 1 (1911), 282.

[3] Since writing this book, Alan I. Marcus has published a monograph on these late nineteenth-century laboratory efforts to understand cancer: Alan I. Marcus, Malignant Growth: Creating the Modern Cancer Research Establishment 1875–1915, (Tuscaloosa AL, 2018).

[4] See John V. Pickstone, Ways of Knowing: A New History of Science, Technology and Medicine (Chicago, 2001).

[5] John V. Pickstone, 'Commentary: From History of Medicine to a General History of "Working Knowledges"', International Journal of Epidemiology, 38 (2009), 646–9, at 647.

[6] This period also saw the development of what Lorraine Daston and Peter Galison call 'mechanical objectivity'—one form of veracity and scientific morality dependent on the use of instruments and machines. Lorraine Daston and Peter Galison, Objectivity (New York, 2007).

The Cancer Problem: Malignancy in Nineteenth-Century Britain. Agnes Arnold-Forster, Oxford University Press (2021).
© Agnes Arnold-Forster. DOI: 10.1093/oso/9780198866145.003.0007

Commentaries on the instrument were replete with sensory metaphors, locating value in the ability of tools and instruments to represent and reveal the body. A late nineteenth-century doctor wrote that medical art 'necessarily develops in the wake of the allied sciences, being dependent upon them for its eyes, its hands and its ears'.[7] For this reason, the author concluded, 'perhaps the most potent factor in the advancement of medicine has been the microscope'.[8] The instrument 'pierced the darkness' and revealed 'long-looked-for-secrets' to 'thousands of eager eyes'.[9] Cells were virgin domain and microscope users were heroic explorers, bringing to light hitherto-undiscovered textures of the body.

However, not everyone was so enthusiastic about the microscope's potential scientific or therapeutic benefits. Despite the instrument's appeal, early micro-scope users confronted considerable scepticism, if not outright hostility, from their colleagues. Critiques circulated around the questionable clarity, veracity, and objectivity of the tool. Eminent anatomists, like Xavier Bichat, made no secret of their disdain for the instrument. A common complaint was that observers were too easily influenced by their assumptions about what they were looking for and what they felt they ought to see.[10] Bichat's anxiety manifested bacteriologist and philosopher Ludwick Fleck's idea that experience and training were required to make sense of the visual chaos that constitutes the microscopic world: 'Direct perception of form requires being experienced in the relevant field of thought. The ability directly to perceive meaning, form, and self-contained unity is acquired only after much experience, perhaps with preliminary training.'[11] Both Bichat and Fleck acknowledged that the microscope did not provide an unmediated 'lens' onto the natural world. Microscopists' doubts did not, however, prevent practi-tioners from turning the instrument to the 'cancer problem'. This chapter thus interrogates the effect of three newly developed theories and practices—cell theory, bacteriology, and parasitology, all intimately associated with the microscope—on late-century ideas about cancer's causes and characteristics.

By the fin de siècle, a network and infrastructure of cancer laboratories and investigation had developed across Europe, North America, and British colonies. The microscope had transformed the ways that cancer was investigated and ushered in a new 'way of knowing' the disease—and, in doing so, the intractable disease exerted its own influence on the shaping of the modern scientific and bureaucratic state. However, this is no straightforward case of medical and scientific 'modernization'. First, the technology's impact on clinical practice was

---

[7] Cyrus Edson, 'The Art of Healing: Marvellous Progress Made in the Science of Medicine', *Los Angeles Times*, 28 January 1900, 4.
[8] Ibid.   [9] Ibid.
[10] L. S. Jacyna, '"A Host of Experienced Microscopists": The Establishment of Histology in Nineteenth-Century Edinburgh', *Bulletin of the History of Medicine*, 75 (2001), 225–53, esp. 229. Ludwick Fleck, *Genesis and Development of a Scientific Fact*, trans. Fred Bradley and Thaddeus J. Trenn (Chicago, 1979), 92.
[11] Fleck, *Genesis and Development of a Scientific Fact*, 92.

limited and the new experimental project did little to alter the incurability of cancer. This observation has been made about Victorian science and medicine more generally. For example, Christopher Lawrence suggests that while British physicians in the second half of the nineteenth century employed a vocabulary 'which routinely invoked science as the foundation of medicine', in fact they 'prescribed for science only a limited role in clinical practice'.[12]

Second, and perhaps most importantly, these new technologies recapitulated ancient ideas about cancer. All three theories—cell theory, bacteriology, and parasitology—were taken up and applied to the disease with enthusiasm, each provided substantial explanatory power and promised therapeutic applications. And yet, despite their close relationship with the microscope and its scientific and progressive associations, all three appealed in part because they depended upon and reconfirmed very old ideas about cancer's causes and characteristics. Thus, while all three shifted the terms and contexts of experimentation and debate, none of them transformed deeply felt beliefs about cancer or impacted clinical management of the disease. By the end of the nineteenth century, cancer was embedded within the new technologies and infrastructure of scientific investigation and being spoken about using language that heralded the 'modern' and promising capacities of fin de siècle biomedicine. And yet these new technologies, institutions, and rhetorical efforts did little to alter the conceptualization of cancer or transform the way it was experienced and treated. This chapter will begin by exploring cell theory, its application to cancer in the mid-nineteenth century, and its contested role in the clinic, before moving on to interrogate bacteriological and then parasitological theories of cancer's causation.

Cell Theory

In 1858, Friedrich Engels wrote to Karl Marx: 'The main thing which has revolutionised the whole of physiology and for the first time made comparative physiology possible is the discovery of the cell—in plants by Schleiden and in animals by Schwann. Everything is a cell.'[13] Accurate in some ways and inaccurate in others (neither Matthias Jakob Schleiden nor Theodor Schwann made any claims to initial 'discovery'), Engels captured the contemporary prevalence and power of 'cell theory'. The idea that there was some structural and functional

---

[12] Christopher Lawrence, '"Incommunicable Knowledge": Science, Technology and the Clinical Art in Britain 1850-1914', *Journal of Contemporary History*, 20 (1985), 503-20, at 504. In contrast, Rosemary Wall suggests that the laboratory and pathologists 'were quickly and routinely used' at elite London and Cambridge hospitals: Rosemary Wall, 'Using Bacteriology in Elite Hospital Practice: London and Cambridge, 1880-1920', *Social History of Medicine*, 24 (2011), 776-95, at 776.

[13] Quoted in L. J. Rather, Patricia Rather, and John B. Frerichs, *Johannes Müller and the Nineteenth-Century Origins of the Tumor Cell Theory* (Baltimore, MD, 1986), 1.

unit—common to all plant and animal organisms—was, according to L. J. Rather, Patricia Rather, and John B. Frerichs, 'part and parcel of the whole history of Western biology'.[14] In the nineteenth century, this unit came to be known as the 'cell' and, as Erwin Ackerknecht argued, cell theory was applied 'with unequalled success' to oncology.[15] Indeed, Lawrence Koblenz suggests 'The structural and functional idea of the cell was the theoretical foundation for the development of modern cancer.'[16] However, as Carsten Timmermann argues, the introduction and reception of cell theory was far less transformative than many contemporaries and historians have suggested.[17]

Cell theory states that all living things are composed of one or more cells, that the cell is the basic unit of life, and that new cells arise from existing cells. Cell theory was developed in Germany in the 1830s by botanists and physiologists including Schleiden, Schwann, Jakob Henle, and Johannes Müller, who used the new, much improved compound microscope with an achromatic lens to launch numerous and sustained enquiries into the unseen structures of living bodies. Müller's pupils, Robert Remak and Rudolf Virchow, refined the Schwann–Schleiden theories into 'a complete set of physiological and pathological concepts and practices'.[18] German texts were rapidly translated into English and cell theory was readily accepted in British medical circles.[19] It offered one cohesive frame through which to interpret all animal and plant processes—both the healthy and the pathological. Thus, Engels was not alone in heralding 'cell theory' as transformative. While not universally accepted, it preoccupied various scientific and medical professionals in Germany, France, Britain, and the United States for much of the late nineteenth century. It created a new biological vocabulary, provoked a proliferation of scientific investigations, and produced new disciplines such as histology and microbiology.

Tumour cell theory, an offspring of normal cell theory, made its debut in a series of papers delivered by Müller in Berlin in 1836, in which he indicated the apparent 'cellular-like' nature of several cancerous growths.[20] In his 1838 monograph, *On the Nature and Structural Characteristics of Cancer and of those Morbid Growths which May Be Confounded With It*, translated into English by Charles West in 1840, Müller observed the same developmental processes in cancerous

---

[14] Rather, Rather, and Frerichs, *Johannes Müller*, 2.

[15] Erwin H. Ackerknecht, 'Historical Notes on Cancer', *Medical History*, 2 (1958), 114–19, at 118.

[16] Lawrence Koblenz, 'From Sin to Science: The Cancer Revolution of the Nineteenth Century' (Columbia University, PhD Thesis, 2013), 361.

[17] Carsten Timmermann, *A History of Lung Cancer: The Recalcitrant Disease* (Basingstoke, 2014), 22–6.

[18] Ibid., 23.

[19] On the reception of Virchow in Britain, see L. S. Jacyna, 'The Romantic Programme and the Reception of Cell Theory in Britain', *Journal of the History of Biology*, 17 (1984), 13–48.

[20] Timothy Lenoir, *The Strategy of Life: Teleology and Mechanics in Nineteenth-Century German Biology* (Chicago, 1989), 143. See also Laura Otis, *Müller's Lab* (Oxford, 2007).

cells that Schwann had witnessed in healthy ones.[21] Müller's monograph set out an intrinsic model of cancer causation: 'The positive characters of carcinoma do not display any thing [sic] heterologous or foreign to healthy organization.'[22] The diseased cells were not alien organic structures or a 'germ' entering the body from without. Instead, they seemed to emerge from the body itself—healthy cells (or cell fragments) transforming into pathological ones. Fundamental units of life turning into fundamental units of death.

Among those who accepted and advocated for tumour cell theory and the intrinsic origin of malignancy there was extensive debate over the precise nature of cancer's cellular causes and characteristics. Müller argued that cells could develop in two ways. They could develop from tiny free nuclei, either within the 'mother' cell (the cell wall of the mother cell dissolving or bursting and thus allowing the 'daughter' cells to exist independently) or *outside* of another, completely developed cell. Or, Müller argued, the nuclei of new cells could form freely in extracellular fluid: 'the germinal cells of carcinoma are formed not from any previously existing fibres, but from a real *seminium morbi*, which develops itself between the tissues of the affected organ'.[23] In contrast, Müller's pupil, Virchow, suggested that the cancerous cell growth constituted a deterioration of healthy tissue or a degeneration of healthy cells. In his book, *Die Cellularpathologie*, published in 1858 and translated into English in 1860, Virchow argued that a pathological process (cancer) had its origins in a healthy one: 'All the cellular types of morbid products must be found in the healthy organism which gives rise to these products. The progeny are always, by nature, directly related to the ancestry that gave them birth.'[24] This idea had almost immediate purchase among the British medical collective. George Southam wrote in 1858: 'There appears, then, no reason to regard the cells found in cancerous growths other than as the ordinary ones formed for the development of healthy tissue.'[25] Similarly, in 1864, Irish surgeon Maurice Henry Collis argued that cancer cells were modified healthy lymph cells.[26]

From the mid-century onwards, case histories of cancer increasingly referred to the use of the microscope. In his 1858 tract on *The Diagnosis of Surgical Cancer*, English ophthalmologist John Zachariah Laurence included descriptions of the 'minute anatomy' of all the published cases.[27] In 1865, Surgeon to the

---

[21] Johannes Müller, *On the Nature and Structural Characteristics of Cancer, and of those Morbid Growths which May Be Confounded With It*, trans. Charles West (London, 1840).
[22] Ibid., 32.   [23] Ibid., 22.
[24] Quoted in E. S. Dunster, 'The Idea of Life, as Deduced from Contemporary Physiology: Virchow-Claude Bernard', *Anthropological Review*, 8 (1870), 49–69, at 59.
[25] George Southam, 'The Nature and Treatment of Cancer: Being the Address in Surgery', *BMJ*, 1 (1858), 4–7, at 6.
[26] Maurice Henry Collis, *On the Diagnosis and Treatment of Cancer and the Tumours Analogous to It* (London, 1864), 3.
[27] For example, the case of six-year-old Susannah Foster, treated for cancer of the eye at University College Hospital in 1853. John Zachariah Laurence, *The Diagnosis of Surgical Cancer*, vol. 2 (London, 1858), 26.

Cancer Hospital (later the Royal Marsden) Thomas Weeden Cooke, stated authoritatively, 'The conflicting theories as to the nature of cancer seem now to be set at rest by the revelations of the microscope, showing that it is... an alteration only in the natural cell-growth.'[28] In his 'Address in Surgery', published in the *British Medical Journal* (*BMJ*) in 1869, Thomas Nunneley argued that the present use of the microscope in the clinical management of cancer was 'almost perfect' and that 'its employment, not only for histological investigations, but in the daily diagnosis of disease and its treatment, has become almost as essential to the scientific practitioner as is the telescope to the astronomer'.[29] Reflecting on recent medical history, in 1864 Collis wrote:

> The combination of microscopic investigation with clinical study has cleared up much that was obscure and unintelligible, and has rendered safe and scientific much that before was empirical in practice. Not only have the means of diagnosis been improved, and treatment rendered more sure, but the results, in a given case, can be predicted with a certainty that we could not have ventured to use a few years ago.[30]

These quotations suggest that in the second half of the nineteenth century the microscope was increasingly used as an aid to diagnosis in cases of cancer.

Histologists viewed magnified tumour tissue to ascertain whether the growth was malignant or benign.[31] Thus, cancer-specific institutions had a new use for 'in-house' laboratories. For example, in the 1890s, the staff of The Middlesex Hospital's cancer ward wrote up a 'Scheme for the Investigation of Cancer' and instituted a Cancer Investigation Committee. They repurposed three rooms for the use of researchers, and set aside the largest room for a 'General Microscopic Laboratory'. They mandated a systematic 'histological examination to be made in every case of Carcinoma or Sarcoma admitted into the Medical, Surgical, or Special Cancer Wards of the Hospital, or dying in the Special of General Wards'.[32] In 1900, the minutes reflected that, for the past year, 'In each case [of cancer] the primary lesion and every secondary formation of new growth [had] been submitted to microscopic examination.'[33]

---

[28] Thomas Weeden Cooke, *On Cancer: Its Allies and Counterfeits* (London, 1865), vii.

[29] Thomas Nunneley, 'Address in Surgery', *BMJ*, 2 (1869), 143–56, at 144.

[30] Collis, *On the Diagnosis and Treatment of Cancer*, 2.

[31] As Ornella Moscucci has pointed out, this was partly because patients began to insist on further proof in the identification of malignancies before they submitted to radical operations, and partly because advocates for such surgeries were more and more anxious to demonstrate that cases 'cured' by operation were indeed cancers. Ornella Moscucci, *Gender and Cancer in England, 1860–1948* (London, 2017), 55.

[32] UCLH Archive, London, 'Scheme for the Investigation of Cancer Finally Amended', Middlesex Hospital Minutes, 15 November 1899.

[33] Ibid.

However, while cell theory provided a seductive explanatory mechanism—and the microscope appeared with increasing frequency in clinical spaces and sources—its influence on therapeutic and diagnostic practice was more ambivalent. Just as some medical men were enthusiastic about the microscope's clinical potential, many other practitioners expressed doubts over the value of the instrument in the clinical identification of cancer and particularly over its ability to act alone. Today, oncology and the microscope are inseparable. Cancer diagnosis, treatment, prognosis, and research are dependent on an instrument that has—not coincidentally—become an icon of modern medicine. The interpretation of the microscopic image of a surgically obtained specimen or 'biopsy'—a term derived from the phrase 'an autopsy of the living'—extracted from a suspicious lesion or neoplasm is the standard and culturally resonant method of cancer diagnosis today. The term 'biopsy' reveals a telling association between the ability of the microscope to lay bare the workings of disease during life and the capacity of post-mortem dissection to reveal pathologies in the dead.[34]

In contrast, the nineteenth-century relationship between malignancy and the microscope was more complex. Not everyone was convinced by the latter's potential scientific or therapeutic benefits, and despite the instrument's appeal, early microscope users confronted considerable scepticism from their colleagues. Even Müller, an early champion of the microscope, was circumspect about its actual utility. His aim in classifying tumours was an eminently practical one. He wanted the physician to be able to distinguish, for purposes of treatment and prognosis, 'benign' tumours from 'malignant' tumours. The diagnostic procedure would have to be one applicable at the bedside or operating table. However, he warned that 'the compound microscope might lead us into partiality and error'.[35] Moreover, he also believed that once the various forms of tumours had been categorized according to their salient microscopic features it would be possible to correlate these features with those ascertainable by the unaided hand and eye. He never intended for the microscope to replace the surgical sensorium.

John Hughes Bennett, another keen advocate for the tool in scientific investigation, was also ambivalent over its therapeutic utility: 'The microscope *alone*— that is, independently of all other kind of observation—can seldom determine in the living subject the presence or absence of Cancer.'[36] Similarly, Alexander Henry called for the 'combination of microscopic investigation with clinical study', and regarded 'the value of the microscope as more scientific than practical'.[37] The microscopic observation was then confirmed by the cancer's clinical trajectory. In 1856, John Zachariah Laurence recorded how a woman had her breast amputated

---

[34] Koblenz, 'From Sin to Science', 327.
[35] Collis, *On the Diagnosis and Treatment of Cancer*, 12.
[36] John Hughes Bennett, *On Cancerous and Cancroid Growths* (Edinburgh, 1849), vii.
[37] Alexander Henry, 'On the Ancient and Modern Doctrines of Cancer', *Association Medical Journal*, 3 (1855), 413–16, at 415.

'for an ordinary scirrhus', and that 'some highly characteristic cancer-cells were observed in the growth' under the microscope.[38] Sure enough, the cancer recurred almost immediately after the operation, demonstrating its own malignancy. However, in this case, the tumour was only analysed *after* it had already been removed—to confirm a diagnosis made through conventional means. This idea continued into the late nineteenth century, even as microscopic accuracy improved. Henry Arnott wrote in 1872: 'The common impression is that these investigations into the minute structure and habits of tumours are more interesting than useful, and that they are not calculated to throw much light upon the question of treatment.'[39] The obstetric physician G. Ernest Herman wrote in 1894: 'I think the value of the microscope in the clinical diagnosis of cancer has been overestimated. The only use of the microscope is to confirm suspicion aroused by the evidence of the unaided senses of sight and touch.'[40]

Indeed, towards the end of the century, detailed individual case histories that described the macro appearance of tumours—the size, shape, smell, colour—continued to feature in journal articles and surgical tracts, while microscopic observations were covered briefly, if at all.[41] Collis, while keen on the diagnostic abilities of the microscope, spoke approvingly of 'texture, feel, colour, and consistence' as guides to cancer classification and identification.[42] He continued to use these unassisted visual and haptic methods of diagnosis, often in place of the microscope. His case notes from the 1860s had much in common with those described in Chapter 1, as they were replete with textural descriptions and comparisons with found objects and organic matter:

> The characteristics of encephaloid are a soft elasticity, often simulating fluctuation, though more frequently resembling the elasticity of a vulcanized india-rubber [sic] ball filled with air; a tendency to irregularity, rounded outline, the lines or curves being abrupt, uneven in length, and mutually intersecting; the entire tumour resembling in shape a potato, Jerusalem artichoke, or truffle.[43]

Thirty years later, Bennett May, Surgeon to the Queen's Hospital in Birmingham, argued that unaided vision was equal to the microscope: 'Can we rely upon the naked-eye appearance of the cut surface? I think so. The fresh cut section of cancer is unmistakable, quite different from the leathery toughness of chronic

[38] John Zachariah Laurence, 'Illustrations of the Pathology of Cancer', *Association Medical Journal*, 4 (1856), 886–7, at 887.

[39] Henry Arnott, *Cancer: Its Varieties, their Histology and Diagnosis* (London, 1872), 76.

[40] G. Ernest Herman, 'An Address on the Early Diagnosis of Cancer of the Cervix Uteri', *BMJ*, 1 (1894), 1009–12, at 1011.

[41] Timmermann, *A History of Lung Cancer*, 24.

[42] Collis, *On the Diagnosis and Treatment of Cancer*, 18.   [43] Ibid., 31.

mammitis.'[44] Thus, while cell theory provided an attractive theoretical framework, contemporaries were unsure about what it could add to the clinical understanding, management, diagnosis, and prevention of cancer.[45]

If, as I suggested at the beginning of this chapter, the microscope appealed in part because it offered a new way of seeing, comprehending, and potentially controlling cancer, why were investigators enthusiastic about the tool in theory but ambivalent in practice? If curing cancer was the goal, why was cell theory and its limited therapeutic utility so popular? The ready acceptance and application of Virchow's theories by British practitioners can be partly explained by pre-existing notions of cancer's causes and characteristics. There was much discussion over what caused a healthy cell to transform into a cancerous one. Many of the proposed 'exciting' causes recapitulated much older cancer concepts, and mid-century enthusiasm for tumour cell theory was dependent on the ability of these new explanatory mechanisms to compliment rather than complicate deeply felt anxieties and ideas. Collis suggested that if the 'normal cells of the tissues of the human body' were 'injured in its birth (so to speak)', either by 'external violence' or irritation or by a 'deficient supply of sound material', they would either 'perish prematurely' or 'develop into some abnormal form'.[46] This reframed an older explanatory mechanism for the causation of cancer in cellular terms. As argued in Chapter 1, throughout the nineteenth century and before, both doctor and patient frequently attributed the origins of malignancy to a moment of physical trauma or a period of physical irritation. Pathologists continued to identify the cause of cancer as 'irritation' on both a macro and microscopic scale. Physician R. H. Meade wrote in 1866: 'The local affection may have been excited by a blow, or some other external cause of irritation.'[47]

Müller, on the other hand, attributed the origin of the cancer cells to a localized 'disposition' of the extra-cellular fluid, the source of which was the 'breakdown of the command of the integrated, whole organism over its parts'.[48] The body's loss of control over its constitutive units not only provoked the initial development of cancer but allowed the tumour to grow uncontrollably: 'the regulated life of the part no longer attains a particular limit'.[49] This equating of cancer with chaotic growth on the one hand, and associating health with ordered cellular development on the other, persisted throughout the second half of the nineteenth century. In his 1874 Goulstonian Lectures, J. F. Payne mirrored Müller's language when he wrote: 'the tumour . . . has no very definite limit, and shows no conformity to rule

---

[44] Bennett May, 'The Ingleby Lectures on the Operative Treatment of Cancer of the Breast', BMJ, 1 (1897), 1335–8, at 1338.

[45] As Jacyna has argued, by about 1900, histological diagnostic techniques served chiefly as an accessory rather than an alternative to the surgeon's own clinical judgement. L. S. Jacyna, 'The Laboratory and the Clinic: The Impact of Pathology on Surgical Diagnosis in the Glasgow Western Infirmary, 1875–1910', Bulletin of the History of Medicine, 62 (1988), 384–406.

[46] Ibid., 8.   [47] R. H. Meade, 'A Few Remarks on Cancer', BMJ, 2 (1866), 94–5, at 95.

[48] Lenoir, The Strategy of Life, 144.   [49] Ibid.

in its shape'.[50] He described how, unlike 'natural' bodily processes, cancer was not governed by discernible laws.

In 1899, Woods Hutchinson, pathologist, clinician, and writer, made Müller and J. F. Payne's dichotomy between health and cancerous chaos explicit. He described the body as the 'cell-state' within which 'we find each organ, every part, strictly subordinated, both in form and function, to the interests of the whole'.[51] He echoed Müller's idea of an 'integrated' bodily whole with command over 'every part'. However, with cases of cancer, 'this relation [or, chain of command] is utterly disregarded'.[52] He compared cancer to political disarray: 'In the body-republic, where we have come to regard harmony and loyalty as the almost invariable rule, we suddenly find ourselves confronted by anarchy and revolt... After forty-fifty, or even sixty years of loyal service, the cells lining one of the tubules of a gland—for instance, of the lip, or tongue, or stomach—begin to grow and increase in number.'[53] However, according to cell theory, this chaos was of the body's own making. Cancer had its origins within the body and it was impossible to predict when the cells might rebel—turning from healthy citizens to revolutionary dissenters. It suggested a fundamental and inherent flaw in human biology, and provoked as much anxiety as calm and clarity. As Hutchinson wrote: 'A man's worst foes are "they of his own household".'[54] The idea that cancer was defined by disorder was an age-old conceptualization and this language found easy application to political commentary.[55] Parliamentarians frequently made use of cancer as a metaphor for social breakdown or revolution. In 1821, an MP argued that poor rates were a 'cancer' and 'it was not for parliament to encourage the growth of an evil so monstrous'.[56] The state, like the body, was vulnerable to rebellion or dissent from within, which could bring either to a destructive apotheosis. Indeed, Johnstone and Baines argue that because of cancer's perceived relationship to the body's building blocks—the mechanisms of cell growth and division—it not only attracted attention from scientists, but was constructed as an arena in which researchers could ponder more fundamental questions about the nature of life itself.[57]

---

[50] J. F. Payne, 'The Goulstonian Lectures on the Origin and Relations of New Growths', *BMJ*, 1 (1874), 293–6, at 293.

[51] Woods Hutchinson, 'The Cancer Problem: Or, Treason in the Republic of the Body', *Contemporary Review*, 76 (1899), 105–17, at 106.

[52] Ibid.

[53] Ibid. See also Paul Weindling, 'Theories of the Cell State in Imperial Germany', in Charles Webster (ed.), *Biology, Medicine and Society 1840–1940* (Cambridge, UK, 1981).

[54] Ibid., 105.

[55] For more on fin-de-siècle cancer metaphors see Agnes Arnold-Forster, '"A rebellion of the cells": cancer, modernity, and decline in fin-de-siècle Britain' in Sally Shuttleworth, Melissa Dickson and Emilie Taylor-Brown (eds.), *Progress and Pathology: Medicine and Culture in the Nineteenth Century* (Manchester, UK, 2020), 173–193.

[56] HC Deb., vol. 4, cc795–6, 19 February 1821.

[57] Emm Barnes Johnstone and Joanna Baines, *The Changing Faces of Childhood Cancer: Clinical and Cultural Visions since 1940* (Basingstoke, 2015), 12.

Bacteriology

Developed in the late nineteenth century, and partially dependent on a series of identifications of pathogenic agents after c.1860, 'germ theory' (or germ theories) suggested that some diseases were caused by specific microscopic beings.[58] Initially framed as a 'bacteriological revolution', the transformative effects of germ theories on the conceptualization and control of disease in the fin de siècle have since been qualified by historians. Nonetheless, by the end of the century there was a new focus on, and enthusiasm for, 'germs' in the pages of medical periodicals and the general-interest press. The observation that cancer played a prominent role in germ theory discourse runs counter to existing historical understandings of both cancer and contagious disease in the late nineteenth and early twentieth centuries.[59] The idea that the twentieth century witnessed an 'epidemiological transition' away from infectious diseases and towards constitutional disorders—with cancer as the emblematic 'modern' malady—manufactures a sharp distinction between cancer and contagion in medical historiography.[60] In 2007 Michael Worboys and Flurin Condrau cited a single reference in the former's *Spreading Germs*, which 'makes it clear that the notion had very few supporters and was anyway short-lived'.[61] While some have critiqued the notion that the Victorian era was a 'period of great epidemics', the idea continues to be prevalent in scholarship and prominent in non-academic imaginings of the nineteenth century. Consequently, nineteenth-century debates surrounding the potentially infectious nature of cancer have escaped historical scrutiny by some of the best-known historians of both cancer and infectious disease.[62] In contrast, ideas about cancer's communicability from person to person, and investigative efforts to isolate and identify a cancer 'germ', were widespread and impacted lay and professional anxieties alike.

Indeed, we can infer that there was something unsatisfying about cell theory for Victorian practitioners, if only because so many of them were drawn to germ theories of malignancy as a viable alternative. The latter theory made explanatory

---

[58] Michael Worboys has implored historians to look at the 'many germ theories of disease'; Michael Worboys, *Spreading Germs: Disease Theories and Medical Practice in Britain, 1865–1900* (Cambridge, UK, 2000), 2.

[59] Recent scholarship on nineteenth-century malignancy does sketch the shape of the 'cancer microbe' debate. However, it tends to narrate it as useful context, or as an interesting anecdote, rather than as central to the construction of cancer, both past and present. For the most detailed and reflective accounts, see Moscucci, *Gender and Cancer in England*; and Timmermann, *A History of Lung Cancer*.

[60] A. Omran, 'The Epidemiological Transition: A Theory of the Epidemiology of Population Change', *Milbank Quarterly*, 83:4 (1971), 731–57.

[61] Flurin Condrau and Michael Worboys, 'Second Opinions: Epidemics and Infections in Nineteenth-Century Britain', *Social History of Medicine*, 20:1 (2007), 147–58, at 148.

[62] Cancer: Robert. A. Aronowitz, *Unnatural History: Breast Cancer and American Society* (Cambridge, UK, 2007); and I. Löwy, *Preventive Strike: Women, Precancer, and Prophylactic Surgery* (Baltimore, MD, 2010). Germ theories: Nancy Tomes, *The Gospel of Germs: Men, Women, and the Microbe in American Life* (Cambridge, MA, 1999); and Worboys, *Spreading Germs*.

promises that were equal to, or better than, those made by cell theory. For not only did germ theories of cancer, like cell theories, coalesce with powerfully felt ideas about the disease's nature, they also offered the opportunity of prevention and epidemic control. Eager practitioners drew comparisons between the manifest successes wrought by germ theories of fever, cholera, and tuberculosis and the potential command and control offered by the application of bacteriology to cancer. There was, therefore, much at stake in the debates over the germ theory of cancer that filled the pages of the periodical and medical press in the fin de siècle.

In the early nineteenth century, miasmatic ideas of disease causation—like those expounded by Edwin Chadwick—identified the origin of epidemics in the atmosphere and environment. Practitioners attributed cholera, diarrhoea, and relapsing fever to the same insanitary aggregate: housing, water, decay, drainage, and dirt (see Chapter 5). From c.1860 onwards, the introduction of Koch's postulates brought a new precision to medical thinking about disease causation and transmission.[63] The resultant 'germ theory' suggested that some diseases are caused not by the general surroundings, but by specific microscopic beings (although, and as shown in Chapter 5, the idea of 'cancer houses' managed to synthesize these two models).[64] Germ theories of disease were less concerned with the mode of transmission and were instead preoccupied with specificity—the idea that certain maladies were caused by certain microorganisms. The tubercle bacillus produces tuberculosis and tuberculosis alone, for example. While the development and acceptance of germ theory was neither as linear nor as clear cut as historians once suggested, by the end of the century there was nonetheless a new focus on, and enthusiasm for, microscopic agents of disease among both professionals and the laity. Crucially, this new zeal had a profound effect on the prevailing debates over the causes, control, and characteristics of cancer.

As with cell theory, germ theory prompted laboratory-based investigations into the microscopic landscape of cancer tissue. Researchers sought to identify and isolate the cancer microbe, cultivate it outside the human body, and then introduce the cultured organism into an experimental animal. If 'successful', the introduced organism would cause an identical form of disease or growth, which would spread through the organs of the new body. The proposed extrinsic origin of cancer thus prompted changes in experimental practices that aimed first to settle the contested question of what agent was responsible, and second, to work

---

[63] Koch's postulates are four criteria used to establish a causative relationship between a microbe and a disease. Koch's postulates are: (1) the microorganism must be found in abundance in all organisms suffering from the disease, but should not be found in healthy organisms; (2) the microorganism must be isolated from the diseased organism and grown in pure culture; (3) the cultured organism should cause disease when introduced into a healthy organism; (4) the organism must be re-isolated from the inoculated, diseased experimental host and identified as being identical to the original specific causative agent. Worboys, *Spreading Germs*, 5.

[64] Worboys, *Spreading Germs*, 2.

out how it spread. As with wider contemporaneous discussions of germ theories, the precise nature of the cancer 'germ' was uncertain.

Some scientists flirted with the idea of a cancer bacillus—likely because of the disease's clinical similarity to tuberculosis. In his 'Morton Lecture on Cancer and Cancerous Diseases', Surgeon to the Queen's Household, Spencer Wells, drew an explicit connection between the potential parity of the two diseases' aetiologies: 'Cases of acute cancerosis or military cancer, analogous to acute tuberculosis or military tubercle, have led to the search for a specific microbe or bacillus.'[65] In 1890, surgeon, microscopist, journalist, and photographer Jabez Hogg wrote: 'we have been steadily drifting towards the more generally accepted opinion, that sooner or later the bacilli of cancer would be discovered by that noble army of younger investigators who are now incessantly at work in this direction'.[66] In 1904 Amédée Borrel in France argued for a viral aetiology of cancer; however, this gained little purchase on the British medical imagination. North American researchers were particularly zealous in their search for a cancer virus, and in 1913 Peyton Rouse discovered the chicken sarcoma virus.[67] In 1908, Danish scientists Vilhelm Ellerman and Oluf Bang demonstrated that leukaemia in chickens was caused by viruses. However, as leukaemia was not yet classified as cancer this observation was not incorporated into contemporary debates on the germ theory of malignancy22.[68] British researchers devoted less time to the viral aetiology of cancer, and much of the evidence to support the notion was collated after the First World War.

In contrast, the search for the cancer bacillus preoccupied the professional community in Britain. Between 1870 and 1910 the *BMJ* alone published over 2,000 articles and letters dealing with the transmission of cancer from person to person and its potential origin outside the human body. There was a comparable level of enthusiasm in the periodical press, whose contributors increasingly spoke of cancer in the language of germ theory. In 1896, the *New York Times* referred to the 'germ theory of the cause of cancer' and presented it as 'held by a large number of specialists in both Europe and this country'. They dismissed the cell theory of cancer as the 'old-style' theory.[69] Public discourse of this kind persuaded an anxious public. In 1913, Mr Richard Boardman wrote to the Rockefeller Institute in New York.[70] He narrated how his wife's aunt had died of cancer ten

---

[65] Spencer Wells, 'The Morton Lecture on Cancer and Cancerous Diseases', *BMJ*, 2 (1888), 1201–5, at 1203.

[66] Jabez Hogg, 'A Characteristic Organism of Cancer', *BMJ*, 2 (1890), 1505–6, at 1506.

[67] Eva Becsei-Kilborn, 'Scientific Discovery and Scientific Reputation: The Reception of Peyton Rous' Discovery of the Chicken Sarcoma Virus', *Journal of the History of Biology*, 43 (2010), 111–57. See also Robin Wolfe Scheffler, *A Contagious Cause: The American Hunt for Cancer Viruses and the Rise of Molecular Medicine* (Chicago, 2019).

[68] Johnstone and Baines, *The Changing Faces of Childhood Cancer*, 30–48.

[69] 'Living Things in Cancers', *New York Times*, 20 September 1896, 9.

[70] Rockefeller Archive, Tarrytown, New York, 'Letter from Mr. Richard Boardman to Dr Simon Flexner', 29 October 1913. 210.3 (4) Business Manager/Subject Files/Cancer 1913–1952.

years earlier. During her last illness, she had slept on two or three different mattresses. One had become stained by the 'drain' from the cancer and had been immediately destroyed. However, two other mattresses remained, upon which she slept during her final days. Both were now in the possession of Mr Boardman's wife. He wrote, 'Mrs. Boardman—like so many other young women . . . has become very much possessed with the fear of germs of every sort.' The mattresses were now a source of great anxiety for his wife—fears that her medical friends refused to allay. Mr Boardman wrote to the Rockefeller Institute to ask 'Whether Mrs. Boardman's fears, of the danger of communication of the disease of cancer from these mattresses, after the space of ten years, has any foundation in fact, under any modern theory on the nature of the disease of cancer?'[71]

Bacteriology not only influenced lay anxieties, but altered the language practitioners used to discuss malignancy, even in the absence of explicit commitment to the germ theory of cancer. Germs were frequently articulated as autonomous individuals. The bacteriologist Jakob Henle said, 'With the epidemic, the causes of the disease *seek out* the individual.'[72] Similarly, metaphors of conquest and colonization permeated medical literature in the late nineteenth century. A French writer in 1885 characterized infection as 'Coming from outside, penetrating the organism like a horde of Sudanese, ravaging it for the right of invasion and conquest.'[73] The close relationship between cancer and bacteriology meant that terms like 'invasion', 'infection', 'diffusion', 'germ', and 'seed'—pre-existing parts of germ theory discourse—infiltrated cancer's vocabulary. As a result, and despite his intellectual commitment to cell theory, the Surgeon to the Cancer Investigation Committee of The Middlesex Hospital in London, J. Bland-Sutton, wrote: 'When the breast is attacked by cancer the cells implicate the lymphatics in the underlying fascia and slowly invade them.'[74]

Charles Ryall, Surgeon to the Cancer Hospital, drew similar comparisons between bacterial disease and cancer—although he stopped short of suggesting that malignancy might be transmitted by an identifiable germ. He compared cancer to pyaemia (malignant septicaemia): 'Some small cancerous growths have a tendency to early formation of metastases, just in the same way that multiple pyaemic abscesses may readily follow an apparently insignificant focus of septic infection.' He described how cancer cells 'invade and infect' the surrounding tissues, and argued that 'these peculiarities of the cancer cell very much remind us of certain infective bacteria'.[75] Just as environmental ideas of cancer's

[71] Ibid.

[72] Quoted in Laura Otis, *Membranes: Metaphors of Invasion in Nineteenth-Century Literature, Science, and Politics* (Baltimore, MD, 2000), 26; emphasis added.

[73] Ibid., 23.

[74] J. Bland-Sutton, 'A Lecture on the Cancer Problem', *The Lancet*, 169 (1907), 1339–45, at 1342.

[75] Charles Ryall, 'The Technique of Cancer Operations, with Reference to the Danger of Cancer Infection', *BMJ*, 2 (1908), 1005–8, at 1005.

causation could fuse with germ theories of disease in debates about 'cancer houses', bacteriological understandings could coalesce with tumour cell theories. Germ theories of cancer evidently appealed to practitioners and the public alike. For some it provided an explanatory mechanism, for others an interpretative framework or new metaphorical language. Moreover, not only could the bacterial origin of cancer explain some of the observed features of the disease, but, as we shall see, it held therapeutic potential and conveyed optimism about the capacity for the medical profession to control cancer.

Various practitioners thought that the discovery of a cancer bacillus would illuminate a range of useful clinical and epidemiological characteristics. Woods Hutchinson suggested that 'the superficial resemblance between cancer and the infections' only encouraged enthusiasm for germ theories of malignancy.[76] In particular, he pointed to the many observable and experiential similarities between cancer and consumption. Both were chronic diseases that caused slow, agonising wasting; both were manifested, in part, by physical growths or tumours; and both were relentless in the face of medical intervention. Moreover, bacteriology could explain why cancer's 'favoured sites are at places which are directly and easily accessible to infective germs'.[77] One proponent of germ theory suggested that

> Wherever cancer grows luxuriantly and rapidly, we find present the chief desiderata for the growth of bacteria, namely moisture, an eminently suitable nutrient medium, a constant temperature... One could hardly imagine a better culture chamber for bacterial growth than the alimentary canal or uterus.[78]

As alluded to, an infective model would also help explain metastasis. As argued in Chapter 5, the existence of a cancer bacillus might explain the geographical distribution of the disease and shed light on the location of 'cancer houses'. Various observers also argued that the children of cancerous or consumptive parents might be congenitally vulnerable to the infective agent: 'The occurrence of cancer in several members of a family after the death of parents from that disease could not be accepted as evidence of heredity; but, on the contrary, could and ought to be accepted as evidence of infection from an obvious source.'[79] Thus,

---

[76] Hutchinson, 'The Cancer Problem', 111.

[77] Alexander Theodore Brand, 'East Yorks and North Lincoln Branch: The Etiology of Cancer', *BMJ*, 2 (1902), 238–42, at 239.

[78] Ibid.

[79] Ibid. Theories of contagion were also more appealing than hereditary explanations: 'As regards cancer, the odds are ten to one that the theory of heredity is a myth, which will vanish before the demonstration of its contagiousness. It is devoutly to be wished that this may prove to be so, since against heredity nothing can be done, while to fight contagion we have science and hygiene', Etienne Burnet, *The Campaign against Microbes*, trans. E. E. Austen (London, 1909), 9.

germ theories could be interpreted in multiple ways and used to explain multiple things—only increasing the concept's appeal.

Germ theories of cancer also held therapeutic potential that cell theories lacked. As will be further discussed in Chapter 7, much nineteenth-century cancer discourse abounded with pessimism, and medical men repeatedly recognized the limits of their knowledge and practice when it came to the 'dread disease'. The *BMJ* argued in 1902: 'If an infectious origin, almost certainly bacterial, were established, the lines on which treatment should be carried out would become clearly defined.'[80] Not only might an 'efficacious bactericide' be found, but 'notification, improved sanitation, including disinfection of houses, cremation of bodies, destruction of dejecta, dressings, etc., by fire, the use of pure drinking water', and so on, might provide useful prophylaxes.[81] Germ theories had, by the end of the nineteenth century, proven themselves effective elsewhere. Woods Hutchinson argued in 1899 that the germ theory of cancer 'has always been a most attractive one, partly on account of the delight of the human mind in assigning concrete, definite causes for phenomena, and partly because of the immensely improved prospects for cure which the discovery of a specific germ would open up'.[82]

However, while germ theories of cancer provided a seductive explanatory mechanism for cancer's causes and characteristics, its impact on clinical practice was more varied and caveated. One reason for this ambivalence was the lack of convincing evidence for the existence of the specific disease agent. Director of the Imperial Cancer Research Fund, Dr E. H. Bashford, claimed to have performed about 10,000 experiments on mice, searching for a cancer microbe.[83] He used this impressive industry to confirm the veracity of his claims that cancer was *not* communicable and that there were no such things as a cancer germ. Bashford was adamant that the experimental evidence gathered 'proved that no analogy existed between cancer and any known form of infective or contagious disease'.[84] Instead, 'future work must, therefore, be directed to ascertaining why cancer arose *de novo*', demonstrating a commitment to cellular pathology.[85]

However, Bashford's dismissal had only a limited effect on the scale of enthusiasm or the scope of research. Non-discovery of the infective agent did little to dampen the debate or dissuade those committed to the germ theory of cancer. Commentators frequently made use of agnostic defences in their analysis of cancer research:

As yet the infective agent of cancer has not been isolated, but neither have those of many other diseases admittedly microbic, so that this must not be used as an

---

[80] Brand, 'East Yorks and North Lincoln Branch', 242.   [81] Ibid.
[82] Hutchinson, 'The Cancer Problem', 111.   [83] Burnet, *The Campaign against Microbes*, 11.
[84] 'Imperial Cancer Research Fund', *BMJ*, 2 (1905), 96–100, at 96.   [85] Ibid.

argument against the theory of the exogenesis of cancer as so many are fond of doing. *Non-discovery and non-existence are not synonymous.*[86]

In a scribbled note to Mr Boardman, the Director of the Rockefeller Institute in New York recognized that 'the medical world has long been trying to find that a cancer is infectious but has not yet obtained satisfactory evidence looking that way'.[87] He admitted the difficulty in confirming non-existence, 'it is usually impossible to prove a negative'.[88]

Nonetheless, non-discovery did dampen the practical applicability of germ theories of cancer and bacteriology had little effect on the clinical management of the disease (aside from in the pursuit of aseptic operations). While many proponents of germ theories for a range of diseases, not just cancer, were enthusiastic about the therapeutic promises of bacteriology, in practice it was immediately successful only in surgery.[89] In 1899, The Middlesex Hospital devoted its largest room for use as a 'Bacteriological and General Microscopic Laboratory' and ordered a 'systematic Bacteriological . . . examination to be made in every case of Carcinoma or Sarcoma admitted into the Medical, Surgical, or Special Cancer Wards of the Hospital'.[90] However, as with histological examinations and the application of cell theory, these investigations took place for the sake of classification and had little bearing on the treatment given to cancer patients. Indeed, clinical experience was a key piece of evidence deployed to disprove the transmissibility of cancer, as surgeons and nurses treating cancer patients never seemed to contract the disease from the sufferer. The turn of the twentieth century saw intense anxiety and debate over hospital infection and the spreading of disease in clinical contexts—yet no British hospital implemented schemes or systems to deal with the potential transmissibility of cancer.[91]

Despite the optimism and future-oriented enthusiasm that located germ theories of cancer in a specific late nineteenth-century context, and much like cell theory, the history of cancer and contagion stretches back much further than the fin de siècle. Bacteriology thus coalesced with powerfully felt ideas about the

[86] Chas. W. Andrews and A. T. Brand, 'Cancer and Its Origin', *BMJ*, 1 (1904), 402; emphasis added.
[87] Rockefeller Archive, Tarrytown, New York, 'Reply from Dr Simon Flexner to Mr. Richard Boardman', 30 October 1913. 210.3 (4) Business Manager/Subject Files/Cancer 1913–1952.
[88] Ibid.
[89] Michael Worboys, 'The Emergence and Early Development of Parasitology', in Kenneth S. Warren and John Z. Bowes (eds.), *Parasitology: A Global Perspective* (New York, 1983), 6.
[90] UCLH Archive, 'Scheme for the Investigation of Cancer'.
[91] The New York Cancer Hospital, founded in 1884, built its wards without corners to enable the free flow of air and the cancer germs it was presumed to carry. Rockefeller Archive, Tarrytown, New York, 'Fourth Annual Report for the Year 1888' (New York Cancer Hospital, Eighth Avenue and 106th Street), 11. In 1913, a *Public Health Report* from the state of New York requested that householders report instances of communicable disease to the Board of Health or health officer. Cancer was included in the list of diseases to be reported alongside bubonic plague, cholera, diphtheria, leprosy, measles, etc. 'North Hempstead, N. Y.: Communicable Diseases. Notification, Placarding, Quarantine, Funerals. Reg. Bd. Of H., June 18, 1912', *Public Health Reports (1896–1970)*, 28 (1913), 1682–3, at 1682.

disease's nature which primed the medical community for the ready acceptance of germ theories of malignancy. Throughout the nineteenth century and before, various commentators suggested that cancer might be caused by an agent entering the body from without and that the disease might be transmissible from person to person. Michael Stolberg has argued that in early modern Europe anxieties over putrid, corrosive secretions, and the often-horrendous smell emanating from cancer victims, raised fears of infection.[92] These concerns bubbled under the surface, rising and falling throughout the eighteenth century. In 1802, the Society for the Investigation into the Nature and Cure of Cancer asked: 'are there any proofs of cancer being a contagious disease?'[93] Attempts to answer this question then recurred periodically in the ensuing half-century. In 1842, 'Dr Watson' from The Middlesex Hospital alluded to 'cases of cancer of the penis in men, whose wives laboured under cancer of the uterus, which would tend to establish the doctrine of its being contagious'.[94] An 1859 *Dictionary of Domestic Medicine* picked up on this theory, and recommended that 'Contact... should be avoided as much as possible; in the intimate relations of husband and wife, especially, whatever the organ or structure affected.'[95] Publications of this kind would have been present in many a middle-class household and likely widely read.

Thus, in 1883, a practitioner could reflect on the powerful hold germ theories of cancer exerted over the public imagination: 'All the world knows what cancer is, and no microscopic analysis will ever persuade men that cancer is anything but the devouring thing, the implacable enemy, that the common eye sees it to be.'[96] Just as each disease had its own pathological arc—initial symptoms, peak suffering, followed by death or resolution—medical writers conceptualized each as having their own intellectual teleology—a period of mystery, innovation, or discovery, followed by effective treatment or prevention (or at the very least, understanding). Cancer had yet to reach that end stage, but the identification of the tubercle bacillus was a promising sign. With contagion, for both professionals and the public 'a clear opportunity was presented for a solution to the cancer problem'.[97] In 1885, *Popular Science Monthly* stated: 'The germ theory appeals to the average mind: it is something tangible; it may be hunted down, captured,

---

[92] Michael Stolberg, 'Metaphors and Images of Cancer in Early Modern Europe', *Bulletin of the History of Medicine*, 88 (2014), 48–74.

[93] Bruce Schoenberg, 'A Program for the Conquest of Cancer: 1802', *Journal of the History of Medicine and Allied Sciences*, 30 (1975), 3–22, at 3. See also Chapter 2.

[94] Dr Watson, 'Course of Clinical Lectures, Delivered at the Middlesex Hospital, Session 1842-3', *Provincial Medical Journal and Retrospect of the Medical Sciences*, 5 (1842), 83–6, at 86.

[95] Spencer Thomson, *A Dictionary of Domestic Medicine and Household Surgery*, 8th edn (London and Glasgow, 1859), 81.

[96] Charles Creighton, 'Address in Pathology: On the Autonomous Life of the Specific Infections', *BMJ*, 2 (1883), 218–24, at 218.

[97] Joan Austoker, *A History of the Imperial Cancer Research Fund 1902-1986* (Oxford, 1988), 16.

colored, [sic] and looked at through a microscope, and then in all its varieties, it can be held directly responsible for so much damage.'[98]

Parasitology

Parasitology is the study of parasites and their hosts. The notion that a living creature might live on, in, or with another species—and that this dependence might cause harm to the host—has been around since at least the eighteenth century. While it only emerged as a scientific discipline in the early twentieth century—propelled by the development of tropical medicine—in the nineteenth century, the study of cestode and trematode parasites was 'well advanced' as the exploration of entozoa or helminthology.[99] Indeed, parasitic theories of cancer causation rivalled both cell theories of the disease and bacteriology in the fin de siècle. Historian John Farley has argued that parasitology and bacteriology developed independently from each other, and that late nineteenth-century British and American scientists failed to develop a generalized parasitic theory of disease that fruitfully exploited connections between parasitology and bacteriology.[100]

However, Michael Worboys has suggested that the rapid acceptance of germ theory was due to the groundwork prepared by work on helminths (a form of parasitic worm) in the mid-century.[101] Moreover, in the case of cancer, there was a concerted uptick in interest in cancer and parasites that coincided with the late nineteenth-century development of germ theories of disease. The press frequently used terms like 'micro-parasitic' and 'germ theory' in the same sentence when covering investigations into the communicability of cancer.[102] Indeed, nineteenth-century medical and scientific specialization was incomplete and it was easy to move from one subject to another. Practitioners spoke of concepts using fluid and ambiguous language, and it is often difficult to differentiate precisely between various aetiological models and disease agents.[103]

Experimenters seeking the cancer parasite inserted pieces of tumour that showed evidence of tiny malignant beings into the bodies of live animals. A report from the German Committee on Cancer Investigation was published in the *BMJ* in 1901: 'Cultures were inoculated into the organs and tissues of animals, especially rabbits, and the results studied histologically.'[104] This practice

---

[98] Quoted in Tomes, *The Gospel of Germs*, 7.
[99] Worboys, 'The Emergence and Early Development of Parasitology', 6.
[100] John Farley, 'Parasites and the Germ Theory of Disease', in Charles E. Rosenberg and Janet Lynne Golden (eds.), *Framing Disease: Studies in Cultural History* (New Brunswick, NJ, 1992).
[101] Worboys, 'The Emergence and Early Development of Parasitology', 6.
[102] 'Living Things in Cancers', 9.
[103] 'At the turn of the century the divisions between pathogenic viruses, bacteria, and protozoa were not clear cut.' Worboys, 'The Emergence and Early Development of Parasitology', 6.
[104] 'The Causation of Cancer', 1281.

was predicated on an old understanding that humans were not the only animals susceptible to cancer: 'When a disease is peculiar to man, experiments are out of the question, science is at a standstill, and despondency takes the place of hope. Fortunately for us, cancer is not the special prerogative of man.'[105] The 1802 thirteen queries asked, 'Are brute creatures subject to any disease resembling cancer in the human body?' By the beginning of the twentieth century, most medical men had settled this question in the affirmative. In 1905, Olt Giessen wrote in the *Journal of Comparative Pathology and Therapeutics*: 'Cancer in domestic animals exactly corresponds histogenetically with that of man.'[106] This piece of good evolutionary luck allowed for extensive experimentation on animals and their tumours. In 1890 Charles A. Balance and Samuel G. Shattock transplanted cancerous tumours into monkeys (most of which died from 'cold'), cats, rabbits, dogs, and sheep.[107] In 1900, Johannes Schuller 'inoculated [a supposed cancer-causing organism] into white mice; subcutaneously it gave rise in two cases to epitheliomatous new growths'.[108] The *BMJ* reported: 'This is the first series of experiments published in which true cancerous new growth has been produced by the inoculation of an isolated organism ... In the new growth forms resembling the "cancer bodies" of human carcinomata were found'.[109]

However, these reports were often contested, with rival practitioners failing to reproduce experiments or witness these 'definite bodies' for themselves. Debates over the communicability of cancer thus increasingly served as an arena in which ideals of 'modern' scientific practice were constructed and contested. In 1912, the *BMJ* called the cancer parasites 'but phantoms'—denigrating scientific observations to the status of mystical apparitions. Those who insisted on the intrinsic origin of cancer used dismissive rhetoric to malign their intellectual opponents. The *BMJ* went on to describe the work of Robert Behla, Director of the Medical Department of the Royal Prussian Statistical Office in Berlin, who 'dogmatically asserts that he has succeeded in cultivating a protozoon ... which he holds to be the true cause of cancer'. The *BMJ* saw these doctrinaire tones as inappropriate for the restrained and empirical scientist—this was an enterprise predicated on observation and evidence, not ideology and belief.[110] As such, Behla's article did not 'inspire confidence' and the journal accused him of obfuscation: '[The text] is overloaded with technical detail to such an extent that the true object of the discussion is hidden from view.'[111] The *BMJ* effectively accused Behla of being an

---

[105] Olt Giessen, 'Cancer in Domestic Animals', *Journal of Comparative Pathology and Therapeutics*, 18 (1905), 278–9, at 278.

[106] Ibid.

[107] Charles A. Balance and Samuel G. Shattock, 'A Note on an Experimental Investigation into the Pathology of Cancer', *Proceedings of the Royal Society of London*, 48 (1890), 397–401.

[108] 'The Parasitic Theory of Cancer', *BMJ*, 2 (1900), 1518.   [109] Ibid.

[110] 'The Parasite of Cancer', *BMJ*, 2 (1912), 1328–9, at 1328.   [111] Ibid.

unreliable witness, an ineffective scientific labourer, and called on his experiments to be 'carefully and thoroughly controlled by capable workers'.[112]

The narrative arc of this version of the parasitic theory of cancer tracked closely to that of bacteriological explanations. However, the physiology and pathology of the proposed cancer parasite was different in crucial ways to that of the proposed cancer bacillus. Some suggested that the cancer cell was itself a parasite. This idea was not only more difficult to prove, but also harder to shed. Henry T. Butlin (1845–1912) was a committed proponent of the idea that cancer consisted of autonomous life and argued that cancer was not *caused* by a parasite, but that cancer *was* a parasite: 'the cancer parasite is the cancer cell'.[113] In this schema, the cancer cell was a form of primitive life—a protozoa. As argued by Andrew Reynolds, in the nineteenth century, protozoology and cell biology 'intersected through the nexus of Darwin's theory of evolution'.[114] The cell was conceptualized as a simple, elementary organism, and a new focus on the amoeba as a scientifically significant object or creature encapsulated a range of evolutionary theories about the community of descent and the rise of complex, orderly creatures from simpler, more primitive ones.[115] Various observers, from Ernst Haeckel to T. H. Huxley, suggested that all animals were descended from a unicellular form, and that probably there was one such ancestor for all animals.[116] These ideas made it possible for Butlin to call cancer cells 'new species of the lowest forms of animals'.[117] The life of the cancerous cell was much the same as that of any other simplistic being—they could grow, travel, and reproduce: 'Let us imagine that, in the growth of the tumour and in the destruction which is occasioned by its growth, masses of cells are detached and carried to distant parts of the body, where they sometimes meet with conditions which are favourable to their maintenance and multiplication.'[118]

Butlin's theory was, therefore, a complex synthesis of cell theory, parasitology, and protozoology. In 1905 he wrote:

I should...once more insist that carcinoma is a parasitic disease, not in the limited sense in which the term appears to have been used of late, as synonymous with infective, but in the larger and wider sense in which it used to be, and should

[112] Ibid.

[113] Henry T. Butlin, 'Two Lectures on Unicellula Cancri: The Parasite of Cancer', BMJ, 2 (1911), 1457–61, at 1457.

[114] Andrew Reynolds, 'Amoebae as Exemplary Cells: The Protean Nature of an Elementary Organism', Journal of the History of Biology, 41 (2008), 307–37, at 307.

[115] See Natasha X. Jacobs, 'From Unit to Unity: Protozoology, Cell Theory, and the New Concept of Life', Journal of the History of Biology, 22 (1989), 215–42.

[116] Marsha L. Richmond, 'Protozoa as Precursors of Metazoa: German Cell Theory and its Critics at the Turn of the Century', Journal of the History of Biology, 22 (1989), 243–76.

[117] Henry T. Butlin, 'Carcinoma is a Parasitic Disease: Being the Bradshaw Lecture Delivered before the Royal College of Surgeons of England', BMJ, 2 (1905), 1565–71, at 1570.

[118] Ibid., 1567.

always be, employed, to express the fact of one organism living at the expense of another organism, each pursuing its otherwise separate and independent existence.[119]

A year later, he argued, 'I shall maintain that the carcinoma cell is an independent organism, like many a protozoon; that it lives a life which is wholly independent and proper to itself.'[120] He quoted Charles Powell White, 'We can say, then, that cancer cells themselves act as parasites. This view will explain all the phenomena of cancer.'[121] Approving reviews in the *BMJ* noted 'Sir Henry Butlin has shown in a striking manner the parallelism that exists between the life and development of different varieties of cancer cells and that of many of the protozoa.'[122] Butlin was not, therefore, alone in thinking of cancer in such terms and his conceptualizations aligned with the plethora of contemporaneous literature that understood the protozoa as a pathological parasite.[123] In 'The Bradshaw Lecture on the Pathology of Cancer', published in 1884, W. S. Savory wrote: 'The structure of cancer and its allies is characterised by the presence of the lowest and simplest of living forms. The so-called cancer-cells—the structural elements of cancer—are the very type of the rudimentary or embryonic form of tissue.'[124]

Butlin's conception of cancer was also like that of the pathologist Charles Creighton. Both Butlin and Creighton understood cancer as an independent creation and Creighton's dependence on Darwinian evolution was clear. He wrote: 'As we have an Origin of Species for animals and plants, it is natural to think of the origin of disease species.'[125] However, the analogy was incomplete. For Creighton, there was a fundamental difference between cancer and living beings: 'In the origin of species, we are dealing with individual things, each with its well-founded, independent life.'[126] In contrast, cancer was 'semi-independent' not 'in absolute independence of the body, but autonomous within it, an *imperium in imperio*'.[127] Creighton encapsulated this tension in a quotation from Paracelsus: 'In such a disease, a man is himself and another; he has two bodies at one time, enclosed the one in the other, and yet he is one man.'[128]

How, then, was cancer supposed to have achieved this precarious status somewhere between dependence and independence? Creighton spoke of an 'acquired autonomy, and of a pre-autonomous stage'.[129] Much like Butlin's *de novo* creation of the cancer cell within the host body, 'the functional disease...acquires the

---

[119] Ibid., 1565.   [120] Ibid., 1566.
[121] Butlin, 'Two Lectures on Unicellula Cancri', 1457.
[122] H. Charlton Bastian, 'The Origin of Cancer and the Origin of Life', *BMJ*, 2 (1911), 1573.
[123] See F. E. G. Cox, 'George Henry Falkiner Nuttall and the Origins of Parasitology and Parasitology', *Parasitology*, 136 (2009), 1389–94; and 'History of Human Parasitology', *Clinical Microbiology Reviews*, 15 (2002), 595–612.
[124] W. S. Savory, 'The Bradshaw Lecture on the Pathology of Cancer', *BMJ*, 2 (1884), 1173–8, at 1175.
[125] Creighton, 'Address in Pathology', 223.   [126] Ibid.   [127] Ibid., 224.   [128] Ibid.
[129] Ibid., 219.

degree of individuality which may be ascribed to a tumour, and that must be the beginning of its life of semi-independence within the body'. Creighton was vague on details of the process—'the pre-autonomous stage is a common disorder of structure and function'[130]—but explicit about the outcome. Following a period of dependence on the host body, cancer then acquired 'the mysterious power of infection'.[131] However, this transition from pre-autonomy to autonomy did not just apply to malignancy. Creighton's main discursive mode was that of analogy and he drew multiple comparisons between tuberculosis and cancer to demonstrate the validity of his theory. Creighton thought both would acquire 'a kind of individuality or independence, and a power to reproduce itself throughout the body'.[132] Indeed, 'If cancer has always been the great popular instance of a disease enjoying a kind of life of its own within the body, consumption hardly yields to it in its relentlessness.'[133]

Both Creighton and Butlin redefined 'infection' to mean the transmission of an intentional disease agent throughout the different textures of the body. In 1883, Creighton claimed that the 'autonomous life of the disease' was 'shown in its infectiveness'.[134] He insisted 'Cancer is an infection, although its infective power does not extend...beyond the individual body in which the disease takes its rise.'[135] In contrast, tuberculosis' infectivity had the capacity to extend beyond corporeal limits and so was 'a more complete example of infection than cancer'. Yet, crucially, cancer still registered on the gradation of 'infectiveness'.[136] That Creighton refers to 'completeness' when talking about the communicability of a disease suggests a sliding-scale model of infectivity rather than a simplistic dichotomy between contagious and non-contagious.

This notion proved compelling not just because it synthesized recent developments in bacteriology, parasitology, protozoology, and cell theory, but because it also recapitulated much older ideas about cancer's aetiology and character. Throughout the nineteenth century, surgeons and physicians observed that cancer could infiltrate the body beyond its initial site, across tissue boundaries or through the blood. Similarly, and from its discovery in the first few decades of the century by George Ernst Stahl and Friedrich Hoffman at the University of Halle in Germany, the lymph and the lymphatic system were stressed as crucial components in the pathogenesis of cancer.[137] In 1844, Walter Hayle Walshe wrote about the 'transmission [of cancer] by the lymphatic or venous system'.[138]

These various mechanisms of metastasis, internal transmission, or internal 'infectivity' were themselves predicated on an even older sense that cancer was a disease with agency. This imagining refracted through society and language,

---

[130] Ibid., 218.   [131] Ibid., 220.   [132] Ibid., 219.   [133] Ibid.   [134] Ibid.

[135] Ibid., 218.   [136] Ibid.

[137] L. J. Rather, *The Genesis of Cancer: A Study in the History of Ideas* (Baltimore, MD, 1978), 30.

[138] Walter Hayle Walshe, *The Anatomy, Physiology, Pathology, and Treatment of Cancer* (Boston, MA, 1844), 88.

appearing in metaphorical discourse of diverse issues. In 1841, an MP claimed: 'The unjust and miserable system of paying wages out of rates—the discouragement of industry, and the premium which was offered to improvidence and sloth—the cancer which has got such a powerful hold of the southern provinces, was gradually *eating* its way to the heart of England.'[139] Metaphors and analogies are rhetorical or analytical techniques, but they also articulate actual scientific and medical understanding.[140] In other words, for these cancer metaphors to 'work' in the political context of parliament, they needed to have some widespread purchase on the collective imagination. That MPs could deploy such language to rhetorical effect was dependent on a general understanding of cancer as possessing active agency, having intention, and being animal-like.

This notion of cancer possessing 'independent vitality' had perhaps an even tighter grip on the imaginations of the early nineteenth-century population than the idea of the communicability of the disease. For centuries, cancer has been conceptualized as a para-parasitical and intentional being—a creature occupying the body and consuming it from within. In her article on malignancy in early modern England, Alanna Skuse describes how, in the seventeenth century, the disease was imagined as 'quasi-sentient, zoomorphising the disease as an eating worm or wolf'.[141] This idea that cancer was an animal, distinct from its host, persisted into the nineteenth century. Cancer was endowed with character, temperament, and disposition—with needs in direct competition with those of the body it inhabited.

In 1817, a doctor at the Middlesex reported on a case of quackery. Mrs Stadden, a miller's wife, had witnessed Mr Ashby, who was supposedly in possession of a remedy for cancer, apply his remedy to the cancerous breast of a woman. Subsequently, 'he extracted eighteen long worms, and about the same number of cancerous reptiles'.[142] While her 'health and spirits' were much improved, the cure was not complete, 'as there are more animalculae to come away'.[143] This cure was later discovered to be a 'fallacy'. Ashby had made the 'cancerous reptiles' 'nestle' in the 'open sores of the poor creatures' who had come to him, desperate for treatment.[144] However, the notion of cancer as a living creature or creatures evidently resonated with an audience keen to have their diseases cured. These old imaginings primed medical men and the laity for the ready acceptance of germ and parasitical theories of cancer and provided them with a rich metaphorical language and intellectual framework with which to comprehend the disease. That

[139]   HC Deb., vol. 56, cc375–451, 8 February 1841; emphasis added.
[140]   See George Lakoff and Mark Johnson, *Metaphors We Live By* (Chicago, 2003).
[141]   Alanna Skuse, 'Wombs, Worms and Wolves: Constructing Cancer in Early Modern England', *Social History of Medicine*, 27 (2014), 632–48, at 632.
[142]   Alexander Shaw, Charles H. Moore, Campbell de Morgan, and Mitchell Henry, *Report of the Surgical Staff of the Middlesex Hospital, to the Weekly Board and Governors, upon the Treatment of Cancerous Diseases in the Hospital, on the Plan Introduced by Dr Fell* (London, 1857), 4.
[143]   Ibid.   [144]   Ibid., 6.

a doctor writing in the 1890s could call cancer 'an independent organism, like many a protozoon; that lives a life which is wholly independent and proper to itself', was as much dependent on recent research into primitive life forms and germ theories of disease as it was on deeply felt conceptualizations of cancer's distinct trajectory within, but not necessarily bounded by, its host body.[145]

Much of Butlin and Creighton's work on cancer was theoretical. They were not preoccupied by practical or therapeutic applications. As with bacteriology, parasitic theories of malignancy had little effect on the clinical management of the disease. Nonetheless, their ideas had a powerful influence on the minds of the lay public. In 1912, the *Washington Post* reflected the opinions of many when it described cancer as 'a phenomenon of independent vitality' that had taken on 'aggressive activity'.[146] However, while Butlin and Creighton put scientific words to widely believed aspects of the disease, such words were restricted in their explanatory capacity. For while this version of the parasitic theory was seductive, it did little to elucidate cancer's aetiology. It might have described its physiology (as an independent life form) and its pathology (its ability to kill its host), but it could not explain its initial appearance. Harking back to explanatory limitations of cell theory: it described the process effectively and meaningfully, but did not answer the fundamental and persistent questions of cancer's cause or cure.

Conclusion

This chapter has explored the impact of cell theory, germ theory, and parasitology on theories and practices pertaining to cancer and its care. It has problematized narratives that suggest cell theories of disease transformed the understanding and diagnosis of cancer, and it has suggested that bacterial and parasitic theories of cancer were enthusiastically taken up by practitioners and professionals in the 1880s and after, although they were never universally accepted. Cell theories of cancer, bacteriological ideas, and parasitological conceptualizations involved extensive laboratory-based investigations into the disease, and all three were closely associated with new technologies (the microscope) and powerful ideas about modern science and medical progress. However, as I have shown, these ostensibly innovative ideas about cancer and its cause had longer histories and none of them could be extracted from much older metaphorical beliefs about what cancer was.

Irrespective of their theoretical models and assumptions, these investigations were part of an effort—like mapping—to make sense of an incurable disease

[145] Butlin, 'Carcinoma is a Parasitic Disease', 1566.
[146] 'Baffling Mystery of Life: Experiments of the Scientists Have so Far Failed to Fathom its Secret', *Washington Post*, 20 October 1912.

without having to come into clinical contact with death. Cell theory, bacteriology, and parasitology had limited influence on clinical practice or therapeutics, and those who investigated tumour cell theories or germ theories of disease could do so with very limited patient interaction. Instead, these were rationalizing efforts—attempts to bring clarity even if they could not bring curability. However, the clarity they brought was also partial. That the medical community could not find the evidence necessary for a consensus on the existence of a cancer microbe (either bacterial or parasitic) frustrated the therapeutic promises of germ theory. The evidence available for cell theories of the disease, and notions that cancer itself constituted a parasite, were perhaps more convincing, but not reassuring. Germ theories of cancer appealed in part because they offered a departure from the troubling idea that cancer cells evolved from the healthy human body. And yet cancer maintained a disconcerting identity and was largely unchanged by these modernizing efforts. Malignancy remained what it had always been: an invasive, semi-independent agent with a tendency towards monstrous growth. Cell theory and parasitology subverted the idea that evolution consisted of the progressive development of order from chaos.

Moreover, what did this idea of the development of independent life indicate about the rationality of the human body and its biological processes? If the healthy could degenerate into the pathological, without warning and without the possibility for reversal, then what did that imply about the inevitability of bodily decline and cancerous suffering? One of the reasons why the three theories so suited the nineteenth-century medical collective was because they articulated in new language an old and deeply felt idea of cancer as an abnormal, chaotic, and uncontrollable rebellion within. For this reason, discussions of cancer cell theory and parasitology worked on multiple registers and operated as proxies for political debates about the state of Victorian society. In Chapter 7 I explore further these connections between cancer and the social body.

7

Making Cancer Modern

From the 1840s onwards, the collection of vital statistics revealed to fretful observers an expanding 'cancer epidemic'. As Chapters 5 and 6 have shown, frustrated by therapeutic impotence and disconcerted by the disease's persistent incurability and increasing incidence, the medical community turned their attention from treatment to cause, prevention, and transmission. While Chapters 5 and 6 looked at practitioners who, using a range of techniques and technologies, attempted to decode the aetiology of cancer and explain and arrest its expansion, the limited success of these efforts prompted some observers to suggest that perhaps the origin of malignancy and the source of the new epidemic could be found in the very fabric of late nineteenth-century British society. If it was not latent in the landscape, nor a waxing and waning infectious disease, then maybe cancer's increasing incidence was a sign of some change in the bodies and lifestyles of the nation and its inhabitants. Perhaps the cause was civilization itself.

It is a well-known and often rehashed trope that cancer today constitutes an unintended consequence of progress, civilization, or modernity. Or, as Charles E. Rosenberg put it, 'the notion that the incidence of much late-twentieth-century chronic disease reflects a poor fit between modern styles of life and humankind's genetic heritage'.[1] However, while Roy Porter called cancer 'the modern disease par excellence' and Siddhartha Mukherjee described it as 'the quintessential product of modernity', they locate that modernity firmly in the twentieth century.[2] Thus, while cancer is widely recognized today as a problem of progress, it is strangely absent from histories of this idea. This chapter goes some way towards rectifying this lacuna by exploring the construction of cancer as a 'disease of civilization' in late Victorian Britain. Attending to these notions adds to our existing understandings of the impact of civilization on nineteenth-century bodies.[3]

Similar debates about the impact of civilization on the integrity of our cells to those that can be found circulating at the end of the twentieth century also appear at the end of the nineteenth. This chapter owes much to recent historiography on

---

[1] Charles E. Rosenberg, 'Pathologies of Progress: The Idea of Civilization as Risk', *Bulletin of the History of Medicine*, 72 (1998), 714–30, at 714.

[2] Roy Porter, *The Greatest Benefit to Mankind: A Medical History of Humanity from Antiquity to the Present* (London, 1999), 574; Siddhartha Mukherjee, *The Emperor of All Maladies: A Biography of Cancer* (New York, 2011), 241.

[3] See A. Omran, 'The Epidemiological Transition: A Theory of the Epidemiology of Population Change', *Milbank Quarterly*, 83 (1971), 731–57.

The Cancer Problem: Malignancy in Nineteenth-Century Britain. Agnes Arnold-Forster, Oxford University Press (2021).

the fin de siècle and its tendency to focus on disciplinary, national, and other micro-history contexts, and examine the period through 'kaleidoscopic edited collections'.[4] Cancer is one such micro history which allows us to not only trace the metanarratives of progress and decline, but also offers us another perspective on well-trodden terrain. While medical historiographical discussions of the impacts of civilization on health tend to emphasize the problems of the young— looking at tuberculosis, venereal disease, and fertility—the history of cancer shows that the early deaths of people who were past breeding age were also seen as highly problematic because of the implications they held for both the biological body and the body politic.

As Daniel Pick argues, the medical community in the fin de siècle experienced a 'move towards a central preoccupation with the economy of the body and the social effects of its reproduction'.[5] This focus on young bodies and birth is unsurprising as the period between 1860 and 1940 witnessed a 'dramatic fall in fertility in British society'.[6] Contemporaries also commented on this central pre-occupation and, in a lecture delivered before the Preventive Medicine Section of the London Congress of the Royal Institute of Public Health in 1905, the physician James Crichton-Browne said: 'Glancing at the subjects of discussion arranged for this section one would infer that preventive medicine is for the young...as for old age, it is practically ignored in our programme.'[7]

In what follows, I will outline the ways in which this perceived 'cancer epidemic' captured the medical and lay imagination and promoted fierce debate in the pages of medical journals, general-interest periodicals, and in parliament. I argue that as with cell theories, and with bacteriological and parasitic ideas of cancer, views of the disease as a product of degeneration and decline—and its construction as a malady of modern life—were readily adopted because of long-standing and flexible disease metaphors.[8] However, this discourse of cancer and degeneration was not the only interpretation of the late nineteenth-century increase in incidence. As I will show, cancer was increasingly perceived as an unintended consequence of public health successes: lower infant mortality, increasing hospitalization, and sanitary reform. At the end of the nineteenth

---

[4] Roy Porter and Mikulas Teich (eds.), *Fin de Siècle and its Legacy* (Cambridge, UK, 1990); Sally Ledger and Scott McCracken (eds.), *Cultural Politics at the Fin de Siècle* (Cambridge, UK, 1990); Sally Ledger and Roger Luckhurst (eds.), *The Fin-de-Siècle: A Reader in Cultural History, c.1880–1900* (Oxford, 2000); Michael Saler (ed.), *The Fin-de-Siècle World* (London, 2015).

[5] Daniel Pick, *Faces of Degeneration: A European Disorder, c.1848–c.1918* (Cambridge, UK, 1989), 6.

[6] Simon Szreter, *Fertility, Class and Gender in Britain, 1860–1940* (Cambridge, UK, 1996), 1. James Crichton-Browne, *The Prevention of Senility and a Sanitary Outlook* (London, 1905), 3.

[7] Crichton-Browne, *The Prevention of Senility*, 3.

[8] Laura Otis, *Membranes: Metaphors of Invasion in Nineteenth-Century Literature, Science, and Politics* (Baltimore, MD, and London, 1999); Susan Sontag, *Illness as Metaphor and AIDS and Its Metaphors* (London, 2013); Michael Stolberg, 'Metaphors and Images of Cancer in Early Modern Europe', *Bulletin of the History of Medicine*, 88 (2014), 48–74. For a broader reflection on metaphors see George Lakoff and Mark Johnson, *Metaphors We Live By* (Chicago, 2003).

century, prominent statisticians and public health experts like John Tatham (Superintendent of Statistics at the General Register Office (GRO) from 1893 to 1909) and Arthur Newsholme (President for the Society of Medical Officers of Health from 1900 to 1901 and Principal Medical Officer for the Local Government Board from 1908 to 1918) claimed that the increasingly efficient and effective medical profession was responsible for the nation's shifting disease profile.

My analysis of these parallel but conflicting constructions of cancer as a pathology of progress reveals how different constituents made use of cancer in their divergent understandings of civilization. This chapter reflects on how cancer was constructed as manifesting national decline, while simultaneously—and somewhat paradoxically—being manufactured as a disease of health. The latter finding suggests that the medical profession's ability to maintain and improve the health, wealth, and well-being of nation and empire generated a late Victorian faith in progress that ran alongside its much-documented preoccupation with the degeneration and decline of British civilization. This chapter begins by looking at the 'global geographies' of cancer that were invoked to demonstrate the epidemic's uneven growth in 'civilized' as opposed to 'uncivilized' countries. It will then explore the different reasons various late nineteenth-century medical men pro-posed to explain this distribution, and will focus on the narratives of bodily decline and social degeneration that thread their way through fin-de-siècle cancer dis-course. I then move on to interrogate the concept of the 'cancer age'—at once a period of life when people were presumed to become particularly vulnerable to the disease and an historical epoch concomitant with imperial decline and over-stretch. Finally, this chapter looks at those public health practitioners and statist-icians who interpreted the cancer epidemic as manifesting medical and social progress.

Degeneration, Decline, and Disease

The second half of the nineteenth century witnessed widespread unease over the perceived 'cancer epidemic' and, by the fin de siècle, this anxiety had escalated. In 1893, Surgical Registrar to The Middlesex Hospital, W. Roger Williams, wrote: 'Examination of the Registrar-General's annual reports shows that the propor-tionate mortality from cancer now is four times greater than it was fifty years ago. No other disease has manifested such a great increase.'[9] In 1899, Assistant Physician to St Thomas's Hospital, Dr J. F. Payne, wrote in the Lancet, 'Of the fact that the mortality from cancer has increased and is increasing I maintain there cannot be the smallest doubt.'[10] The non-medical press, too, frequently invoked

---

[9] W. Roger Williams, 'The Question of the Increase of Cancer', BMJ, 2 (1893), 1450–1, at 1450.
[10] J. F. Payne, 'A Lecture on the Increase on Cancer', The Lancet, 154 (1899), 765–70, at 765.

melodramatic language to impress upon the public the gravity of the cancer epidemic. In 1895, physician and inventor of the clinical thermometer, Clifford Allbutt, commented in the *Contemporary Review*: 'There is a bitter cry that cancer is on the increase.'[11] In 1907, the *New York Times* stated: 'The cancer problem is assuming more and more menacing proportions ... we are doing nothing to hold cancer in check as a cause of mortality.'[12] Even the fashion magazine *Vogue* despaired: 'It is sad news indeed that cancer is increasing at such a rate that it begins to rival the white plague—as tuberculosis is called—in the number of its victims.'[13]

This new 'cancer epidemic' prompted an array of rival explanatory models and investigative strategies, including spatial configurations of the disease on a global scale. In Chapter 5, I showed how the nineteenth century saw a reconceptualiza-tion of cancer as a disease of locality and environment. It was plotted and arranged on maps of the United Kingdom, with its varying incidence correlated and connected to different geographical features. Alfred Haviland endeavoured to uncover the reasons for cancer's increase and he located the epidemic in the English landscape.[14] While Haviland did not associate cancer with degeneration, this reconceptualization of cancer as a disease of place chimed with the self-consciously international character of fin-de-siècle cancer investigation. Thus— and in part because science and medicine were key components of British imperial expansion—by the closing decades of the century, a dynamic and interactive network of scientists and doctors were working in colonial contexts. Men like W. Renner, Medical Officer of Freetown, Sierra Leone, and Sir William MacGregor, Lieutenant-Governor of British New Guinea, compiled data, obser-vations, and anecdotes about cancer incidence in their respective indigenous populations and reported them back to the metropole.[15] London-based journals like the *British Medical Journal* (*BMJ*) and *The Lancet* acted as nexuses of cancer information, sent in from across the British Empire. This information fed into conceptual cartographies of cancer that covered the globe. While I have not come across visual, physical maps of cancer incidence across the British Empire, commentators theoretically plotted populations on a gradient—from immune to

---

[11] Clifford Allbutt, 'Nervous Diseases and Modern Life', *Contemporary Review*, 67 (1895), 210–31, at 215.
[12] 'Cancer Deaths Increasing: Porter Says the Malady is Assuming Menacing Proportions', *New York Times*, 5 November 1907, 1.
[13] Comparing cancer to consumption—the archetypal romantic tragedy of the fin de siècle—would have had a powerful impact on readers and cemented the supposed increase in the incidence of cancer in the imaginations of the middle classes. 'Cancer Increasing at an Alarming Rate', *Vogue*, 15 April 1909, 726.
[14] Alfred Haviland, *The Geographical Distribution of Heart Diseases and Dropsy, Cancer in Females and Phthisis in Females, in England and Wales* (London, 1875).
[15] William MacGregor, 'Some Problems of Tropical Medicine', *The Lancet*, 2 (1900), 1055–61; W. Renner, 'The Spread of Cancer among the Descendants of the Liberated Africans or Creoles of Sierra Leone', *BMJ*, 2 (1910), 587–9.

cancer riddled—with sub-Saharan African communities at one end and Anglo-Saxon or Teutonic races at the other: 'Observation has shown that cancer has a certain geographical distribution. It prevails extensively in some parts of the globe, and is scarcely known in others.'[16]

This 'mapping' suggested that England and its Anglo-Saxon inhabitants suffered the greatest burden: 'Englishmen may be regarded as unfortunate; for within the geographical area of these islands cancer asserts largely its malignant and fatal influence.'[17] In contrast, cancer incidence in British colonies was low, even non-existent. In 1906, the *BMJ* reported, 'There can be no doubt that cancer in natives of British Central Africa is of the utmost rarity. Repeated efforts made by Government medical officers throughout the country for some time past have so far resulted in the discovery of but a single case.'[18] The situation in Sierra Leone was similar: 'Cancer as a disease is very rare among the aborigines...I would rather not say that the aborigines are immune from the disease, but that the disease is rare among them.'[19] Dr A. J. Craigen, writing from Port Moresby in New Guinea in 1905, reported 'that during his stay of nearly four years in the Possession he has not yet seen a single case of cancer among the native population'.[20] The disease was also rare in Ceylon.[21] Cancer rates were slightly higher in Hong Kong: 'The returns made to the Registrar-General show that the total number of deaths among the Chinese in the period 1895–1904 was 11, giving an annual death-rate from cancer of 4.45 per 100, 000 of population.'[22] However, as Dr Francis Clark, Acting Principal Civil Medical Officer, pointed out, this compared 'very favourably with the death-rate from the same cause in England'.[23] These colonial observations of cancer proved troubling to social and medical commentators. Not only was the disease on the increase, but the epidemic seemed to be confined to nations that were conventionally understood as biologically, culturally, and economically superior.

English people were more susceptible to cancer than their colonized communities and they were also more vulnerable than their European neighbours. The *BMJ* wrote in 1903: 'In considering countries as a whole it appears that the disease is more common in rich countries such as England, France, Holland, and Bavaria, while the lowest rates are among the poorer nations, Italy and Ireland.'[24] As with the broader empire, cancer was not thought to be increasing at equal rates in England, Scotland, Wales, and Ireland. Celts were believed to be more prone to cancer than their Anglo-Saxon or Teutonic counterparts: 'Certain races seemed to have a great susceptibility than others to cancer, a tendency especially marked

---

[16] Hugh P. Dunn, 'The Increase of Cancer', *Pall Mall Gazette*, 12 May 1884.   [17] Ibid.
[18] 'Cancer in the Colonies', *BMJ*, 1 (1906), 812–13, at 812.
[19] Renner, 'The Spread of Cancer', 588.   [20] 'Cancer in the Colonies', 812.   [21] Ibid., 813.
[22] Ibid., 812.   [23] Ibid.
[24] 'A Comparative Statistical Study of Cancer Mortality. V. General Summary (Concluded)', *BMJ*, 1 (1903), 1154–6, at 1154.

among peoples of Teutonic or Scandinavian origin, while an exceptionally low mortality was most often noted among Celtic or Sclavonic [sic] peoples.'[25] The *BMJ* published data comparing cancer rates in Ireland favourably with rates in England: 'In the eleven years 1877–87 the annual death-rate from cancer in England and Wales among persons aged upwards of 25 years was 1,188 per million; and the rate increased steadily year by year from 1,079 in 1877 to 1,331 in 1887. In Ireland, on the other hand, the mean annual rate in the same eleven years, at the same ages, was only 828 per million.'[26]

Army surgeon William Hill-Climo did not believe that this uneven distribution was coincidental. He argued that the increasing death rate from cancer in all European countries, and in the United States of America could not be 'ascribed to local or accidental causes' but must instead be 'sought for in the growth of new conditions...common to all the affected countries, which the people themselves have produced'.[27] The new epidemic was a product of 'new conditions'—and they were conditions of the societies' own making. Hill-Climo's comments relied upon, and in turn confirmed, pervasive contemporary anxieties over the degeneration and decline of 'civilized' societies and the inherent dangers of modernity. Coupled with the observed rise in cancer incidence, global geographies of cancer fed into anxieties about the unintended costs of civilization. The cancer epidemic and its uneven distribution prompted people to explore a key tension in modern medicine and society. Cancer was a terrible disease—synonymous with death and decline—and yet it seemed to predominate in communities marked otherwise by progress and civilization.

The idea of degeneracy, hereditary or otherwise, suffused fin-de-siècle culture and the discourse of Europe's urban elite—and with it the idea that prosperity, industrialization, and urbanization brought with them a plethora of physical and emotional complaints. Neither the 'natural' triumph of the 'civilizing' imperial Western powers, nor the stability of the racial order, were guaranteed. In 1892, physician, author, and social critic Max Nordau published his famous text, *Degeneration*, and in 1896 the zoologist E. Ray Lankester wrote: 'Degeneration is a necessary accompaniment of progress.'[28] He was one of many writers negotiating theories of degeneration at the turn of the twentieth century. This body of literature dealt with the 'apparent paradox' that civilization itself 'might be the catalyst of, as much as the defence against, physical and social pathology'.[29] Thus, this discourse of cancer and degeneration aligned with widespread understandings

---

[25] Ibid.

[26] 'Recorded Cancer Mortality in England and Ireland', *BMJ*, 1 (1889), 1240–1, at 1240.

[27] William Hill-Climo, 'Cancer in Ireland: An Economic Question', *Empire Review*, 6 (1903), 410–16, at 410.

[28] E. Ray Lankester, 'The Present Evolution of Man', *Fortnightly Review*, 66 (1896), 408–15; Max Nordau, *Degeneration*, trans. George L. Moss (Lincoln, NE, and London, 1993).

[29] Pick, *Faces of Degeneration*, 11.

of social and somatic decline in late nineteenth-century Europe and North America. These were societies preoccupied with inheritance, atavism, evolution, and eugenics, and the cancer story can be mapped on to these anxieties.[30]

The notion that civilization was disease-causing was in part dependent on a nineteenth-century version of biological anthropology that structured strict and impermeable boundaries between different races. A socio-cultural evolutionary viewpoint characterized British anthropology after c.1860 and infiltrated a range of academic pursuits and public conversations.[31] Scholarship into this area is extensive and the historical narratives are complex; however, cancer theorists were drawing on a variety of overlapping concepts that formed the vocabulary of the fin-de-siècle bourgeoisie. These concepts included ideas about the diversity of humankind and its maintained relationship with biblical assumptions, the positivistic and naturalistic study of the progress of civilization, a tradition of Anglo-Saxon racialism and ideas about inherent Teutonic superiority, and broader notions of biological racial determinism.[32] Racialization of populations structured rigid hierarchies between colonizers and colonized, and between different European communities. Thus, this period witnessed a concretization of racial distinctions and a heightened commitment of the importance of *biology* in dictating behaviours and tendencies. This coincided with, and was causally linked to, an increasingly rapacious and fretful imperialism.

It was, therefore, a hallmark of late nineteenth-century anthropology that race rested on material facts—'it is no arbitrary idea, no abstraction'.[33] The idea that certain races were inherently more or less vulnerable to certain diseases was a common concept in Victorian medicine. In his 1883 'Address in Pathology', the parasitologist Charles Creighton wrote that smallpox was 'peculiarly an African disease'. This particularity was a biological one— 'the loathsomeness, the peculiar odour, and the no less peculiar scars of small-pox, might of themselves suggest another skin than ours'.[34] Practitioners toyed with the idea that cancer was also a product of inherent biology—born of 'Other' flesh. Surgeon Leo Loeb reflected 'whether those differences in the cancer morbidity are primarily questions of race or whether they are due to the external conditions under which the races live'.[35] However, for most commenters, cancer was less a product of the civilized *body*,

---

[30] See Edwards Chamberlin and Sander L. Gilman (eds.), *Degeneration: The Dark Side of Progress* (New York, 1985); Stephen J. Gould, *The Mismeasure of Man* (New York and London, 1981); Wendy Kline, *Building a Better Race: Gender, Sexuality, and Eugenics from the Turn of the Century to the Baby Boom* (Berkeley, CA, 2001); Pauline M. H. Mazumdar, *Eugenics, Human Genetics and Human Failings: The Eugenics Society, its Sources and its Critics in Britain* (London, 1992); and George W. Stocking, *Race, Culture and Evolution: Essays in the History of Anthropology* (Chicago, 1982).

[31] George W. Stocking, *Victorian Anthropology* (London, 1991), 45.   [32] Ibid.

[33] Houston Stewart Chamberlain, *The Foundations of the Nineteenth Century*, trans. John Lees (New York, 1968), 318.

[34] Charles Creighton, 'Address in Pathology: On the Autonomous Life of the Specific Infections', *BMJ*, 2 (1883), 218–24, at 221.

[35] Leo Loeb, 'The Cancer Problem', *Interstate Medical Journal*, 17 (1910), 376–91, at 376.

and more of the civilized *way of living*. Director of the Imperial Cancer Research Fund (ICRF), E. F. Bashford, insisted that there was nothing intrinsic in the bodies of Black people that made them immune to cancer—nor, as some people suggested, had they been infected by contact with cancer-carrying colonialists—but rather it was due to their conditions of life.[36] He wrote:

> I venture to assert that the prevalence of cancer among the negroes of America was not brought about contact with cancer-infested white men...Cancer was inherent in the negroes when they were shipped from their native Africa, where it probably existed as it still does to-day, in natives removed from civilisation.[37]

There was, therefore, something 'carcinogenic' in civilized habits.

Dangerous Diets

Some suggested that the increasing incidence of the disease in civilized nations was because their societies had departed from nature and 'natural' ways of living. Drawing on a new, late nineteenth-century preoccupation with the relationship among food, wealth, poverty, and disease, the idea that certain diets could make populations prone to cancer was widespread at the end of the nineteenth century.[38] For example, eating was central to ideas about the civilized versus the uncivilized lifestyle. Hill-Climo wrote in 1903: 'there is a strong presumption that it is the food which is at fault'.[39] This correlation could take many forms. James Braithwaite suggested in the *BMJ* that cancer was caused by an 'excess of salt in the diet'.[40] Similarly, a pair of colonial doctors claimed that tea drinking was to blame for an increase in incidence in New Zealand.[41] There was also a popular strand of thought that located the cause of cancer—and its increased incidence—in the consumption of meat, and various doctors, food scientists, and social commentators—including the founder of the popular cereal brand, John Harvey Kellogg—advocated for vegetarianism as a preventative measure against malignancy, as well as against a whole range of other maladies:

[36] E. F. Bashford, 'An Address Entitled Are the Problems of Cancer Insoluble?', *BMJ*, 2 (1905), 1507–11, at 1510.

[37] Ibid.

[38] Agnes Arnold-Forster, 'The Pre-History of the Paleo Diet: Cancer and Dietary Innovation in Nineteenth-Century Britain', in David Gentilcore and Matthew Smith (eds.), *Proteins, Pathologies, and Politics* (London, 2018).

[39] Hill-Climo, 'Cancer in Ireland', 411.

[40] James Braithwaite, 'Excess of Salt as a Cause of Cancer', *BMJ*, 2 (1902), 1376–7, at 1376.

[41] P. W. Hislop and P. Clennell Fenwick, 'Cancer in New Zealand', *BMJ*, 2 (1909), 1222–5, esp. 1225.

During the last 45 years the writer has had unusual opportunities for observation in relation to the influence of a non-flesh dietary upon the occurrence of cancer. Of many thousands of flesh-abstainers with whom he has been acquainted, he has known during this period of only four cases of cancer in persons who had been for a long time flesh abstainers... There can be no doubt that among the thousands of persons under observation who escape the disease, as the writer believes through flesh abstaining, there must have been a considerable number who were especially susceptible to cancer because of heredity and who were able to overcome this special susceptibility by a non-flesh dietary.[42]

Cancer-causing diets seemed to cluster around the civilized end of the spectrum, whereas communities that seemed relatively immune tended to eat uncivilized, simple foods. Uncivilized people were less vulnerable to malignancy because they lived in harmony with the natural world and pursued simple, abstemious habits. Uncivilized communities tended to avoid decadent or artificial food, tracked closely to nature, and so avoided cancer. Surgical Registrar to The Middlesex Hospital, W. Roger Williams, wrote in 1902:

The reputation of Egypt for comparative immunity from cancer is well founded... The conditions of existence are unfavourable to the development of cancer. If I am asked to define these conditions, it may be answered that they comprise extreme frugality in living; open-air existence, and last—but not least—an alimentation which includes but little animal food.[43]

The low incidence of cancer in Egypt could be explained by its inhabitants' uncivilized lifestyles—its stable cancer epidemic was a product of the country's static relationship with nature and its stationary position on the gradient of societal progress. However, changing diets were also used to explain the shifting shapes of national or regional cancer epidemics. For example, Hill-Climo mulled over the relatively low, but nonetheless rising, cancer incidence in Ireland. For while the disease was less common among Celtic communities than its English counterparts, it nonetheless appeared to be increasing: 'It is clear that two questions require to be investigated; the first is that cancer has steadily increased in Ireland during the past forty years, and the second is that the mortality is much lower than in England and in Scotland.'[44] His answer to both these questions, 'paradoxical as it may appear', was the *poverty* of the Irish people'.[45] Commenters

---

[42] John Harvey Kellogg, *The New Dietetics, What to Eat and How: A Guide to Scientific Feeding in Health and Disease* (Battle Creek, MI, 1921), 793.
[43] W. Roger Williams, 'Cancer in Egypt and the Causation of Cancer', *BMJ*, 2 (1902), 917.
[44] Hill-Climo, 'Cancer in Ireland', 413.
[45] Ibid.; historian Ian Miller has explored the vexed question of diet in post-famine Ireland, although he neglected the role Ireland played in conceptualizations of cancer, consumption, and civilization. Ian

from Linnaeus to Lapouge suggested European populations could be separated along biological lines. Like their northern Celtic counterparts, people from the Mediterranean were understood as physically inferior—'Homo Alpinus' rather than 'Homo Europaeus'—and seen as closer in quality to the less-civilized races of warmer climes. Northern Italians sometimes said that Calabria evoked Africa; the South was cast as a form of 'other' world.[46] The Irish were similarly racialized, caricatured in the British press with simian noses, long upper lips, huge projecting mouths, and sloping foreheads.[47]

Hill-Climo harked back to an imagined, pre-lapsarian phase in Irish history: 'Before the Irish famine the Irish lived on oatmeal porridge, potatoes, eggs and milk, with fish and home-cured bacon occasionally.'[48] He believed that this simpler, less decadent diet was less likely to initiate cancer but lamented that the Irish had lost touch with their wholesome culinary past: 'Now, cheap American bacon and flour pancakes cooked in bacon fat, Indian meal porridge sweetened with chemically-coloured beet sugars, and boiled tea are the stable food commodities of the people.'[49] This quotation reveals a complex coalescing of anxieties over food, cancer, national borders, and imperial coherence. Some were concerned by the potentially pathological results of importing refrigerated meat to the British Isles from overseas dominions and other countries. In 1897, the MP for Dorset North, Mr Wingfield-Digby, proclaimed in the House of Commons that 'the consumers of frozen meat were liable to cancer and other terrible diseases'.[50] This anxiety was in part a product of an increased awareness of food as a vector for disease—for example, contemporary concerns that contaminated milk communicated typhoid.[51] Hill-Climo shared in this specific anxiety over meat and argued that 'cancerous diseases...are caused by the long-continued consumption of unwholesome animal food'.[52] Although it was unclear what he thought had corrupted this animal food—was it something inherent in the animal-ness of the product, its overseas passage, or its foreignness? In their review of Hill-Climo's argument, the *BMJ* was deeply unimpressed that 'such an important medical proposition' had been first printed 'in a lay journal, in which it cannot be conveniently subjected to skilled criticism'.[53] They recognized the impact such a

Miller, *Reforming Food in Post-Famine Ireland: Medicine, Science, and Improvement, 1845–1922* (Manchester, 2014).
[46] Pick, *Faces of Degeneration*, 114.
[47] L. P. Curtis, *Apes and Angels: The Irishman in Victorian Caricature* (Washington, DC, 1971), 29.
[48] 'Cancer in Ireland: An Economical Question', *BMJ*, 2 (1903), 1544.   [49] Ibid.
[50] HC Deb., vol. 48, cc677–711, 7 April 1897.
[51] See Jacob Steere-Williams, 'The Perfect Food and the Filth Disease: Milk-Borne Typhoid and Epidemiological Practice in Late Victorian Britain', *Journal of the History of Medicine and Allied Sciences*, 65 (2010), 514–45; and Keir Waddington, 'The Dangerous Sausage: Diet, Meat and Disease in Victorian and Edwardian Britain', *Cultural and Social History*, 8 (2011), 51–71.
[52] Hill-Climo, 'Cancer in Ireland', 1544.
[53] 'Cancer in Ireland: An Economical Question', 1544.

claim could make on the imaginations of the *Empire Review*'s middle-class readership. While they were damming about the veracity of Hill-Climo's claims, the damage had been done.

The bacon, porridge, and tea that Hill-Climo was worried about were all foreign products, imported into Ireland across expanses of land and sea. He was distressed at the 'want of variety' in the food and its unwholesomeness. He argued that the imported flour was 'inferior' and 'wanting in freshness'.[54] This could reveal a generic anxiety over anything alien and introduced from elsewhere. However, it is telling that he noted that the process by which these goods had arrived in Ireland was dependent on 'modern economic conditions'. He blamed technological change, claiming that the shift in diet had 'been facilitated by steam transport'.[55] Hill-Climo was evidently troubled by the possibility that communication and transport technologies—the very fabric of British success and imperial dominion—could be the source of its undoing. The departure by the Irish from their 'natural' diets, facilitated by technologies that imported civilization and its attendant consumables from countries like the United States of America, had made these people vulnerable to cancer.

This theme recurred throughout medical writing at the end of the nineteenth century and was accompanied by an anxiety over the appropriateness of importing diet and lifestyles to indigenous communities. W. Renner wrote about the Creole populations of Sierra Leone: 'The descendants of the liberated Africans.' He claimed that there was an increase in cancer among them, in contrast with the disease's 'apparent rarity among the aborigines in the colony and in the hinterland of Sierra Leone'.[56] Renner's argument was that this was due to the influences of European civilization and the adoption of the 'European mode of living': 'The existence of cancer and other malignant growths among the creoles, and its absence or rarity among the aborigines, are due in my opinion to the civilised habits of, and the civilising influences operating upon, the former, and to the primitive mode of living of the latter.'[57] Renner was concerned that changes in lifestyle were making the Creoles more prone to cancer:

> The creoles have adopted the mode of living, the food and dress, of the Europeans—have to a great extent discarded the simple food of their forefathers, have been craving for and indulging in preserved and imported foreign food—have substituted the European for the natural African environment, and entailed on themselves in their eager pursuit for wealth and luxury the anxieties and worries incidental to civilization and consequent liability to premature decline.[58]

Cancer accompanied a societal departure from nature.

---

[54] Hill-Climo, 'Cancer in Ireland', 414.   [55] Ibid., 413.
[56] Renner, 'The Spread of Cancer', 588.   [57] Ibid.   [58] Ibid.

This sentiment was echoed by Sir William MacGregor in *The Lancet*: 'For nine and a half years I never saw a case of cancer in British New Guinea, but at the end of that time there occurred an example of encephaloid cancer of the tibia in the person of a Papuan who had for seven or eight years lived practically a European life.'[59] W. Roger Williams made parallel arguments about African and Native Americans:

In their native habitat negroes appear to be almost exempt from cancer. Transplanted to the United States, and living there in slavery—with hard work and frugal diet—cancer was not common among them, although they then became subject to it. Since the abolition of slavery, however, and the altered habits thus entailed, the United States negroes have become almost as prone to cancer as their white neighbours.[60]

Similarly, 'The North American Indians were in their natural state exempt from cancer; but, in proportion as they have adopted civilised ways of living, they have become increasingly prone to cancer.'[61]

Renner framed his analysis as concern for the well-being of the Creole population. However, it can instead be read as an invective against populations deviating from their 'proper' and 'natural' state of existence. In 'their eager pursuit for wealth and luxury', the Creoles were subverting the hierarchy inherent in the British Empire's system of rulers and ruled and suffering increased rates of cancer as a result. Renner was reflecting commonly held views at the end of the nineteenth and beginning of the twentieth centuries. His concerns manifested widespread beliefs about the deterministic powers of landscape, environment, and locale in constructing bodies and habits, as well as the danger inherent in living in conflict with your surroundings and outside the bounds of your 'natural' means. However, Renner was clearly ambivalent about the changing living conditions of the Creoles. Increased cancer incidence was obviously problematic, but it had somehow become implicated in the British Empire's civilizing mission.

In these debates about changing diets, lifestyles, and cancer incidence, some commentators used animals as a proxy for human variance. This comparative exercise rested on the assumption that cancer was the same disease in both humans and animals.[62] Animal health was used as a metaphor for the cancer scale, emphasizing the causal relationship between the disease and civilization. Wild animals were discursively connected to 'wild' or 'uncivilized' peoples and

---

[59] MacGregor, 'Some Problems of Tropical Medicine', 1059.

[60] Williams, 'Cancer in Egypt', 917.   [61] Ibid., 917.

[62] Olt Giesson wrote in the *Journal of Comparative Pathology and Therapeutics*: 'Cancer in domestic animals exactly corresponds histogenetically with that of man.' Olt Giessen, 'Cancer in Domestic Animals', *Journal of Comparative Pathology and Therapeutics*, 18 (1905), 278–9, at 278.

parallels drawn between 'civilized' man and domesticated creatures: 'Cancer is by no means an uncommon disease among the domesticated animals, while in wild animals and uncivilized man it is rare.'[63] W. Roger Williams claimed: 'I have never met with a single instance of cancer in any wild animal in a state of nature, and I know of no duly authenticated case of the kind that has ever been recorded in the literature of the subject.'[64] Animals living in 'a state of nature' were immune whereas those under human control were more vulnerable. If you brought a wild creature into a domestic context—a farm or a zoo, for example—its vulnerability to cancer increased. Williams wrote: 'It is, of course, well known that wild animals that have been kept long in confinement may be thus affected.'[65] In this context, care and intrusion had pathological potential and artificial environments might be carcinogenic (a term invented at the beginning of the twentieth century). All three case studies—Ireland, Sierra-Leone, and domesticated animals—demonstrated that imported modernity was damaging to the health of the uncivilized. This conclusion fed into discourses of decadence and degeneration. It confirmed the idea that as humans (and creatures) moved further from their intended style of life—customs, diet, relationship with nature—they were increasingly susceptible to the ravages of cancer.

This explanatory model—that negatively correlated 'nature' and the natural with cancer—was powerful if paradoxical. It chimed with widespread contemporary anxieties over the dangers inherent in industrialized, artificial, and urban life. Much has been written about the late nineteenth-century preoccupation with 'diseases of modern life'.[66] There was widespread anxiety about the negative influence of civilization on the minds and bodies of the urban bourgeoisie. Dr James Crichton-Browne spoke in 1860 of the 'velocity of thought and action' now required, and of the stresses imposed on the brain forced to process in a month more information 'than was required of our grandfathers in the course of a lifetime'.[67] Charles E. Rosenberg has argued that concern for the 'psychic dangers of an artificial and emotionally fevered life' had become conventional by the mid-century.[68] Commentators observed an increase in diseases from worry, overwork, mental or physical strain, excess, self-abuse, stimulants, and narcotics. They diagnosed neurosis, hysteria, and melancholy on a mass scale, and articulated modern, urban life as inherently risky. However, this conclusion was seemingly at odds with the claims of the domestic map-makers surveyed in Chapter 5, who

[63] Dunn, 'The Increase of Cancer'.

[64] W. Roger Williams, 'Cancer in Wild Animals', *The Lancet*, 154 (1899), 1194.   [65] Ibid.

[66] See Sally Shuttleworth, Melissa Dickson, and Emilie Taylor-Brown (eds.), *Progress and Pathology: Medicine and Culture in the Nineteenth Century* (Manchester, 2020) This book includes my chapter '"A Rebellion of the Cells": Cancer, Modernity, and Decline in Fin-de-Siècle Britain'.

[67] See https://diseasesofmodernlife.org/, accessed 25 August 2017.

[68] Rosenberg, 'Pathologies of Progress', 718.

found cancer to be most common in areas of bucolic beauty—not the over-crowded, fast-paced metropolis.[69]

We are, however, dealing with different communities of medical men, scientists, and social commentators. While they might have been writing at the same time, and shared the same broader professional space, they held competing, even contradictory views. The men just described were, as with any nineteenth-century medical practitioner, invested in invoking cancer in support of their own aims and ideologies. The disease's easy inclusion in the discourses of degeneration and the dangers of artifice reveal the power of cancer and its ability to act as proxy for a range of socio-cultural debates. Cancer was, it seems, a meaningful 'example' for practitioners eager to convince others of the unintended costs of civilization to use. That is not to say, however, that cancer's relationship with this broader fin-de-siècle debate was easy or simplistic. There were facets to the correlation between civilization and malignancy that were specific to cancer and its peculiar characteristics. While the historiography about the cultural, scientific, and medical discourses of the period has tended to highlight the problems of youth, the increasingly fraught and prevalent idea that cancer was a disease of senescence reveals a late nineteenth-century preoccupation with the premature deaths of people past their childbearing years that has hitherto gone unrecognized.

The 'Cancer Age'

An association between age and cancer is present in eighteenth-century tracts and treatises. It was the subject of one of the Society and Institution for Investigating the Nature and Cure of Cancer's thirteen queries (see Chapter 2).[70] Query eleven asked, 'Is there any period of life absolutely exempt from the attack of this disease?' Sir Thomas Bernard answered: 'It seems to be generally admitted to be most frequent in old or advanced in age.'[71] The disease was seen as particularly threatening to post-menopausal women.[72] Irish surgeon Walter Hayle Walshe extended this claim in the 1840s: 'the mortality [from cancer] goes on steadily

[69] Anthropologist Erin O'Connor argues that while Victorian physicians understood cancer as a disease of modernity, they forged 'strong linguistic associations between breast cancer and urban culture'. While I agree that in the second half of the nineteenth century, 'the language of cancer began to be filled with the very words and phrases that were being used to describe the special problems arising from England's massive, rapid, and deeply troubling economic growth', I suggest that observers were as interested in the rural as they were in the urban. Erin O'Connor, *Raw Material: Producing Pathology in Victorian Culture* (Durham, 2000), 61 and 63.

[70] See Chapter 2, 'Incurability and the Clinic'.

[71] Thomas Bernard, 'Extract from an Account of the Institution for Investigating the Nature and Cure of Cancer', in *Reports of the Society for Bettering the Condition and Increasing the Comforts of the Poor*, vol. 3 (London, 1802), 388.

[72] Thomas Denman, *Observations on the Cure of Cancer; with some Remarks upon Mr Young's Treatment of that Disease* (London, 1816), 43.

increasing with each succeeding decade, until the eightieth year'.[73] In the 1870s, surgeon and pathologist James Paget made a similar claim: 'Cancer is a disease of degeneracy, the frequency of which increases as the years increase.'[74] With the increasing anxiety over rising cancer rates after c.1880, 'the peculiar age-incidence' of the disease attracted new attention.[75]

E. F. Bashford argued that the cancer-causing qualities of civilization were, paradoxically, its ability to procure and maintain long life. He suggested 'civilised man's responsibility for the occurrence of cancer in native races...was in all probability limited to providing them with an opportunity for reach the "cancer ages"'.[76] Medical men and social commentators had similar conversations about animal cancer. Unlike wild animals, for whom 'the struggle for existence' constrained their life expectancies, those domesticated animals—particularly 'pet dogs and cats and horses'—who were allowed to 'attain old age' were increasingly susceptible to cancer.[77] Bashford wrote: 'Man's responsibility in regard to domestic animals may, for all we know to the contrary, be limited to the provision of opportunities for reaching the cancer age.'[78] While some people found this encouraging and developed a positive narrative around the concept of the 'cancer age' (discussed in 'Progress and Fin de Siècle Medical Optimism'), others saw something more sinister.

The concept of the 'cancer age'—the period of life when people were presumed to become particularly vulnerable to the disease—was pregnant with meaning for the late nineteenth-century observer. There were clear parallels to be drawn between a healthy body ultimately succumbing to disorder, and a prosperous nation or empire suffering inevitable deterioration. As Hutchinson lamented: 'To a twelfth of us who have passed the age of forty it is indeed a riddle of the Sphinx, for unless we solve it, it will destroy us.'[79] In a climate of widespread anxiety over the vigour of empire and concerns over imperial overstretch, 'life-cycle' metaphors were increasingly used to reflect on the waxing and waning of empires, past and present.[80] In 1907, the *Contemporary Review* began an article:

---

[73] Walter Hayle Walshe, *The Nature and Treatment of Cancer* (London, 1846), 149.

[74] Quoted in Hugh P. Dunn, 'An Inquiry into the Causes of the Increase of Cancer (Continued)', *BMJ*, 1 (1883), 761–3, at 761.

[75] E. F. Bashford, 'The Investigations of the Imperial Cancer Research Fund', *BMJ*, 2 (1906), 1554–5, at 1554.

[76] Bashford, 'An Address Entitled Are the Problems of Cancer Insoluble?', 1509.

[77] E. F. Bashford, 'The Problems of Cancer', *BMJ*, 2 (1903), 127–9, at 128.   [78] Ibid.

[79] Woods Hutchinson, 'The Cancer Problem: Or, Treason in the Republic of the Body', *Contemporary Review*, 76 (1899), 105–17, at 105.

[80] This was exacerbated by the failings of the British Army during the Boer War in South Africa (1899–1902), where they faced near defeat at the hands of a force that was barely trained. Ornella Moscucci, 'Gender and Cancer in Britain, 1860–1910: The Emergence of Cancer as a Public Health Concern', *American Journal of Public Health*, 95 (2005), 1312–21, at 1318.

It is a question which has been often discussed, and to which men's minds have often turned of late, whether States and nations have, like individual men, their necessary periods of infancy, childhood, adolescence, and old age, to be followed, in the one case as in the other, by death, which is the end of all.[81]

The author continued the 'life-cycle' analogy and peppered his article with medical metaphors: 'It is quite certain that States are liable to something which we may without any strained analogy call disease.' He described nations who had succumbed to 'fierce attacks of fever', 'raving madness', or who had 'died of over-work'.[82]

This was a clever rhetorical apparatus, but it also hinted towards a practical and prevalent concern over the possibility that disease might undermine a great empire. In the early 1900s, the fight against cancer became closely identified with Britain's imperial interests. Mirroring developments in other Western countries, the British debate over the quality of national stock and the future of the 'imperial breed' invigorated anxiety over chronic disease and its negative effects on the imperial labour force. That cancer primarily affected the mature elements of the population had dire potential consequences. Unlike tuberculosis, 'the special foe of the young', cancer attacked 'mature lives in full bearing, which represents society's greatest capital in the share of work and energy'.[83] The cancer epidemic, and its specific age profile, encouraged a new, concerted effort on behalf of state and state-sanctioned institutions to eradicate the disease. Encouraged by the idea that perhaps the British Empire might be entering its senescence and thus its 'cancer age', in 1902, an MP tabled the appointment of a Royal Commission on Cancer along 'similar lines to that which has been appointed to inquire in Tuberculosis'.[84] Philanthropic support for cancer research and treatment in Britain came from men who were playing a key role in the colonial exploitation of mineral resources in South Africa. Julius Wernher, of Wernher, Beit & Co., was instrumental in establishing the ICRF in 1902 (conversely, however, the ICRF's head was convinced that the cancer epidemic was only 'apparent' and interpreted it as a positive indictment of social medicine and public health).[85]

---

[81] Thomas Hodgkin, 'The Fall of the Roman Empire and its Lessons for Us', *Contemporary Review*, 1 January 1898, 51.

[82] Ibid.

[83] Etienne Burnet, *The Campaign against Microbes*, trans. E. E. Austen (London, 1909), 1; the *BMJ* stated in 1903: 'There is no problem in pathology that more urgently calls for solution than the causation of cancer; nor is there any of greater importance in preventive medicine, for the disease seeks its victims not among those whose lives are, in an economic sense, of no value, but in the main among those whose productive power and usefulness to the community are at their highest.' 'The Cure of Cancer', *BMJ*, 1 (1903), 1327–8, at 1327.

[84] HC Deb., vol. 101, cc799–800, 24 January 1902.

[85] Moscucci, 'Gender and Cancer in Britain', 1318.

The cancer epidemic, and its specific age profile, had implications not just for the state of nation and empire, but also for ideas about the body and its internal logic. Just as biological metaphors appeared in political rhetoric, political metaphors entered biological conceptualizations. As shown in Chapter 6, cancer was defined as a disease of 'anarchic' cells that threatened the internal stability of the British state. Hutchinson described the malady as 'a rebellion of the cells'.[86] French physician Etienne Burnet styled the disease in similar terms: 'When a cancer is discovered in the body, anarchy may have been said to have arisen in the community, and everything is in confusion.'[87] This is a declinist narrative of the body—hitherto governed by order and progress, now entropy takes over and descends into chaos. Drawing on cell theory, these evocative descriptions personify the cancer cell: 'In a cancer we have cells and nothing but cells, which refuse to explain why they have left their places, and have much less the air of policemen than the suspicious demeanour of vagabonds.'[88] In this metaphor, the cells are agents of degeneration—*in* them and *by them* diseases are made.

Thus, cancer increasingly signalled to a troubled medical profession that perhaps disease—specifically degenerative diseases of cancer's type—might be an essential element of the human body—and, by extension—an unavoidable component of modern society. Thus, the 'cancer age' was a troubling indication that perhaps this period of British civilization was concomitant with chronic and incurable disease. Cellular models of malignancy—mapped on to social and political discourse—suggested that both bodies and states might reach a natural limit. Latent in late nineteenth-century cancer discourse was a version of planned obsolescence, a modernist notion that objects (or maybe bodies) had mechanisms for collapse built in to allow for the successive intervention of new models (or new selves/civilizations).[89] The body held within it the apparatus of its own decline: 'Cells are the bricks of which the Metazoan edifice is constructed, but that edifice is also the manufactory for their construction, and the laboratory for their destruction.'[90] In 1912, cytologist Charles E. Walker wrote about the body in terms of 'destiny' and pre-determined futures: 'Apparently all the somatic or body cells are destined to disintegrate within a limited space of time.'[91] Cancer was, according to the philosopher P. Topinard, a 'necessary evil'—a fundamental, even essential, component of the civilized body and the civilized society.[92]

[86] Hutchinson, 'The Cancer Problem', 106.   [87] Burnet, *The Campaign against Microbes*, 2–3.
[88] Ibid., 4.
[89] Henry Berry, *From Revolution to Fads: The Progress of Modernity* (Bloomington, IN, 2001), 206–11.
[90] 'Review: The Microscope in Medicine, by Lionel S. Beale', *American Naturalist*, 16 (1882), 500–4, at 503.
[91] Charles Walker, 'Theories and Problems of Cancer: Part III', *Science Progress in the Twentieth Century (1906–1916)*, 7 (1912), 223–8, at 224.
[92] P. Topinard, 'The Social Problem (Concluded)', *The Monist*, 9 (1898), 63–100, at 70.

Progress and Fin de Siècle Medical Optimism

In 1893, George King and Arthur Newsholme published a thirty-three-page article entitled 'On the Alleged Increase of Cancer' in the *Proceedings of the Royal Society of London*.[93] The introduction sculpted the shape and profile of the debate in the late nineteenth century: 'During the last few years the minds of medical men and of the general public has been exercised over the rapid and striking increase in the mortality from cancer, as shown by the statistics contained in the Registrar-General's Annual Reports.'[94] However, they were there to offer a rebuttal. They presented a careful consideration of the GRO's data and summarized many of the key critiques of the supposed increase in the incidence of cancer. Their rebuttal suggests that while many understood the increase in incidence as manifesting national and imperial decline, equal numbers took the cancer epidemic as only 'apparent'—a product of statistical error and demographic changes. Indeed, at the end of the nineteenth century prominent statisticians and public health experts like John Tatham, George King, and Arthur Newsholme all claimed that improved public health practices and an increasingly efficient and effective medical profession was responsible for the nation's shifting disease profile. Cancer was increasingly presented as a disease of health—of individual body, the body politic, and the state.

These men put forward an alternative causal link between civilization and increased cancer incidence. For them, the cancer epidemic did not accord to the well-travelled terrain of societal degeneration and decline, but instead manifested medical progress and improvement. Just as the fin-de-siècle debate over the causes and implications of the 'cancer epidemic' acted as proxy for a broader conversation about imperial overstretch and decline, it was also a stand-in for a discussion about the past, present, and future of medicine and its contributions to society. The idea that the nineteenth century had witnessed a transformation in the efficacy and humanity of British medicine and society was widespread. The fin de siècle was, therefore, a moment of simultaneous reflection and prediction. Medical men looked back on a distant past of barbarism and a recent history of rapid scientific progress. At the same time, they looked forward, and laced their rhetoric with optimism and utopianism. This period was, therefore, conceptualized as a turning point in medical theory and practice. While those preoccupied with degeneration and decline imagined the end of the nineteenth century as the 'old age' of the British nation and empire, those who proclaimed the progress and advance of medical science and practice thought of the period as 'the childhood of the world'.[95] As before, such 'life-cycle' metaphors were common. Cyrus Edson

---

[93] George King and Arthur Newsholme, 'On the Alleged Increase of Cancer', *Proceedings of the Royal Society of London*, 54 (1893), 209–42.
[94] Ibid., 209.   [95] 'Recent Advances in Medicine', *Science*, 17 (1891), 170–1, at 171.

wrote in the *Los Angeles Times*: 'Physicians who practiced at an earlier period look back to it, as men remember their childhood, in wonderment at their former ignorance, and the men and women who submitted to the treatment of those days are sometimes lost in amazement at the feats accomplished by modern practitioners.'[96]

In 1891, *Science* painted a familiar portrait of historic failure and present progress and improvement: 'Emancipated from the thralldom of authority in which it was fast bound for centuries, medicine has progressed with extraordinary rapidity, and even within the present generation has undergone a complete revolution.'[97] The nineteenth century was repeatedly framed—by both professionals and the laity—as a period that had seen unique scientific, public health, and therapeutic progress. An article published in the *Ladies' Cabinet* stated: 'Truly this may be called "the iron age": and is it not fast approaching to "the golden" one? How fast and earnest are the efforts which philanthropists have, for the last twenty of thirty years, been making to ameliorate the mental and bodily sufferings of their fellow creatures!'[98] It proclaimed that 'there is no class of men more thoughtfully and *actively* benevolent than those belonging to the medical profession'.[99] J. W. Byer wrote in 1901:

> It is, therefore, only natural that we should seize upon the present as a suitable time to look backwards, and to ask how have obstetric medicine and gynaecology advanced during the nineteenth century, a period more fertile in the results of scientific research than that of almost all the years that have gone before.[100]

Regius Professor of Medicine at the University of Oxford, William Osler, turned from past, to present, to future in his 1906 work *Science and Immortality*. He described the recent history of progress: 'Within the lifetime of some of us, Science—physical, chemical, and biological—has changed the aspect of the world, changed it more effectively and more permanently than all the efforts of man in all preceding generation. The control of physical energies, the biological revolution, and the good start which has been made in a warfare against disease, were the three great achievements of the nineteenth century, each one of which has had a profound and far-reaching influence on almost every relationship in the life of man.'[101] However, he acknowledged that the 'warfare against disease' was only just beginning and positioned himself at the beginning of a new period in

---

[96] Cyrus Edson, 'The Art of Healing: Marvelous Progress Made in the Science of Medicine', *Los Angeles Times*, 28 January 1900, 4.

[97] 'Recent Advances in Medicine', 170.

[98] Valentine Bartholomew, 'Dr Fell versus Cancer', *Ladies' Cabinet*, 1 November 1856, 268.

[99] Ibid.

[100] J. W. Byer, 'Introductory Remarks by the President on Puerperal Fever, Uterine Cancer, and the Falling Birth Rate', *BMJ*, 2 (1901), 941–3, at 941.

[101] William Osler, *Science and Immortality* (London, 1906), 13–14.

medical history: 'We have entered another century in an attitude of tremulous expectation, and with a feeling of confidence.'[102] As *Science* had stated in the previous decade, any progress would be 'gradual', and while medical men might suffer 'many disappointments', society must not be impatient, as 'science moves but slowly, slowly creeping from point to point'.[103] The article was, nonetheless, optimistic about the future: 'Some of the brightest hopes of humanity are with the medical profession. To it, not to law or theology, belong the promises. Disease will always be with us, but we may look forward confidently to the time where epidemics shall be no more, when typhoid shall be as rare as typhus, and tuberculosis as leprosy.'[104]

To an extent, this vision of medical triumph reflected a reality. The late Victorian and Edwardian periods witnessed a decline in mortality—particularly from infectious diseases—attributed by Thomas McKeown to rising living standards and increases in per capita nutritional consumption and by Simon Szreter to an 'expansion in health infrastructure', albeit in the absence of advanced medical or clinical technology.[105] This climate of self-satisfied enthusiasm primed the medical community to interpret the increase in cancer incidence as a positive indictment of their practice and profession. Specific causes for the cancer epidemic were found, particularly by public health practitioners, in improved public health intervention, increased life expectancy, reduced infant mortality, better health surveillance, and more accurate diagnosis. In 1907, Dr John Tatham of the GRO reflected on the achievements of public health practice over the last half-century in the *Supplement to the Sixty-Fifth Annual Report of the Registrar-General*: 'That the state of the public health in England and Wales has greatly improved in recent years is attested by the steady decrease of mortality that has taken place since the passing of the first Public Health Act [in 1848].'[106] In his coverage of the 1881–90 'Registrar-General's Decennial Supplement in the Journal of the Royal Statistical Society', Noel A. Humphreys was emphatic: 'The report displays unmistakable evidence of satisfactory health progress in England and Wales during the ten years with which it deals.'[107] Tatham recorded in his 'Supplement': 'In the decennium under present consideration an average annual saving of 540 lives has been achieved in each million of the population of England and Wales.'[108] Many of these lives saved belonged to infants. The increase in life

---

[102] Ibid., 14.   [103] 'Recent Advances in Medicine', 171.   [104] Ibid.

[105] Simon Szreter, 'The Importance of Social Intervention in Britain's Mortality Decline c. 1850–1914: A Re-Interpretation of the Role of Public Health', *Social History of Medicine*, 1 (2012), 1–38, at 37.

[106] John Tatham, 'Letter to the Registrar-General on the Mortality in England and Wales in the Period of Ten Years 1891–1900', in *Supplement to the Sixty-Fifth Annual Report of the Registrar-General of Births, Deaths, and Marriages in England and Wales, 1891–1900, Part One* (London, 1907), x.

[107] Noel A. Humphreys, 'The Registrar-General's Decennial Supplement, 1881–90', *Journal of the Royal Statistical Society*, 59 (1896), 543–6, at 544.

[108] Tatham, 'Letter to the Registrar-General', lxxi.

expectancy was attributed to the falling death rate. The 'Supplement' displayed 'unmistakable evidence of satisfactory health progress in England and Wales during the ten years with which it deals'.[109] Indeed, an undercurrent of optimism and self-satisfaction—verging occasionally on utopianism—ran through fin-de-siècle medical writing.

This optimism could be invoked in reinterpretations of the 'cancer age'. While many commenters assessed the rise in cancer incidence as 'real', for some it manifested neutral or even positive things about British society and statecraft. Rather than a troubling indication of imperial decline, it was instead proof of significant public health successes—longer life expectancies and a reduction in infant mortality. The increased likelihood that a child would survive to adulthood was taken as a potential cause for inflated cancer rates: 'It is now necessary to proceed to the consideration of the general mortality amongst the infant popula-tion, and its bearing upon the increase of cancer.'[110] Surgeon Hugh P. Dunn went on to remind that reader 'that for some time there has been a notable reduction in the death-rate in early life, which in England has been almost maintained'. Such a reduction 'has resulted in swelling the ranks of those who survive the exigencies of early life and pass to adult age'.[111] Thus, Dunn suggested an inverse relationship between infant and cancer mortality: 'It would appear that there are good grounds for believing that there is some connection between the infantile mortality on the one hand, and the cancer mortality on the other.'[112]

In slight contrast, others argued that the 'cancer epidemic' was only 'apparent'. The GRO—committed to health statistics as a means of social measurement and management—suggested that the perceived increase in cancer incidence was a result of improved health surveillance (circumventing the problem of clinical management). This surveillance came—or so they said—in the form of better diagnostic abilities, increased hospitalization, and more comprehensive and accurate death certification. In the decennial supplement to the sixty-fifth annual report, Tatham reminded readers: 'It must be borne in mind . . . that the increase of cancer mortality shown in the table is, to some extent, and probably to a large extent, due to the more favourable opportunities of correct diagnosis which have become available in recent years.'[113] Thus, just as those men described in 'Degeneration, Decline, and Disease' and 'Dangerous Diets' were invested in invoking cancer in support of their ideologies of imperial decline and national degeneration, public health practitioners were eager to marshal cancer as evidence for their professional success.

With better diagnostic techniques and improved skill, medical men were making it 5appear as though cancer was increasing. King and Newsholme agreed,

[109] Humphreys, 'The Registrar-General's Decennial Supplement', 544.
[110] Dunn, 'An Inquiry into the Causes of the Increase of Cancer', 762.   [111] Ibid.   [112] Ibid.
[113] Tatham, 'Letter to the Registrar-General', cii.

and argued that the increase in cancer incidence was because the medical community had improved in their investigative ability—that deaths previously attributed to other causes, or not explained at all, were now being correctly assigned to cancer: 'The increase in cancer is only apparent and not real, and is due to improvement in diagnosis and more careful certification of the causes of death.'[114] Tatham gave a detailed example of the impact of incorrect diagnosis on the recorded rates of cancer:

> To the total mortality from *cancer or malignant disease*, 6,353 deaths, of which 5,255 had been originally attributed to tumour, 574 to stricture of oesophagus, 42 to haemorrhage, 30 to dyspepsia, and 22 to atrophy; whilst 70 deaths had been certified as from surgical causes, without further specification.[115]

That the increase in incidence could be explained by improved detection was proven by 'the fact that the whole of the increase has taken place in inaccessible cancers difficult to diagnosis, while accessible cancer easily diagnosed has remained practically stationary'.[116] In other words, the increase in cancer incidence recorded in the reports was not uniform. Instead, it was predominantly among cancers affecting internal organs—cancers that had long evaded the detection of the medical profession.

This distinction between 'accessible' and 'inaccessible' cancers was also used to explain discrepancies in the disease's rate of increase in men and women. King and Newsholme claimed that cancer had increased 'in such greater proportion among males'.[117] This was because 'cancer of the special female organs [breasts and genitals]'—those 'most easy of all to diagnose'—had remained stable.[118] Breast cancer had, throughout the nineteenth century, predominated in cancer tracts, treatises, and cases primarily because it was the most visible, tangible, and detectable.[119] The rise in cancers of organs hidden from view was interpreted as the result of improved diagnostic techniques and the increase in post-mortem dissection. Another commenter observed a similar trend in animal cancers: 'A difficulty met with in mankind presents itself in animals in augmented form; cancer in animals is only likely to be recognised during life if it be situated on the visible, readily accessible portions of the body; cancer of the internal organs is only likely to come rarely under observation, viz. at necropsies.'[120] However, this conclusion by public health practitioners and statisticians contradicted their contemporaries working in the clinic who, even into the twentieth century, maintained ambivalence over their ability to accurately diagnose cancer.

---

[114] King and Newsholme, 'On the Alleged Increase of Cancer', 228.
[115] Tatham, 'Letter to the Registrar-General', lxxi.
[116] King and Newsholme, 'On the Alleged Increase of Cancer', 228.   [117] Ibid., 223.
[118] Ibid.   [119] See the Introduction and Chapter 1.
[120] Bashford, 'The Problems of Cancer', 6.

Moreover, there is little evidence to suggest that more people were dying in hospitals at the end of the nineteenth century than they had at the beginning. Instead, much of the perceived increase in incidence was likely more to do with 'more careful certification' than 'improvement in diagnosis'. This was a success of surveillance, not therapeutic mastery.

Indeed, Tatham wrote in 1907: 'In the early years of the last half century a considerable portion of the residents in remote parts of England and Wales died without medical care, and that consequently their deaths were registered as not certified.'[121] That whole swathes of the population were insufficiently monitored artificially reduced the numbers who were recorded as dying of cancer. He attributed the increase in cancer rates directly to legislative innovations that extended the arm of the medical professions: 'The Birth and Death Registration Act, which imposed upon medical practitioners the duty of formally certifying the cause of death of their patients, was not passed until 1874.'[122] For Tatham, this date was a watershed mark in the British cancer epidemic. The defining feature of the disease for this public health practitioner was an expansion in the healing profession's reach. In equating 'medical care' with the ability to certify death (just as they retrospectively diagnosed cancer with mortality—see Chapters 1, 2, and 3), Tatham made clear that he considered this extension a positive innovation.

The presumed improvements in diagnosis and inspection also explained the discrepancies between cancer rates in England and in other, 'less civilized' countries. King and Newsholme attributed the relatively low rates of cancer in Ireland to 'deficient medical attendance'.[123] In such a 'poor country', most inhabitants could not afford hospital attention and would thus escape death certification. Moreover, 'owing to the poverty of the patients and consequently of the medical attendants, the average skill of the general practitioners over large tracts in Ireland is less than in Scotland and England, and this again would lead to defective diagnosis'.[124] Other commenters agreed: 'The discrepancy between the recorded incidence of cancer in England and Wales, and Ireland, exists also in the extent to which cancer is recorded in the hospitals of the two countries.'[125] Autopsies were 'performed with minimal frequency in Irish hospitals, whereas in English hospitals they add largely to the certified number of deaths from cancer'.[126]

Thus, various commentators argued for an inverse relationship between a population's general health and its cancer incidence. In his short essay, 'An Inquiry into the Causes of the Increase of Cancer', surgeon Hugh P. Dunn wrote: 'By means of the enforcement of sanitary laws, the health of the community, as a whole, is immeasurably better than in the days of a civilisation which,

---

[121] Tatham, 'Letter to the Registrar-General', vii.   [122] Ibid.
[123] King and Newsholme, 'On the Alleged Increase of Cancer', 221.   [124] Ibid.
[125] E. F. Bashford, 'Real and Apparent Differences in the Incidence of Cancer', *Transactions of the Epidemiological Society of London*, 26 (1907) 43–77.
[126] Ibid.

though necessarily advancing, was yet in a primitive condition.'[127] Public health intervention inflated the cancer epidemic in two ways. First, it protected the population, allowing them to live longer and so expanded the proportion who contracted cancer. Second, it subjected people to greater surveillance which increased the amount of malignancy detected and recorded. Public health intervention was a marker and a necessary condition of progress. It lengthened lives, averted death from disease, and increased the incidence of cancer. Dunn suggested 'A high general mortality would be associated with a low cancer one.'[128] This mapped on to the conclusions of the cancer cartographers in Chapter 5 who argued the disease prevailed in healthful, bucolic, and rural regions of the country. Hutchinson was succinct in his analysis of the question of cancer and national health: 'Paradoxical as it may sound, [cancer's] greater prevalence is a symptom of increasing longevity and vigour on the part of the community. Cancer is the price paid for longer life.'[129] Dunn went even further: 'As far as statistics are capable of showing, the cancer-rate of a country may generally be accepted as the index of its healthiness.'[130] The cancer epidemic thus demonstrated that the English were better at surveying their population, better at governance, and had a more sophisticated state apparatus than their European counterparts. This all constituted a prime example of Victorian mental gymnastics—turning the tragedy of cancer into a triumph of Anglo-Saxon civilization.

Conclusion

To some extent, this chapter has incorporated cancer into a well-trodden narrative of late- century preoccupation with degeneration and decline. Together, these various contexts and sources of evidence suggested to anxious observers that civilization—rather than an agent of medical progress—was, instead, the cause of the 'cancer epidemic'—the country's greatest pathological foe. Contemporaries began to conceptualize cancer as a 'pathology of progress': 'civilisation appears to be the cause of this disease'.[131] Mapping the global distribution of cancer had suggested that Black people—biologically inferior in every other way—were almost immune to the disease. Cancer incidence subverted the conventional hierarchy between colonizers and colonized and found in 'savage' lifestyles a fundamental redeeming feature. Moreover, cancer increasingly signalled to a

---

[127] Dunn, 'An Inquiry into the Causes of the Increase of Cancer', 708.   [128] Ibid., 762.
[129] Hutchinson, 'The Cancer Problem', 115.
[130] Dunn, 'An Inquiry into the Causes of the Increase of Cancer', 762; the *New York Daily Tribune* likewise wrote in 1890: 'Cancer is not a disease due to misery, to poverty, to bad sanitary surroundings, to ignorance or to bad habits, but on the contrary, a disease afflicting the cultured, the wealthy and the inhabitants of salubrious localities.' 'Enlarging the Hospital to Relieve Cancer Victims', *New York Daily Tribune*, 20 July 1890.
[131] 'Academy of Sciences, Paris', *Provincial Medical & Surgical Journal*, 8 (1844), 237–9, at 238.

troubled medical profession that perhaps disease (specifically degenerative diseases of cancer's type) might be an essential element of the human body and, by extension, an unavoidable component of modern society. Thus, cancer was particularly troubling to fin-de-siècle observers as it both challenged widely held notions of Anglo-Saxon superiority and fed into discourses of degeneration that were then reaching their zenith.

However, these melodramatic lamentations on the cancer-causing effects of civilization were only one aspect of the landscape. There were powerful counter-arguments to this negativity: peaks to the emotional troughs. Cancer was increasingly perceived as an unintended consequence of public health successes: lower infant mortality, increasing hospitalization, sanitary reform, and greater surveillance of bodies in life and after death. These competing narratives of the cancer epidemic's implications for late Victorian society and bodies coexisted and it is difficult to tell which more accurately represents the public health reality. It is tempting to deny that the 'cancer epidemic' ever even existed. While anxieties about malignancy's burden on society were certainly both profound and productive, the arguments made by the epidemic's detractors are compelling. In part, because they tend to be presented in a more rational rhetorical style—without the histrionics which people like Woods Hutchinson were so fond. One of the jobs of the historian is perhaps to determine which of the many stories people in the past told about their respective epochs is the closest to reality.

However, I am wary of making such pronouncements. Partly because I have no more knowledge at my disposal than the medical men and social commentators writing in the fin de siècle, and partly to avoid a pitfall common to many assessments of historical cancer rates. As argued at both the beginning of this chapter and in the Introduction to this book, cancer's relationship to modernity has often been asserted and only rarely scrutinized. This supposed relationship is both metaphorical—cancer manifests something troubling about progress, civilization, and industrial society—and epidemiological—the disease incidence is supposed to have increased into the twentieth century. This book was always more concerned with the metaphorical than the epidemiological, but one thing that is clear is that knowing the numerical burden of cancer has never been straightforward and continues to challenge public health professionals today. We cannot say with certainty how many people lived with and died from cancer in twentieth-century Britain, any more than we can do so for the nineteenth.

Conclusion

Cancer Then and Now

In the nineteenth century, cancer's incurability was not just an obstacle to overthrow, but a galvanizing and intellectually provocative idea that shifted medicine, health care, and professional identity in profound and lasting ways. It enabled the construction of professional credentials and community values; turned hospitals into places for treating 'terminal' illness; made possible the invention of new forms and rationales of intervention; and brought into being certain modes of investigating the disease such as mapping, the microscope, and discourses of progress and decline. For surgeons, scientists, and social commentators, cancer's incurability was an invaluable opportunity to demonstrate the power and promise of their respective investigative techniques.

Much of this intellectual and practical creativity was driven by optimism—a quality central to the ideals and ideologies of modern medicine. The inevitability of scientific and clinical progress became fundamental to the ideologies of nineteenth-century surgeons and physicians in part because cancer's incurability left them little space for anything else. Without a current cure, those who encountered the relentless suffering of malignancy in the clinic turned their attentions to the future and relied on subsequent generations of medical men to elucidate and eradicate the 'dread disease'. And yet, one hundred years after Dorothy Bullock from Chapter 1 died on The Middlesex Hospital cancer ward, the *Pall Mall Gazette* reported:

> Cancer...stands almost alone as a disease which increases with our prosperity, and while our health laws are raising the standard of public health, the mortality from cancer stands forth as a blot upon the results, detracting in part at least from the measure of the success which has thus far been obtained.[1]

Thus, while cancer had been key to the construction of a chief ideology of modern medicine—a commitment to the teleology of medical discovery and the progressive nature of scientific knowledge—it also undermined that same belief. Cancer's persistent incurability caveated the confidence of medicine and its practitioners.

---

[1] Hugh P. Dunn, 'The Increase of Cancer', *Pall Mall Gazette*, 12 May 1884.

The Cancer Problem: Malignancy in Nineteenth-Century Britain. Agnes Arnold-Forster, Oxford University Press (2021).
© Agnes Arnold-Forster. DOI: 10.1093/oso/9780198866145.003.0009

Malignancy made the Sisyphean labours of that community manifest—'for what is gained at one period of life is to a considerable extent lost at another'.[2] By the beginning of the twentieth century, the promises made by the medical men a century before remained unfulfilled. In 1903, the *British Medical Journal* (*BMJ*) lamented that while 'in past ages a vast amount of time and intellectual energy was spent in the search for the elixir of life'; now, 'the hope of discovering the secret of making the body immortal has long been given up'.[3]

Malignancy's persistent and growing threat to the body politic and the body corporeal, demonstrated the futile promises of the early nineteenth-century practitioners—those men who believed that by bringing the disease inside the hospital walls they were setting it on an irreversible trajectory towards therapeutic success. The futility of nineteenth-century medical efforts showed that cancer— despite all its rationalization by modern and innovative technologies—was resistant to improvement. This process made cancer into the archetypal modern malady—at once tied to Western civilization and necessitating the full technical arsenal of biomedicine—and the intractable and untameable foe—one that evoked our basest fears and anxieties of suffering and death.

This identity was—crucially—only possible once cancer was confirmed as an incurable illness that wreaked havoc on both body and nation. This construction took place in two cancer-specific institutions, established in 1792 and 1802 respectively. 'Construction' is the right word. Not only did it happen in specific built environments, but 'incurable' was not just a biological observation but a flexible category that was made and deployed to suit various professional, personal, and intellectual ends. For some, cancer and its incurability was a something to overcome—a challenge posed to a newly effectively and newly professionalized medical collective. For others, it was a powerful tool in aid of surgical professionalization and the development of new categories of intervention. For opponents to factions within the 'regular' medical and surgical professions who were committed to its intractability, cancer's incurability was a fatal flaw—a chink in the orthodox armour through which alternative remedies could pierce and persuade patients eager for an effective remedy for the 'dread disease'. For public health practitioners, sanitary reformers, medical map-makers, cell theorists, bacteriologists, parasitologist, social commentators, and statisticians, cancer's incurability was an invaluable opportunity to demonstrate the power and promise of their respective tools and technologies. And for those watching their bodies—or the bodies of others—being consumed from the inside out (or the outside in), incurability was an emotionally and physically traumatic experience—a troubling reminder of everyone's inevitable death and decline.

---

[2] Ibid.   [3] 'The Cure of Cancer', *BMJ*, 1 (1903), 1327–8, at 1327.

The nineteenth century *made* cancer. In Chapter 1, I demonstrated how The Middlesex Hospital and its co-institutions confirmed and constructed cancer as a 'local' disease, identifiable through surgical touch and skilled observations; as a malady with an implacable tendency towards growth and spread; and as an incurable illness with a dire prognosis. And I have shown how the nineteenth century made cancer *in its own image*. In Chapter 1, I argued that this hospitalization gave the care of the disease new legitimacy, tied it closely to the investigative and charitable projects of the metropolitan medical elite, and provided cancer with a presence in London's built environment. Cancer's new incurable status had great emotional, political, and rhetorical power. Practitioners used this status to establish their professional identities with characteristics such as humanity, restraint, and intellectual nuance; they used it to articulate a professional chronology and progressive teleology.

Just as cancer was made, the disease exerted its own influence on the medical world around it. In Chapter 3, I examined how just as surgery became the most rational of cancer treatments, 12its role as a curative enterprise was rapidly contested. In response, practitioners reconstructed cancer surgery as palliative—designed to ameliorate suffering—rather than curative. Palliative surgery both responded to the needs and demands of patients, and was an effort to intervene in cases otherwise beyond the reach of medical care. In this way, thinking with cancer has allowed us to reconsider nineteenth-century notions of therapeutic success, efficacy, and failure. Chapter 4 picked up on this thread of patient agency, and explored the wider ramifications of conflict between professional expectation and lay demand in mid-nineteenth-century cancer therapeutics. Despite financial and geographical constraints, patients made choices and selected from a vibrant medical marketplace. Key to their decision-making process—and essential to the advertising strategies of a whole range of practitioners—was the promise to cure an incurable disease without the knife.

This conflict over the curability of cancer continued into the second half of the nineteenth century, as did anxieties over the therapeutic limitations of regular medical and surgical practice. Throughout the century, elite elements of the medical community continued to construct cancer as incurable. This incurability continued to be levied as a differentiating factor between groups of practitioners, and it continued to form part of the self-expression and maintenance of medical authority. Cancer's stagnancy at the turn of the twentieth century prompted some observers to return to an explicitly eighteenth-century understanding of medical care and cure. The *BMJ* argued in 1913:

We have now learnt the lesson taught by David Pitcairn, who died as long ago as 1800. Asked his opinion of a certain book on fevers, he replied: 'I do not like fever curers; we may guide fever—we cannot cure it. What would you think of a pilot who attempted to quell a storm? Either position is absurd. We must steer the ship as well as we can in a storm and in a fever. We can only employ patience and judicious measures to meet the difficulties of the case.' As medicine has become more scientific it has become more humble. The sacerdotal dogmatism which used to prevail among doctors has now been banished from the ward.[4]

While this new circumspection worked to effectively denigrate their predecessors and rival 'quacks' and itinerants, it did not provide a viable therapeutic schema that could effectively replace 'heroic' remedies or adversarial treatments. Non-intervention did not work with cancer—the incurable, unresolvable, intractable malady.

In the mid-century, this continued therapeutic futility coincided with a new interest in the vital statistics of the nation and the systematic collection of data pertaining to birth, marriages, and causes of death to produce a new anxiety. Not only was cancer incurable, but it appeared to be increasing in incidence. In response, some practitioners turned their attentions elsewhere to elucidate the evasive malady. The continued therapeutic futility provoked a diversification of investigative efforts and elements of the medical community refocused on cancer's aetiology, pathology, and transmission. In Chapter 5, I argued that vital statistics offered both a challenge and an opportunity to the medical community. In response, scientific and medical practitioners formulated new approaches to the 'cancer problem'—they moved away from investigating potential *cures* for cancer, and instead focused on potential *causes*: landscapes, rebellious cells, microscopic beings, and modernity. In doing so, they reconfigured cancer as a disease of space, and specifically, rural space. I suggested that unlike sanitary map-makers, Alfred Haviland was not preoccupied by the threat of urban 'civilization' and industrial overcrowding. Instead, cancer maps overwhelmingly represented the countryside.

Moreover, while geographical conceptualizations of malignancy and the plotting of its incidence persisted into the fin de siècle and beyond, mapping was a highly adaptable medium and increasingly presented a range of aetiological models of disease—geographical, environmental, and bacteriological. In Chapter 6, I explored some of these aetiological models in more detail. I interrogated the impact of cell theory, germ theories, and parasitology on ideas and practices pertaining to cancer and its care. This book has problematized narratives that suggest cell theories of disease transformed the understanding and diagnosis of cancer and instead suggested that bacterial and parasitic theories of malignancy were enthusiastically taken up by practitioners and professionals in the 1880s and after, although they were never universally accepted. I also argued that the three theories suited the nineteenth-century medical collective because they articulated, in new language, old and deeply felt ideas about cancer as abnormal,

---

[4] 'Mockers at Medicine', *BMJ*, 1 (1913), 1234–45, at 1235.

chaotic, and semi-independent from the host body. Moreover, these discussions of cancer cell theory and parasitology operated as proxies for political debates about the state of Victorian society.

Finally, Chapter 7 further interrogated this relationship between cancer and Victorian society and incorporated the disease into a much-told story of a late-century preoccupation with degeneration and decline. I showed how practitioners and the public conceptualized cancer as a 'pathology of progress'—an unintended cost of civilization. The disease's association with old age enabled parallels to be drawn between a healthy body ultimately succumbing to disorder and a prosperous nation or empire suffering inevitable deterioration. However, cancer was also increasingly perceived as a product of public health successes like lower infant mortality, increasing hospitalization, sanitary reform, and greater surveillance of bodies in life and after death. If fin-de-siècle public health practitioners and statisticians could transform the 'cancer epidemic' into a positive indictment of their profession and achievements with relative ease, clinicians found it more difficult to reflect with confidence on the recent history of the disease. Indeed, just associating cancer with the reduction of infectious diseases and the improvements of public health did little to eradicate its many and various negative and traumatic meanings and implications.

As Chapter 7 demonstrated, the fin de siècle was both end and a beginning. It contained within it the promises of the next century and the failings and triumphs of the previous. Much of the optimism of the late nineteenth century was, therefore, directed towards the next century, the twentieth. Today, more than half of us will live or die in the 'kingdom of the sick' ruled by cancer.[5] The disease is a commonplace if catastrophic part of modern life. Yet, there is a paradox in our modernity being so marked by a malady that we neither fully understand nor can effectively treat. Cancer is *the* diagnosis you do not want to be given, and for many people it has become synonymous with death. It is now a near-universal experience—with almost everyone having been treated for cancer, living with cancer, dying from cancer, or caring for someone with cancer. Cancer forces the historian to come face to face with the inevitable facts of death, disease, and decline, and to situate those facts historically. To analyse texts that describe acute suffering, or to read the words of the dying, is an emotional labour as much as an intellectual one. In the time it has taken me to write this book, and the PhD thesis before it, two people very close to me were diagnosed with cancer and one of them died. This labour is, therefore, thrown into sharper relief because cancer's power is undimmed. It continues to form part of all our lives and our encounters with it are both quotidian and earth-shattering.

---

[5] Susan Sontag, *Illness as Metaphor and AIDs and Its Metaphors* (London, 2013).

In this historical moment—the one we are all living through—we will all encounter cancer. Whether in our own bodies, in the bodies of those we love, or, if we are lucky, just in the social, cultural, and political landscape we all traverse. It is, therefore, almost impossible to research and write a history of cancer without reflecting on its contemporary life. At various points in this book, I have made arguments that prompted me to reappraise the twenty-first-century disease. That, for example, nineteenth-century surgeons constructed a new category of surgical palliation suggests that the language we use to talk about cancer today—the language of remission—obscures the essentially palliative nature of most of the treatments doctors now deploy. Nineteenth-century critiques of William Halsted's 'three-year' watershed could equally be applied to the oncologists, researchers, and cancer organizations who now use an obfuscating array of statistics and rates of recurrence to elide the precariousness of cancer survivorship. We know that 'cancer survival' in Britain in 2011 was set at 50 per cent, but this statistic refers to the likelihood of a person diagnosed surviving for ten years or more.[6] If someone is treated for cancer, but dies of that same illness eleven years later—does that still count as survival? And who is defining these terms? Cancer Research UK acknowledges the liminal phase that cancer 'survivors occupy': 'Unfortunately, it isn't usually possible for doctors to say for certain that cancer has been cured. They can't definitely say that it will never come back. Living with this uncertainty is one of the most difficult things about having had cancer.'[7]

Uncertainty coupled with fear reifies cancer as a disease that, even today, necessitates a violent response. As I argued in the Introduction, we tend to locate the emergence of cancer as the 'dread disease' in the middle of the twentieth century, when even cancer organizations portrayed the disease as 'an insidious, dreadful, relentless invader'.[8] In 1957, the physician and cancer educationalist George W. Crile blamed those cancer organizations for having 'fashioned a devil out of cancer'. Crile lamented that they 'have bred in a sensitive public a fear that is approaching hysteria. They have created a new disease, cancerophobia, a contagious disease that spread from mouth to ear. It is possible that to-day cancerophobia causes more suffering than cancer itself.'[9] This was an astute observation, but Crile misidentified the source of the phobia. As I have shown, 'cancerophobia' existed in the nineteenth century, and provoked a new type of adversarial, surgical palliation, that targeted cancer with violence, even as a measure of last resort.

---

[6] 'Survival Statistics', http://www.cancerresearchuk.org/about-cancer/what-is-cancer/understanding-cancer-statistics-incidence-survival-mortality#survival, accessed 19 August 2017.

[7] 'Why Some Cancers Come Back', http://www.cancerresearchuk.org/about-cancer/what-is-cancer/why-some-cancers-come-back, accessed 19 August 2017. See also Robert A. Aronowitz, *Risky Medicine: Our Quest to Cure Fear and Uncertainty* (Chicago, 2015).

[8] Quoted in Joanna Bourke, *Fear: A Cultural History* (London, 2015), 234.   [9] Ibid.

For many people, cancer remains incurable. Not only is survivorship effected by site, stage, and type—it is also scandalously structured by class, gender, nationality, and race. Many people—even those living in major cities in the Global North—continue to *perceive* cancer as incurable even if effective treatments are available. In 2013, an article about the racial gap in breast cancer diagnosis by Tara Parker-Pope started with an anecdote:

> After her doctors told her two months ago that she had breast cancer, Debrah Reid, a 58-year-old dance teacher, drove straight to a funeral home. She began planning a burial with the funeral director and his wife, even requesting a pink coffin.[10]

For Debrah, cancer was just not a disease that you could survive. The nineteenth-century notion of cancer's incurability has had a lengthy legacy. This fear continues to propel men and women into radical treatment, and those who decide otherwise are remarked upon as outliers. In her lyrical account of her breast cancer, *The Undying*, poet Anne Boyer describes her treatments—more toxic than the disease itself—by making clear their very real nature as poisons:

> To administer the medicine [Adriamycin], the oncology nurse...must dress in an elaborate protective costume...The medicine destroys tissues if it escapes the veins: it is sometimes considered too dangerous to everyone and everything else to administer by drip. It is rumoured, if spilled, to melt the linoleum on a clinic floor.[11]

If twenty-first-century readers recoil at my descriptions of arsenic and acid used as cancer treatments in the nineteenth century, then they should take a walk through their local chemotherapy ward.

The very word, 'cancer', affects the decisions patients make with respect to treatment options—it persuades people into surgery even when the evidence to support its utility is limited. Zehra B. Omer, from Massachusetts General Hospital in Boston, and colleagues surveyed 394 healthy women without a history of breast cancer to examine the impact of terminology used to describe ductal carcinoma in situ (DCIS) on treatment decisions. Women were presented with three scenarios describing DCIS as non-invasive breast cancer, breast lesion, or abnormal cells, and they then chose between three treatment options (surgery, medication, or active surveillance). Depending on the terminology used, significantly more

---

[10] Tara Parker-Pope, 'The Cancer Divide: Tackling a Racial Gap in Breast Cancer Survival', *New York Times*, 20 December 2013.
[11] Anne Boyer, *The Undying: A Meditation on Modern Illness* (New York, 2019), 57.

women changed their preference from a surgical to non-surgical option. The authors concluded that the terminology used to describe DCIS 'has a significant and important impact on patients' perceptions of treatment alternatives'.[12] What does treatment mean—then as now? The very concept of effective therapy is, in some ways, evasive. All treatment is palliative in that it only delays the inevitable death. We all live in a liminal phase, punctuated by periodic diseases. Most that do not kill us, and one that does. Indeed, part of cancer's significance as a disease is bound up in the ways that it helps to define, or set boundaries around, therapeutic effectiveness (where 'effectiveness' also suggests palliation). Cancer emphasizes a way of understanding medicine that calls out a part of its modern logic to which we have tried hard not to attend. That is not to say there is no difference between cures and palliative care, but I want to suggest that they might be more closely associated—more situated on a continuum—than we like to concede. Modern medicine has these 'blind spots' built into it so that we can all pretend certain things—to serve important social, political, and professional functions—without having to confront the realities of our own mortality and the ultimate futility of intervention. While, as René Dubos suggested, modern medicine promises 'perfect health and happiness' as 'birthrights of men', the epidemiology and incurability of cancer reveals that 'complete freedom from disease and from struggle is almost incompatible with the process of living'. Dubos cautions against the 'inappropriate and dangerous expectations' of 'medical utopias', and instead suggests that 'threats to health are inescapable accompaniments of life'.[13]

This tension between the promises of modern medicine and the incurability of cancer persists, and malignancy continues to appeal to 'modern-day quackery' in part because it exposes people to the myths of 'medical utopias'. Indeed, various scholars have observed the rise of what they call a 'new medical pluralism', and in 2000 the House of Lords Select Committee on Science and Technology called for measures to 'ensure that the public are protected from incompetent and dangerous practitioners', as interest in complementary and alternative medicines increases.[14] Some of these alternatives have been incorporated into orthodox practice with the development of 'integrative oncology'—the use of interventions such as hypnosis, herbal remedies, or massage to alleviate suffering and 'complement' more radical treatments like chemotherapy. However, cancer quackery 'remains a flourishing and lucrative business' today, and treatments like the Gerson Therapy are infamous for promising to effect a complete cure with coffee

[12] Zehra B. Omer, E. Shelley Hwang, Laura J. Esserman, Rebecca Howe, and Elissa M. Ozanne, 'Impact of Ductal Carcinoma in Situ Terminology on Patient Treatment Preferences', *JAMA Internal Medicine*, 173 (2013), 1830–1.

[13] René Dubos, *Mirage of Health: Utopias, Progress and Biological Change* (New York, 1959), 29.

[14] House of Lords Select Committee on Science and Technology, 21 November 2000, https://publications.parliament.uk/pa/ld199900/ldselect/ldsctech/123/12301.htm, accessed 20 April 2020.

enemas and a diet of vegetables.[15] The appeal of these alternatives is obvious. It depends on the manifest failures of orthodox medicine to both affect a *complete* cure for cancer, but also on its inability to acknowledge the limitations to the faculty's craft.

However, it is not just Victorian therapeutics that have refracted through the subsequent centuries. The notion of carcinogenic landscapes and environments became common parlance in mid-twentieth-century cancer discourse. Cell theory remains the primary paradigm for understanding cancer and even today infectious agents are responsible for almost one in six cases of malignancy worldwide.[16] Moreover, the idea that cancer is an independent agency with the capacity for growth, spread, and even communication runs latent in our twenty-first-century imaginings. In 2017, after Senator John McCain announced his glioblastoma diagnosis (a form of brain cancer), he received messages of support and sympathy from across the political spectrum, many of which drew on an ingrained language and traded on an adversarial model of the cancer experience. President Barack Obama tweeted: 'John McCain is an American hero & one of the bravest fighters I've ever known. Cancer doesn't know what it's up against. Give it hell, John.'[17] Obama was not alone in drawing on McCain's military background, weaving his martial history into his medical present and positioning cancer as an identifiable and malevolent foe.

Finally, the two conceptualizations of cancer explained in Chapter 7 resonate with persistent, twenty-first-century understandings of the disease. Cancer continues to be conceptualized as a disease of health or as a disease of affluence. Health and affluence are, in both common-sense parlance and professional discourse, frequently understood as coterminous. Or at least one begets the other. The sixth United Nation's (UN's) millennium development goal (a roadmap for poverty reduction formulated in 2000) is concerned with infections only—the ailments of poverty. Combatting chronic disease is not part of what the UN calls its 'universal framework for development'.[18] Frequently, contagious maladies are conceptualized as disease of poverty, whereas chronic illnesses—cancer in particular—are seen as diseases of wealth. While this identification has come under scrutiny by epidemiologists and public health researchers, it continues to predominate in imaginings of the disease and holds particular sway in certain alternative 'health and wellness' circles.

[15] 'Gerson Therapy', https://www.cancerresearchuk.org/about-cancer/cancer-in-general/treatment/complementary-alternative-therapies/individual-therapies/gerson, accessed 31 January 2020.

[16] Catherine de Martel, Jacques Ferlay, Silvia Franceschi, Jérôme Vignat, Freddie Bray, David Forman, and Martyn Plummer, 'Global Burden of Cancer's Attributable to Infections in 2008: A Review and Synthetic Analysis', *The Lancet*, 13:6 (2012): 607–15.

[17] Agnes Arnold-Forster, 'Metaphors and Malignancy in Senator McCain's Cancer Diagnosis', *Nursing Clio*, July 2017.

[18] 'Good Health and Well-Being', http://www.undp.org/content/undp/en/home/sustainable-development-goals/goal-3-good-health-and-well-being.html, accessed 26 August 2017.

Similarly, cancer as a disease of 'degeneration' continues as a trope of modern medical critique. Multiple elements of our contemporary style of living are deemed pathological. Our diets, work patterns, and leisure choices are all potential causes of cancer. Medical publications and journalistic commentary alike invert the seemingly self-evident narrative of linear progress towards our current health status. Historian Charles E. Rosenberg marshals various examples from the press in the 1990s that together emphasize the identification of late twentieth-century chronic disease as manifesting disharmony between the human body, developed in accordance with a bucolic, hunter-gatherer existence, and our modern ways of living.[19] For example, an essay published in the New Yorker in 1998 lamented: 'In the past thirty years the natural relationship between our bodies and our environment—a relation that was developed over thousands of years—has fallen out of balance.'[20] While Rosenberg acknowledges that these arguments feature in nineteenth-century discourse on health, disease, progress, and decline, he does not recognize that twenty-first-century debates about cancer were constructed by Victorian commenters, both professional and lay.

Cancer remains prominent in our public discourse—culture, politics, and social commentary—and in our individual imaginings of disease and death. Indeed, it has become symbolic of death itself. And yet, as this book has shown, and contrary to what historians and journalists have hitherto supposed, these characteristics of the 'dread disease' were produced more than a century ago. It was in the nineteenth century, therefore, that cancer acquired the symbolic, politicized status it maintains today. Finally, while cancer may be 'the quintessential product of modernity'—it is a 'modernity' forged in the nineteenth century.[21] And yet, while it came to be conceptualized as a disease of civilization in a way that reflected the complexities of 'civilization' as a concept in fin-de-siècle Britain, its continued power as a frame of reference can be attributed to its malleability as a concept. Cancer is representative of modern biomedicine and yet continues to undermine its claims.

[19] Charles E. Rosenberg, 'Pathologies of Progress: The Idea of Civilization as Risk', Bulletin of the History of Medicine, 72 (1998), 714–30.
[20] Malcolm Gladwell, 'Annals of Medicine: The Pima Paradox', New Yorker, 2 February 1998, 56.
[21] Siddhartha Mukherjee, The Emperor of all Maladies: A Biography of Cancer (New York, 2011), 241.

Bibliography

Archival Material

Hansard

- HC Deb., vol. 21, cc911–31, 23 February 1812
- HL Deb., vol. 21, cc1166–8, 5 March 1812
- HC Deb., vol. 35, cc100–43, 29 January 1817
- HC Deb., vol. 4, cc795–6, 19 February 1821
- HC Deb., vol. 19, cc470–595, 9 May 1828
- HC Deb., vol. 1, cc655–5, 23 November 1830
- HC Deb., vol. 33, cc1227–36, 31 May 1836
- HC Deb., vol. 34, cc8–117, 3 June 1836
- HC Deb., vol. 53, cc1236–307, 5 May 1840
- HC Deb., vol. 56, cc375–451, 8 February 1841
- HC Deb., vol. 57, cc460–509, 22 March 1841
- HC Deb., vol. 63, cc1320–64, 7 June 1842
- HC Deb., vol. 70, cc15–85, 16 June 1843
- HC Deb., vol. 91, cc952–1032, 19 April 1847
- HC Deb., vol. 100, cc696–743, 22 July 1848
- HC Deb., vol. 104, cc1260–89, 4 May 1849
- HC Deb., vol. 141, cc779–867, 10 April 1856
- HC Deb., vol. 156, cc378–90, 31 January 1860
- HC Deb., vol. 184, cc943–71, 17 July 1866
- HC Deb., vol. 200, cc1607–86, 11 April 1870
- HC Deb., vol. 230, cc1333–71, 12 July 1876
- HC Deb., vol. 252, cc333–422, 24 May 1880
- HC Deb., vol. 261, cc288–375, 12 May 1881
- HC Deb., vol. 269, cc462–526, 11 May 1882
- HC Deb., vol. 274, cc1206–87, 10 November 1882
- HC Deb., vol. 314, cc105–48, 27 April 1887
- HL Deb., vol. 335, cc1194–219, 6 May 1889
- HC Deb., vol. 41, cc304–10, 2 June 1896
- HC Deb., vol. 56, cc479–527, 19 April 1898
- HC Deb., vol. 101, cc799–800, 24 January 1902
- HC Deb., vol. 118, cc247–56, 18 February 1903
- HC Deb., vol. 132, cc321–71, 21 March 1904

Johns Hopkins University Archive, Baltimore, Maryland, USA
- Box No. 32, Folder No. 8, 12448, Case Note, Surgical No. 25282, 1910.
- Box No. 33, Folder No. 5, 12632, Statistical Study of Cases of Carcinoma of the Breast Admitted to the Johns Hopkins Hospital, June 1889 to June 1902.

- Patient Correspondence from 'JHH Cases of Carcinoma of the Breast, 1895–1920', Letter to Dr Halsted, 18 June 1914.
- Patient Correspondence from 'JHH Cases of Carcinoma of the Breast, 1895–1920', Letter to Dr Halsted, 7 July 1914.
- Patient Correspondence from 'JHH Cases of Carcinoma of the Breast, 1895–1920', Letter from Dr Halsted, 1 October 1914.

Rockefeller Archive, Tarrytown, New York, USA

- 1225 (7) John D. Rockefeller Papers/Financial Materials/V14 Charities Index Cards/ Skin and Cancer Hospital (New York) 1884–1890
- 189 (24) Medical Interests/Memorial Hospital 1900–1930
- 199.31: Rockefeller University Records, Corporation, Biography, Frederick T. Gates
- 210.3 (4) Business Manager/Subject Files/Cancer 1913–1952
- IV YBI.101, Box 68, Folder 606, American Society for the Control of Cancer, 1913–1917
- Box 2, Folder 31, Hayes Martin Collection, Cancer Therapy, Cancer Cures, 1884, 1921
- Correspondence with Simon Flexner, 1907–1918
- 'Fourth Annual Report for the Year 1888' (New York Cancer Hospital, Eighth Avenue and 106th Street)

UCLH Archive, London, UK

- 'The Cancer Investigation Committee', Middlesex Hospital Minutes, 12 January 1900
- 'The Cancer Investigation Committee', Middlesex Hospital Minutes, 1 June 1900
- 'The Cancer Investigation Committee', Middlesex Hospital Minutes, 19 December 1900
- 'The Cancer Investigation Committee', Middlesex Hospital Minutes, 20 May 1901
- 'The Cancer Investigation Committee', Middlesex Hospital Minutes, 4 November 1901
- 'The Cancer Investigation Committee', Middlesex Hospital Minutes, 31 January 1902
- 'The Cancer Investigation Committee', Middlesex Hospital Minutes, 4 February 1902
- 'The Cancer Investigation Committee', Middlesex Hospital Minutes, 22 May 1902
- 'The Cancer Investigation Committee', Middlesex Hospital Minutes, 3 November 1902
- 'The Cancer Investigation Committee', Middlesex Hospital Minutes, 2 April 1903
- 'The Cancer Investigation Committee', Middlesex Hospital Minutes, 28 October 1903
- 'Cancer Registers', 1870–1871
- 'Cancer Registers', 1887–1891
- Cancerous Patients Register, 1829–1846
- Case Notes from the Cancer Ward at the Middlesex Hospital, 1805–1838
  - 'Dorothy Bullock', 1805
  - 'Hannah Cressford', 1805
  - 'Jane Barnes', 1805
  - 'Mary Gardner', 1805
  - 'Ann Manisty', 1806
  - 'Eliza Moore', 1806
  - 'Eloy Wilmot', 1806
  - 'Hannah Delamere', 1806

- 'Martha Moore', 1806
- 'Martha Oliver', 1806
- 'Mary Townly', 1806
- 'Sarah Camphire', 1806
- 'Ann Jeffries', 1807
- 'Eleanor Shopman', 1807
- 'Jane Roberts', 1807
- 'Mrs. Ward', 1807
- 'Susan Squires', 1807
- 'Susan Wagner', 1807
- 'Anne Brine', 1808
- 'Mary Bowy', 1808
- 'Mary Cummins', 1808
- 'Mary Dunkley', 1808
- 'Sarah Lackland', 1808
- 'Sarah Oldman', 1808
- 'Ann Saftwell', 1809
- 'Martha Are', 1809
- 'Mrs Carman', 1809
- 'Susan Bennet', 1809
- 'Ann Darney', 1810
- 'Mary Glover', 1810
- 'Mary Mocha', 1810
- 'Lydia Dettmer', 1811
- 'Mary Dawon', 1811
- 'Mary Herbert', 1811
- 'Mary Morrison', 1811
- 'Sarah McMurdy', 1811
- 'Sarah Weeder', 1811
- 'Sophia Othen', 1811
- 'Ann Dibbins', 1812
- 'Judith Williams', 1812
- 'Eliza Willis', 1813
- 'Sarah Moore', 1813
- 'Ann Aberley', 1814
- 'Ann Beazley', 1814
- 'Ann Bradley', 1814
- 'Charlotte Skinnor', 1814
- 'Dina Hayes', 1814
- 'Jane Bassney', 1814
- 'Susan Hackney', 1814
- 'Theo Alon', 1814
- 'Sarah Hill', 1816
- 'Barbara Dewes', 1824
- 'Ann Sharp', 1825
- 'Hannah Thirlowe', 1825
- 'Ann Dawson', 1826
- 'Elizabeth Jones', 1826

- 'Ann James', 1828
- 'Ann Smith', 1830
- 'Caroline Wilson', 1831
- 'Mary Spillman', 1838
- 'Of Trying Dr Otto Schmidt's Treatment upon Cancer Patients in the Middlesex Hospital', 26 November 1903.
- 'Scheme for the Investigation of Cancer Finally Amended', Middlesex Hospital Minutes, 15 November 1899
- 'System of Admission of Patients', 1875–1892
- 'Weekly Board Meeting', Middlesex Hospital Minutes, 29 November 1791
- 'Weekly Board Meeting', Middlesex Hospital Minutes, 10 January 1792

Printed Primary Sources

Abernethy, John, *Surgical Observations on Tumours* (London, 1811).

Alison, William Pulteney, *Dissertation on the State of Medical Science: From the Termination of the Eighteenth Century to the Present Time* (London, 1834).

Allbutt, Clifford, 'Nervous Diseases and Modern Life', *Contemporary Review*, 67 (1895), 210–31.

Andrews, Chas. W., and Brand, A. T., 'Cancer and Its Origin', *BMJ*, 1 (1904), 402–3.

Anon., *Rules and Order of the General Infirmary at Leeds* (Leeds, 1771).

Anon., 'Editorial Article', *The Observer*, 18 June 1791.

Anon., 'Classified Ads', *Lloyd's Evening Post*, 20 January 1792.

Anon., 'Classified Ad 5', *The Observer*, 21 April 1799.

Anon., 'Obituaries', *The Times*, 16 October 1801.

Anon., 'Classified Ad 5', *Manchester Guardian*, 29 September 1821.

Anon., 'Recent Deaths', *Wesleyan-Methodist Magazine*, October 1823.

Anon., 'The Body Medical', *The Lancet*, 21 (1833), 31–2.

Anon., *Report of the Leeds Board of Health, MDCCCXXXIII* (Leeds, 1833).

Anon., 'Living Dissection', *Satirist, and the Censor of the Time*, September 1835.

Anon., 'Means of Checking the Operations of Quacks', *The Lancet*, 1 (1835–6), 946–9.

Anon., 'Classified Advertisement', *Manchester Guardian*, 18 August 1838.

Anon., 'Dr Elliotson's Experiments in "Mesmerism" at the House of Mr. Wakley with Two Girls Deceiving', *The Lancet*, 36 (1838), 805–14.

Anon., 'Academy of Sciences, Paris', *Provincial Medical & Surgical Journal*, 8 (1844).

Anon., 'Advertisements & Notices', *Leeds Mercury*, 24 February 1844.

Anon., 'Chester Assizes: Accusation of Manslaughter Against One of "Graham's Own". Quack Plasters for Cancer. Trial at Chester, before Mr. Baron Gurney', *The Lancet*, 44 (1844), 382–3.

Anon., 'Classified Ad 7', *Manchester Guardian*, 4 May 1844.

Anon., 'Court and Fashionable', *John Bull*, 20 July 1844.

Anon., 'All May be Cured by Holloway's Ointment', *Berrow's Worcester Journal*, 23 April 1846.

Anon., *Woman and her Diseases, from the Cradle to the Grave: Adapted Exclusively to her Instruction in the Physiology of her System and all the Diseases of her Critical Periods* (New York, 1847).

Anon., 'Quarterly Return of Deaths in the Parish of St. Martin-in-the-Fields, *Medical Officer for Health Report for St Martin-in-the-Fields*' (London, 1856).

Anon., 'The Cancer Ward of Middlesex Hospital', *The Observer*, 13 April 1857.

Anon., 'The Middlesex Hospital and Treatment of Cancer', *The Lancet*, 69 (1857), 128.

Anon., 'The Black Doctor', *The Observer*, 8 January 1860.

Anon., 'Quacks Abroad and At Home', *BMJ*, 1 (1860), 52–3.

Anon., 'Advertisements & Notices', *Hull Packet and East Riding Times*, 5 April 1867.

Anon., 'Multiple News Items', *Bradford Observer*, 11 March 1869.

Anon., 'Strange Charge of Manslaughter at Leeds', *Bradford Observer*, 11 March 1869.

Anon., 'Cancer Cures', *BMJ*, 1 (1873), 650–1.

Anon., 'Review: The Microscope in Medicine, by Lionel S. Beale', *American Naturalist*, 16 (1882), 500–4.

Anon., 'The Defeated Ennerdale Railway', *The Spectator*, 21 July 1883.

Anon., 'The Increasing Fatality of Cancer', *BMJ*, 1 (1883), 969–71.

Anon., 'Recorded Cancer Mortality in England and Ireland', *BMJ*, 1 (1889), 1240–1.

Anon., 'Enlarging the Hospital to Relieve Cancer Victims', *New York Daily Tribune*, 20 July 1890.

Anon., 'The Mattei Cancer Cure', *Woman's Herald*, 17 January 1891.

Anon., 'Recent Advances in Medicine', *Science*, 17 (1891).

Anon., 'A "Cancer Curer"', *BMJ*, 1 (1895), 158.

Anon., 'Living Things in Cancers', *New York Times*, 20 September 1896.

Anon., 'Cancer in Relation to the Dwelling', *BMJ*, 2 (1898), 1571–2.

Anon., 'The Influence of Locality on the Prevalence of Cancer', *BMJ*, 1 (1899), 812–13.

Anon., 'Clerical Errors', *BMJ*, 2 (1900), 1733.

Anon., 'The Parasitic Theory of Cancer', *BMJ*, 2 (1900), 1518.

Anon., 'The Causation of Cancer', *BMJ*, 1 (1901), 1281–2.

Anon., 'Malaria a Cure for Cancer', *New York Times*, 7 April 1902.

Anon., 'Alfred Haviland, M.R.C.S.', *BMJ*, 1 (1903), 1522.

Anon., 'Cancer in Ireland: An Economical Question', *BMJ*, 2 (1903), 1544.

Anon., 'A Comparative Statistical Study of Cancer Mortality. V. General Summary (Concluded)', *BMJ*, 1 (1903), 1154–6.

Anon., 'The Cure of Cancer', *BMJ*, 1 (1903), 1327–8.

Anon., 'Imperial Cancer Research Fund', *BMJ*, 2 (1905), 96–100.

Anon., 'Cancer in the Colonies', *BMJ*, 1 (1906), 812–13.

Anon., 'Cancer Deaths Increasing: Porter Says the Malady is Assuming Menacing Proportions', *New York Times*, 5 November 1907.

Anon., 'Cancer Houses: Does the Disease Infect our Dwellings?', *The Observer*, 8 September 1907.

Anon., 'Cancer Houses: Infection or Coincidence? Disease-Haunted Buildings', *Times of India*, 1 October 1907.

Anon., 'A Prophet of Quackery', *BMJ*, 1 (1907), 644–5.

Anon., 'Cancer Increasing at an Alarming Rate', *Vogue*, 15 April 1909.

Anon., 'Baffling Mystery of Life: Experiments of the Scientists Have so Far Failed to Fathom Its Secret', *Washington Post*, 20 October 1912.

Anon., 'The Parasite of Cancer', *BMJ*, 2 (1912), 1328–9.

Anon., 'Mockers at Medicine', *BMJ*, 1 (1913), 1234–5.

Anon., 'North Hempstead, N. Y.: Communicable Diseases. Notification, Placarding, Quarantine, Funerals. Reg. Bd. Of H., June 18, 1912', *Public Health Reports (1896–1970)*, 28 (1913), 1682–3.

Anon., 'Logic and Disease', *The Spectator*, 11 April 1914.

Anon., 'France', *BMJ*, 1 (1933), 716–17.

Anon., 'Secret Surgery, and the "Mystery Men" of the Middlesex', *The Lancet*, 69 (1957), 358.

Anon., 'Soil and Stomach Cancer', *BMJ*, 1 (1965), 1–2.

Arnott, Henry, *Cancer: Its Varieties, their Histology and Diagnosis* (London, 1872).

Ashbury Smith, Joseph, 'On the State of the Medical Profession in England, and on Quackery in the Manufacturing Districts', *The Lancet*, 63 (1854), 402–3.

Balance, Charles A., and Shattock, Samuel G., 'A Note on an Experimental Investigation into the Pathology of Cancer', *Proceedings of the Royal Society of London*, 48 (1890), 392–403.

Bartholomew, Valentine, 'Dr Fell versus Cancer', *Ladies' Cabinet*, 1 November 1856.

Bartlett, Elisha, *An Essay on the Philosophy of Medical Science* (Philadelphia, PA, 1844).

Bashford, E. F. 'The Problems of Cancer', *BMJ*, 2 (1903), 127–9.

Bashford, E. F., 'An Address Entitled Are the Problems of Cancer Insoluble?', *BMJ*, 2 (1905), 1507–11.

Bashford, E. F., 'The Investigations of the Imperial Cancer Research Fund', *BMJ*, 2 (1906), 1554–5.

Bashford, E. F., 'Real and Apparent Differences in the Incidence of Cancer', *Transactions of the Epidemiological Society of London*, 26 (1907), 43–77.

Bashford, E. F., 'Cancer, Credulity, and Quackery', *BMJ*, 1 (1911), 1222–30.

Bastian, H. Charlton, 'The Origin of Cancer and the Origin of Life', *BMJ*, 2 (1911), 1573.

Bell, Charles, *Surgical Observations; Being a Quarterly Report of Cases in Surgery; Treated in the Middlesex Hospital, in the Cancer Establishment, and in Private Practice* (London, 1816).

Bernard, Thomas, 'Extract from an Account of the Institution for Investigating the Nature and Cure of Cancer', in *Reports of the Society for Bettering the Condition and Increasing the Comforts of the Poor*, vol. 3 (London, 1802).

Bland-Sutton, J., 'A Lecture on the Cancer Problem', *The Lancet*, 169 (1907), 1339–45.

Bourgery, J. M., *Iconografia d'Anatomia Chirurgica e di Medicina Operatoria* (Florence, 1841).

Braithwaite, James, 'Excess of Salt as a Cause of Cancer', *BMJ*, 2 (1902), 1376–7.

Braithwaite, James, 'Cancer Mortality', *BMJ*, 1 (1903), 1289.

Brand, Alexander Theodore, 'East Yorks and North Lincoln Branch: The Etiology of Cancer', *BMJ*, 2 (1902), 238–42.

Buchan, William, *Domestic Medicine; or A Treatise on The Prevention and Cure of Diseases, by Regimen and Simple Medicines* (London, 187?).

Burnet, Etienne, *The Campaign against Microbes*, trans. E. E. Austen (London, 1909).

Burney, Frances, 'Account from Paris of a Terrible Operation', in *Journal Letter to Esther Burney* (London, 1812).

Butlin, Henry T., 'A Clinical Lecture on Halsted's Operation for Removal of Cancer of the Breast', *BMJ*, 2 (1898), 1665–8.

Butlin, Henry T., 'Carcinoma is a Parasitic Disease: Being the Bradshaw Lecture Delivered before the Royal College of Surgeons of England', *BMJ*, 2 (1905), 1565–71.

Butlin, Henry T., 'Two Lectures on Unicellula Cancri: The Parasite of Cancer', *BMJ*, 2 (1911), 1457–61.

Byer, J. W., 'Introductory Remarks by the President on Puerperal Fever, Uterine Cancer, and the Falling Birth Rate', *BMJ*, 2 (1901), 941–3.

Cadogan, William, *A Dissertation on the Gout, and all Chronic Diseases, Jointly Considered, as Proceeding from the Same Causes; what those Causes are; and a Rational and Natural Method of Cure Proposed. Addressed to all Invalids* (London, 1772).

Carmichael, Richard, *An Essay on the Effects of Carbonate, and other Preparations of Iron, upon Cancer: With an Inquiry into the Nature of that and other Diseases to which it Bears a Relation* (Dublin, 1809).

Chadwick, Edwin, *Report on the Sanitary Conditions of the Labouring Population of Great Britain: A Supplementary Report on the Results of a Special Inquiry into the Practice of Internment in Towns* (London, 1843).

Chamberlain, Houston Stewart, *The Foundations of the Nineteenth Century*, trans. John Lees (New York, 1968).

Collis, Maurice Henry, *On the Diagnosis and Treatment of Cancer and the Tumours Analogous to it* (London, 1864).

Cooper, Bransby Blake, *Lectures on the Principles and Practice of Surgery* (London, 1851).

Cooper, Samuel, *The First Lines of the Practice of Surgery: Designed as an Introduction for Students, and a Concise Book of Reference for Practitioners*, vol. 1, 4th edn (London, 1819).

Cowan, Charles, *The Danger, Irrationality, and Evils of Medical Quackery; Also, The Causes of Its Success; The Nature of Its Machinery; The Amount of Government Profits; With Reasons Why It Should Be Suppressed: And an Appendix containing the Composition of Many Popular Quack Medicines: Addressed to all Classes* (London, 1839).

Creighton, Charles, 'Address in Pathology: On the Autonomous Life of the Specific Infections', *BMJ*, 2 (1883), 218–24.

Crichton-Browne, James, *The Prevention of Senility and a Sanitary Outlook* (London, 1905).

Denman, Thomas, *Observations on the Cure of Cancer, with some Remarks upon Mr. Young's Treatment of that Disease* (London, 1816).

Dickson, Samuel, *The 'Destructive Art of Healing': A Sequel to the 'Fallacies of the Faculty'* (London, 1856).

Dunn, Hugh P., 'An Inquiry into the Causes of the Increase of Cancer', *BMJ*, 1 (1883), 708–10.

Dunn, Hugh P., 'An Inquiry into the Causes of the Increase of Cancer (Continued)', *BMJ*, 1 (1883).

Dunn, Hugh P., 'The Increase of Cancer', *Pall Mall Gazette*, 12 May 1884.

Dunn, Hugh P., 'English Experience with Cancer', *Popular Science Monthly*, 36 (1885).

Dunster, E. S., 'The Idea of Life, as Deduced from Contemporary Physiology: Virchow-Claude Bernard', *Anthropological Review*, 8 (1870), 49–69.

Edson, Cyrus, 'The Art of Healing: Marvelous Progress Made in the Science of Medicine', *Los Angeles Times*, 28 January 1900.

Elliotson, John, *Cure of a True Cancer of the Female Breast with Mesmerism* (London, 1848).

Engledue, William Collins, 'Introductory Remarks', in John Elliotson, *Cure of a True Cancer of the Female Breast with Mesmerism* (London, 1848).

Erichsen, John Eric, 'Clinical Lectures Delivered at University College Hospital', *BMJ*, 1 (1860), 279–81.

Fell, J. Weldon, *A Treatise on Cancer, and Its Treatment* (London, 1857).

Fergusson, William, *A System of Practical Surgery* (London, 1846).

Gaylord, H. G., 'Evidences that Infected Cages are the Source of Spontaneous Cancer Developing among Small Caged Animals', *BMJ*, 2 (1906), 1555–8.

Giessen, Olt, 'Cancer in Domestic Animals', *Journal of Comparative Pathology and Therapeutics*, 18 (1905), 278–9.

Glover, Robert M., *On the Philosophy of Medicine, on Quackery, &c. Being the Last of a Course of Lectures Delivered in the School of Medicine, Newcastle-upon-Tyne* (London, 1851).

Gosse, Philip Henry, *A Memorial of the Last Days on Earth of Emily Gosse* (London, 1857).

Graham, George, *Fourth Annual Report of the Registrar-General* (London, 1841).

Graham, George, 'Statistical Nosology', in George Graham, *Fourth Annual Report of the Registrar-General* (London, 1841).

Graham, George, 'Causes of Death in England and in Each Division and County in 1851', in George Graham, *Fourteenth Annual Report of the Registrar-General* (London, 1855).

Graham, George, *Fourteenth Annual Report of the Registrar-General* (London, 1855).

Graham, Thomas J., *Practical Observations on the Cure of Cancer, Illustrated by Numerous Cases of Cancer in the Breast, Lip, and Face; which Have Been Cured by a Mild Method of Treatment, that Immediately Alleviates the Most Agonizing Pain* (London, 1824).

Green, Charles E., *The Cancer Problem: A Statistical Study* (London, 1909).

Green, Charles E., *The Cancer Problem: A Statistical Study*, 2nd edn (London, 1912).

Halsted, William, 'The Results of Operations for the Cure of Cancer of the Breast Performed at the Johns Hopkins Hospital from June, 1889, to January, 1894', *Annals of Surgery*, 20 (1894), 497–555.

Haviland, Alfred, *The Nature and Treatment of Cancer* (London, 1844).

Haviland, Alfred, *Climate, Weather, and Disease: Being a Sketch of the Opinions of the Most Celebrated Ancient and Modern Writers* (London, 1855).

Haviland, Alfred, *The Sanitary Regulations of Ancient Rome* (London, 1855).

Haviland, Alfred, 'Abstracts of Lectures on the Geographical Distribution of Disease in England and Wales: One', *BMJ*, 2 (1871), 453–4.

Haviland, Alfred, 'Abstracts of Lectures on the Geographical Distribution of Disease in England and Wales: Two', *BMJ*, 2 (1871), 573–5.

Haviland, Alfred, *The Geographical Distribution of Heart Diseases and Dropsy, Cancer in Females and Phthisis in Females, in England and Wales* (London, 1875).

Haviland, Alfred, *Geology in Relation to Sanitary Science* (London, 1879).

Haviland, Alfred, *Scarborough as Health Resort: Its Physical Geography, Geology, Climate and Vital Statistics* (London, 1883).

Haviland, Alfred, *A Paper on the Influence of Clays and Limestones on Medical Geography; Illustrated by the Geographical Distribution of Cancer among Females, in England and Wales* (London, 1891).

Haviland, Alfred, *The Geographical Distribution of Heart Diseases and Dropsy, Cancer in Females and Phthisis in Females, in England and Wales*, 2nd edn (London, 1892).

Hayle Walshe, Walter, *The Anatomy, Physiology, Pathology, and Treatment of Cancer* (Boston, MA, 1844).

Henniker, Brydges P., 'Deaths from Several Zymotic and Other Causes, and Inquest Cases, in the Divisions, Counties, and Districts of England', in *Forty-Second Annual Report of the Registrar-General* (London, 1881).

Henry, Alexander, 'On the Ancient and Modern Doctrines of Cancer', *Association Medical Journal*, 3 (1855), 413–16.

Henry, David, and Nichols, John (eds.), 'Deaths', *Gentleman's Magazine: and Historical Chronical*, August 1788.

Herman, G. Ernest, 'An Address on the Early Diagnosis of Cancer of the Cervix Uteri', *BMJ*, 1 (1894), 1009–12.

Highmore, A., *Pietas Londinensis: The History, Design, and Present State of the Various Public Charities in and Near London* (London, 1814).

Hill-Climo, William, 'Cancer in Ireland: An Economic Question', *Empire Review*, 6 (1903), 410–16.

Hislop, P. W., and Clennell Fenwick, P., 'Cancer in New Zealand', *BMJ*, 2 (1909), 1222–5.

Hodgkin, Thomas, 'The Fall of the Roman Empire and Its Lessons for Us', *Contemporary Review*, 73 (1898), 70.

Hogg, Jabez, 'A Characteristic Organism of Cancer', *BMJ*, 2 (1890), 1505–6.

Hughes Bennett, John, *On Cancerous and Cancroid Growths* (Edinburgh, 1849).

Humphreys, Noel A., 'The Registrar-General's Decennial Supplement, 1881–90', *Journal of the Royal Statistical Society*, 59 (1896), 543–6.

Hunt, Leigh, Fonblanque, Albany William, and Forster, John (eds.), 'Obituary', *The Examiner*, 13 November 1858.

Hunter, John, *Lectures on the Principles of Surgery* (Philadelphia, PA, 1839).

Hutchinson, Woods, 'The Cancer Problem: Or, Treason in the Republic of the Body', *Contemporary Review*, 76 (1899), 105–17.

Jackson, Arthur, 'An Address on the Incidence of Cancer', *BMJ*, 2 (1899), 1465–7.

Johnson, James, *Practical Researches on the Nature, Cure, and Prevention of Gout, in all its Open and Concealed Forms; Partly Translated and Condensed from the French of Guilbert and Hallé; with a Critical Examination of some Celebrated Remedies and Modes of Treatment Employed in this Disease* (London, 1819).

Jouve, Henri, *Thèse pour Le Doctorat en Médecine sur La Topographie et La Contagion du Cancer* (Paris, 1897).

Kellogg, John Harvey, *The New Dietetics, What to Eat and How: A Guide to Scientific Feeding in Health and Disease* (Battle Creek, MI, 1921).

King, George, and Newsholme, Arthur, 'On the Alleged Increase of Cancer', *Proceedings of the Royal Society of London*, 54 (1893), 209–42.

Lankester, E. Ray, 'The Present Evolution of Man', *Fortnightly Review*, 66 (1896).

Laurence, John Zachariah, 'Illustrations of the Pathology of Cancer', *Association Medical Journal*, 4 (1856), 886–7.

Laurence, John Zachariah, *The Diagnosis of Surgical Cancer* (London, 1858).

Lloyd Jones, E., 'The Topographical Distribution of Cancer', *BMJ*, 1 (1899), 813–15.

Loeb, Leo, 'The Cancer Problem', *Interstate Medical Journal*, 17 (1910), 376–91.

Lynn Thomas, J., 'A Note upon a Case of Cancer in the Right Breast "Cured" by the Cardigan "Cancer Curers": The Aftermath: A Danger-Signal to the Public', *BMJ*, 2 (1908), 1676–8.

MacGregor, William, 'Some Problems of Tropical Medicine', *The Lancet*, 2 (1900), 1055–61.

MacLachlan John T., and Wardman-Wilbourne, E., 'The Cancer Problem', *BMJ*, 1 (1911), 282.

May, Bennett, 'The Ingleby Lectures on the Operative Treatment of Cancer of the Breast', *BMJ*, 1 (1897), 1335–8.

Meade, R. H., 'A Few Remarks on Cancer', *BMJ*, 2 (1866), 94–5.

Moore, Charles H., *The Antecedents of Cancer* (London, 1865).

Müller, Johannes, *On the Nature and Structural Characteristics of Cancer, and of those Morbid Growths which May Be Confounded with it*, trans. Charles West (London, 1840).

Nooth, James, *Observations on the Treatment of Scirrhous Tumours, and Cancers of the Breast* (London, 1804).

Nordau, Max, *Degeneration*, trans. George L. Moss (London, 1993).

Nunneley, Thomas, 'Address in Surgery', *BMJ*, 2 (1869), 143–56.

Osler, William, *Science and Immortality* (London, 1906).

Owen, Isambard, 'Reports of the Collective Investigation Committee of the British Medical Association: Geographical Distribution of Rickets, Acute and Subacute Rheumatism, Chorea, Cancer, and Urinary Calculus in the British Islands', *BMJ*, 1 (1899), 113–16.

Pancoast, Joseph, *A Treatise on Operative Surgery Comprising a Description of the Various Processes of the Art, including all the New Operations; Exhibiting the State of Surgical Science in Its Present Advanced Condition* (Philadelphia, PA, 1856).

Parker, Langston, *The Treatment of Cancer Diseases by Caustics* (London, 1856).

Parsons, Usher, *Cancer of the Breast* (Providence, RI, 1849).

Payne, J. F., 'The Goulstonian Lectures on the Origin and Relations of New Growths', *BMJ*, 1 (1874), 474–5.

Payne, J. F., 'A Lecture on the Increase on Cancer', *The Lancet*, 154 (1899), 765–70.

Pearson, John, *Practical Observations on Cancerous Complaints: With an Account of some Diseases which Have Been Confounded with the Cancer* (London, 1792).

Pearson, Karl, 'On "Cancer Houses" from the Data of the Late Th. Law Webb, M.D.', *Biometrika*, 8 (1912), 430–5.

Plimmer, H. G., 'The Parasitic Theory of Cancer', *BMJ*, 2 (1903), 1511–15.

Pope, Thomas, 'On Cancer', *Association Medical Journal*, 3 (1855), 859–60.

Power, D'Arcy, 'Cancer Houses and their Victims', *BMJ*, 1 (1894), 1240.

Renner, W., 'The Spread of Cancer among the Descendants of the Liberated Africans or Creoles of Sierra Leone', *BMJ*, 2 (1910), 587–9.

Robertson, J. Argyll, *Excision of the Eyeball in Cases of Melanosis, Medullary Carcinoma, and Carcinoma: With Remarks* (London, 1844).

Rodman, John, *Practical Explanation of Cancer in the Female Breast* (London, 1818).

Rowley, William, *A Treatise on the Management of Female Breasts during Childbed; and Several New Observations on Cancerous Diseases*, 2nd edn (London, 1790).

Ryall, Charles, 'The Technique of Cancer Operations, with Reference to the Danger of Cancer Infection', *BMJ*, 2 (1908), 1005–8.

Savory, W. S., 'The Bradshaw Lecture on the Pathology of Cancer', *BMJ*, 2 (1884), 1173–8.

Scarpa, Antonio, *Remarks and Practical Results of Observation on Scirrhus and Cancer*, trans. by James Briggs (London, 1822).

Sheild, A. Marmaduke, 'The "Cure" of Cancer by Operation', *The Lancet*, 147 (1896), 801–2.

Simons, Robert J., 'A Cancer House', *BMJ*, 1 (1909), 275–6.

Simpson, James Young, *Cases of Excision of the Cervix Uteri for Carcinomatous Disease* (Dublin, 1846).

Skinner, Henry Burchstead, *The Female's Medical Guide and Married Woman's Adviser: Containing a Description of the Causes, Symptoms and Cure of Diseases Peculiar to Females, whether Married or Single, from Early Childhood to Old Age, such as Retention, Suppression and Cessation of Menses, Difficult and Irregular Menstruation, Pregnancy, Its Indications and Attendant Diseases, Miscarriage or Abortion, Midwifery, the Turn of Life, Causes and Cure of Barrenness, and Female Complaints Generally. The Whole Adapted to the Private Use of Families* (Boston, MA, 1849).

Snow, John, *On the Mode of Communication of Cholera*, 2nd edn (London, 1855).

Southam, George, 'The Nature and Treatment of Cancer: Being the Address in Surgery', *BMJ*, 1 (1858), 4–7.

Southam, George, *The Nature and Treatment of Cancer: Being the Address in Surgery Read before the 25th Meeting of the British Medical Association, Held at Nottingham July 1857* (London, 1858).

Spencer Wells, T., *Cancer Cures and Cancer Curers* (London, 1860).

Tatham, John, 'Letter to the Registrar-General on the Mortality in England and Wales in the Period of Ten Years 1891–1900', in *Supplement to the Sixty-Fifth Annual Report of the Registrar-General of Births, Deaths, and Marriages in England and Wales, 1891–1900, Part One* (London, 1907).

Thomson, Spencer, *A Dictionary of Domestic Medicine and Household Surgery*, 8th edn (London and Glasgow, 1859).

Urquhart, Alexander, 'Notes on Recent Cancer Mortality in the Thames Valley', *BMJ*, 1 (1904), 825–6.

Velpeau, Alfred-Armand, *A Treatise on Cancer of the Breast and of the Mammary Region*, trans. W. Marsden (London, 1856).

Walford, Edward, *Old and New London*, vol. 4 (London, 1878).

Walker, Charles, 'Theories and Problems of Cancer: Part III', *Science Progress in the Twentieth Century (1906–1916)*, 7 (1912), 223–8.

Ward Richardson, Benjamin, *Diseases of Modern Life* (London, 1876).

Watson, Dr, 'Course of Clinical Lectures, Delivered at the Middlesex Hospital, Session 1842–3', *Provincial Medical Journal and Retrospect of the Medical Sciences*, 5 (1842), 83–6.

Weeden Cooke, Thomas, *On Cancer: Its Allies and Counterfeits* (London, 1865).

Wells, Spencer, *Cancer Cures and Cancer Curers* (London, 1860).

Wells, Spencer, 'The Morton Lecture on Cancer and Cancerous Diseases', *BMJ*, 2 (1888), 1201–5.

Whitbread, Samuel, 'Address: To the Governors of the Middlesex Hospital', in Samuel Young, *Minutes of Cases of Cancer and Cancerous Tendencies Successfully Treated by Mr. Samuel Young* (London, 1815).

Williams, W. Roger, 'The Question of the Increase of Cancer', *BMJ*, 2 (1893), 271–2.

Williams, W. Roger, 'Cancer in Wild Animals', *The Lancet*, 154 (1899), 1194.

Williams, W. Roger, 'Cancer in Egypt and the Causation of Cancer', *BMJ*, 2 (1902), 917.

Williams, W. Roger, *The Natural History of Cancer: With Special Reference to Its Causation and Prevention* (London, 1908).

Young, Samuel, *An Inquiry into the Nature and Action of Cancer; with a View to the Establishment of a Regular Mode of Curing that Disease by Natural Separation* (London, 1805).

Secondary Sources

Ackerknecht, Erwin H., 'Historical Notes on Cancer', *Medical History*, 2 (1958), 114–19.

Ackerknecht, Erwin H., *Medicine at the Paris Hospital, 1794–1848* (Baltimore, MD, 1967).

Ackerknecht, Erwin H., 'A Plea for a "Behaviorist" Approach in Writing the History of Medicine', *Journal of the History of Medicine*, 22 (1967), 211–14.

Anderson, Benedict, *Imagined Communities: Reflections on the Origin and Spread of Nationalism* (London, 1991).

Arnold-Forster, Agnes '"A rebellion of the cells": cancer, modernity, and decline in fin-de-siècle Britain' in Sally Shuttleworth, Melissa Dickson and Emilie Taylor-Brown (eds.),

Progress and Pathology: Medicine and Culture in the Nineteenth Century (Manchester, UK, 2020), 173–193.

Arnold-Forster, Agnes, 'The Pre-History of the Paleo Diet: Cancer and Dietary Innovation in Nineteenth-Century Britain', in David Gentilcore and Matthew Smith (eds.), *Proteins, Pathologies, and Politics* (London, 2018).

Arnold-Forster, Agnes, 'Gender and Pain in Nineteenth-Century Cancer Care', *Gender and History*, https://doi.org/10.1111/1468-0424.12468.

Arnold-Forster, Agnes, 'Resilience in Surgery', *British Journal of Surgery*, https://doi.org/10.1002/bjs.11493.

Arnold-Forster, Agnes, 'A Small Cemetery: Death and Dying in the Contemporary British Operating Theatre', *Medical Humanities*, http://dx.doi.org/10.1136/medhum-2019-011668 .

Aronowitz, Robert A., *Unnatural History: Breast Cancer and American Society* (Cambridge, UK, 2007).

Aronowitz, Robert A., 'The Converged Experience of Risk and Disease', *Milbank Quarterly*, 87 (2009), 417–42.

Aronowitz, Robert A., *Risky Medicine: Our Quest to Cure Fear and Uncertainty* (Chicago, 2015).

Austoker, Joan, *A History of the Imperial Cancer Research Fund 1902–1986* (Oxford, 1988).

Barker, Hannah, 'Catering for Provisional Tastes: Newspapers, Readership and Profit in Late Eighteenth-Century England', *Historical Research*, 69 (1996), 42–61.

Barker, Hannah, 'Medical Advertising and Trust in Late Georgian England', *Urban History*, 36 (2009), 379–98.

Barnes, Emm, 'Caring and Curing: Paediatric Cancer Services since 1960', *European Journal of Cancer Care*, 14 (2005), 373–80.

Barnes, Emm, 'Captain Chemo and Mr. Wiggly: Patient Information for Children with Cancer in the Late Twentieth Century', *Social History of Medicine*, 3 (2006), 501–19.

Barnes, Emm, 'Between Remission and Cure: Patients, Practitioners and the Transformation of Leukaemia in the Late Twentieth Century', *Chronic Illness*, 3 (2007), 253–64.

Barnes, Emm, 'Cancer Coverage: The Public Face of Childhood Leukaemia in 1960s Britain', *Endeavour*, 32 (2008), 10–15.

Barnes Johnstone, Emm, and Baines, Joanna, *The Changing Faces of Childhood Cancer: Clinical and Cultural Visions since 1940* (Basingstoke, 2015).

Barrett, Frank A., 'Alfred Haviland's Nineteenth-Century Map Analysis of the Geographical Distribution of Diseases in England and Wales', *Social Science and Medicine*, 46 (1998), 767–81.

Barrett, Frank A., 'Ginke's 1792 Map of Human Diseases: The First World Disease Map?', *Social History of Medicine*, 50 (2000), 915–21.

Barry, J., and Jones, C. (eds.), *Medicine and Charity before the Welfare State* (London, 1991).

Becsei-Kilborn, Eva, 'Scientific Discovery and Scientific Reputation: The Reception of Peyton Rous' Discover of the Chicken Sarcoma Virus', *Journal of the History of Biology*, 43 (2010), 111–57.

Berkowitz, Carin, 'Charles Bell's Seeing Hand: Teaching Anatomy to the Senses in Britain, 1750–1840', *History of Science*, 52 (2014), 377–400.

Berkowitz, Carin, *Charles Bell and the Anatomy of Reform* (Chicago, 2015).

Berry, Henry, *From Revolution to Fads: The Progress of Modernity* (Bloomington, IN, 2001).

Boddice, Rob (ed.), *Pain and Emotion in Modern History* (Basingstoke, 2014).

Bound Alberti, Fay (ed.), *Medicine, Emotion and Disease, 1700–1950* (Basingstoke, 2006).

Bound Alberti, Fay, 'Bodies, Hearts, and Minds: Why Emotions Matter to Historians of Science and Medicine', *Isis*, 100 (2009), 798–10.

Bound Alberti, Fay, *Matters of the Heart: History, Medicine, and Emotion* (Oxford, 2010).

Bourke, Joanna, 'Pain: Metaphor, Body, and Culture in Anglo-American Societies between the Eighteenth and Twentieth Centuries', *Rethinking History*, 18 (2014), 475–98.

Bourke, Joanna, *The Story of Pain* (Oxford, 2014).

Bourke, Joanna, *Fear: A Cultural History* (London, 2015).

Bracegirdle, Brian, *A History of Microtechnique: The Evolution of the Microtome and the Development of Tissue Preparation*, 2nd edn (Lincolnwood, IL, 1986).

Bradbury, Savile, *The Microscope: Past and Present* (Oxford, 1968).

Bradbury, Savile, and L'Estrange Turner, Gerard, *Historical Aspects of Microscopy* (Cambridge, UK, 1967).

Brandstrom A., and Tedebrand L. G. (eds.), *Society and Health during the Demographic Transition* (Stockholm, 1988).

Brieger, Gert H., 'Bodies and Borders: A New Cultural History of Medicine', *Perspectives in Biology and Medicine*, 47 (2004), 402–21.

Brown, Michael, 'Medicine, Quackery and the Free Market: The "War" against Morison's Pills and the Construction of the Medical Profession, c.1830–c.1850', in Mark S. R. Jenner and Patrick Wallis (eds.), *Medicine and the Market in England and Its Colonies* (Basingstoke, 2007).

Brown, Michael, 'Medicine, Reform and the "End" of Charity in Early Nineteenth-Century England', *English Historical Review*, 124 (2009), 1353–88.

Brown, Michael, *Performing Medicine: Medical Culture and Identity in Provincial England, c. 1760–1850* (Manchester, 2011).

Brown, Michael, 'Surgery and Emotion: The Era before Anaesthesia', in Thomas Schlich (ed.), *The Palgrave Handbook of the History of Surgery* (Basingstoke, 2017).

Brown, P. S., 'Social Context and Medical Theory in the Demarcation of Nineteenth-Century Boundaries', in W. F. Bynum and Roy Porter, *Medical Fringe and Medical Orthodoxy 1750–1850* (London, 1987).

Brunton, Deborah, 'Willan, Robert (1757–1812)', in *Oxford Dictionary of National Biography* (Oxford, 2004).

Burchardt, Jeremy, *Paradise Lost: Rural Idyll and Social Change in England since 1800* (London, 2002).

Burney, Ian, *Bodies of Evidence: Medicine and the Politics of the English Inquest, 1830–1926* (Baltimore, MD, 1999).

Burnham, John C., *How the Idea of Profession Changed the Writing of Medical History* (London, 1998).

Bynum, Caroline, 'Why all the Fuss about the Body? A Medievalist's Perspective', *Critical Inquiry*, 22 (1995), 1–33.

Bynum, W. F., *Science and the Practice of Medicine in the Nineteenth Century* (Cambridge, UK, 1994).

Bynum, W. F., and Porter, Roy, *Medical Fringe and Medical Orthodoxy 1750–1850* (London, 1987).

Bynum, W. F., and Porter, Roy, *Medicine and the Five Senses* (Cambridge, UK, 2005).

Cantor, David, *Cancer in the Twentieth Century* (Baltimore, MD, 2008).

Cantor, Geoffrey, 'Young, Thomas (1773–1829)', in *Oxford Dictionary of National Biography* (Oxford, 2004).

Cavallo, S., 'Charity, Power and Patronage in Eighteenth-Century Hospitals: The Case of Turin', in Lindsay Granshaw and Roy Porter (eds.), *The Hospital in History* (London, 1991).

Chamberlin, F. Edwards, and Gilman, Sander L. (eds.), *Degeneration: The Dark Side of Progress* (New York, 1985).

Chartier, R., and Corsi, P. (eds.), *Science et Langues en Europe* (Paris, 1996).

Clark, David, 'From Margins to Centre: A Review of the History of Palliative Care in Cancer', *Lancet Oncology*, 8 (2007), 430–38.

Clark, David, *To Comfort Always: A History of Palliative Medicine since the Nineteenth Century* (Oxford, 2016).

Classen, Constance, 'Engendering Perception: Gender Ideologies and Sensory Hierarchies in Western History', *Body & Society*, 3 (1997), 1–19.

Classen, Constance (ed.), *The Book of Touch* (Oxford, 2005).

Classen, Constance, *The Deepest Sense: A Cultural History of Touch* (Urbana, IL, 2012).

Clay, Reginald S., *The History of the Microscope: Compiled from Original Instruments and Documents, up to the Introduction of the Achromatic Microscope* (London, 1932).

Clow, Barbara, *Negotiating Disease: Power and Cancer Care, 1900-1950* (Montreal, 2001).

Clow, Barbara, 'Who's Afraid of Susan Sontag? Or, the Myths and Metaphors of Cancer Reconsidered', *Social History of Medicine*, 14 (2001), 293–12.

Coley, N. G., 'Home, Sir Everard, First Baronet (1756-1832)', in *Oxford Dictionary of National Biography* (Oxford, 2004).

Condrau, Flurin, and Worboys, Michael, 'Second Opinions: Epidemics and Infections in Nineteenth-Century Britain', *Social History of Medicine*, 20 (2007), 147–58.

Cooter, Roger, 'The Turn of the Body: History and the Politics of the Corporeal', *Arbor*, 186 (2010), 393–405.

Corfield, Penelope J., *Power and the Professions in Britain 1700-1850* (London, 1995).

Cox, F. E. G., 'History of Human Parasitology', *Clinical Microbiology Reviews*, 15 (2002), 595–12.

Cox, F. E. G., 'George Henry Falkiner Nuttall and the Origins of Parasitology and Parasitology', *Parasitology*, 136 (2009), 1389–94.

Crook, Paul D., *Darwin's Coat-Tails: Essays on Social Darwinism* (London, 2007).

Cubitt, G. (ed.), *Imagining Nations* (Manchester, 1998).

Cunningham, Andrew, and Williams, Perry (eds.), *The Laboratory Revolution in Medicine* (Cambridge, UK, 1992).

Curtis, L. P., *Apes and Angels: The Irishman in Victorian Caricature* (Washington, DC, 1971).

Daston, Lorraine, and Galison, Peter, *Objectivity* (New York, 2007).

Daunton, Martin J. (ed.), *Charity, Self-Interest and Welfare in the English Past* (New York, 1996).

Demaitre, Luke, 'Medieval Notions of Cancer: Malignancy and Metaphor', *Bulletin of the History of Medicine*, 72 (1994), 609–37.

Denney, Peter, 'Looking Back, Groping Forward: Rethinking Sensory History', *Rethinking History*, 15 (2011), 601–16.

Dixon, Thomas, '"Emotion": The History of a Keyword in Crisis', *Emotion Review*, 4 (2012), 338–44.

Dubos, René, *Mirage of Health: Utopias, Progress and Biological Change* (New York, 1959).

Duden, Barbara, *The Woman Beneath the Skin: A Doctor's Patients in Eighteenth-Century Germany*, trans. Thomas Dunlap (London, 1991).

Duerden Comeau, Tammy, 'Gender Ideology and Disease Theory: Classifying Cancer in Nineteenth Century Britain', *Journal of Historical Sociology*, 20 (2007), 158–81.

Dyck, Erika, and Fletcher, Christopher, 'Introduction: Healthscapes: Health and Place among and between Disciplines', in Erika Dyck and Christopher Fletcher (eds.), *Location Health: Historical and Anthropological Investigations of Health and Place* (London, 2011).

Dyck, Erika, and Fletcher, Christopher (eds.), *Location Health: Historical and Anthropological Investigations of Health and Place* (London, 2011).

Eaton, S. Boyd, Konner, Melvin, and Shostak, Marjorie, 'Stone Agers in the Fast Lane: Chronic Degenerative Diseases in Evolutionary Perspective', *American Journal of Medicine*, 84 (1988), 739–49.

Epstein, J. E., 'Writing the Unspeakable: Fanny Burney's Mastectomy and the Fictive Body', *Representations*, 16 (1986), 131–66.

Eyler, J., *Victorian Social Medicine: The Ideas and Methods of William Farr* (Baltimore, MD, 1979).

Eyler, J., 'The Conceptual Origins of William Farr's Epidemiology: Numerical Methods and Social Thought in the 1830s', in Abraham M. Lilienfeld (ed.), *Times, Places, and Persons* (Baltimore, MD, 1980).

Farley, John, 'Parasites and the Germ Theory of Disease', in Charles E. Rosenberg and Janet Lynne Golden (eds.), *Framing Disease: Studies in Cultural History* (New Brunswick, NJ, 1992).

Fisher, D. R., 'Whitbread, Samuel (1764–1815)', in *Oxford Dictionary of National Biography* (Oxford, 2004).

Fissell, Mary E., 'The Disappearance of the Patient's Narrative and the Invention of Hospital Medicine', in R. French and A. Wear (eds.), *British Medicine in an Age of Reform* (London, 1991).

Fissell, Mary E., *Patients, Power and the Poor in Eighteenth-Century Bristol* (Cambridge, UK, 1991).

Fleck, Ludwick, *Genesis and Development of a Scientific Fact*, trans. Fred Bradley and Thaddeus J. Trenn (Chicago, 1979).

Foucault, Michel, *The Birth of the Clinic: An Archaeology of Medical Perception* (London, 1973).

French, R., and Wear, A. (eds.), *British Medicine in an Age of Reform* (London, 1991).

Gallagher, James, 'Cancer "Tidal Wave" on Horizon, Warns WHO', *BBC News*, 4 February 2014, http://www.bbc.co.uk/news/health-26014693, accessed 21 April 2020.

Gardner, K. E., *Early Detection: Women, Cancer, and Awareness Campaigns in the Twentieth-Century United States* (Chapel Hill, NC, 2006).

Gavrus, Delia, 'Men of Dreams and Men of Action: Neurologists, Neurosurgeons, and the Performance of Professional Identity, 1920–1950', *Bulletin of the History of Medicine*, 85 (2011), 57–92.

Gilbert, Pamela K., *Mapping the Victorian Social Body* (Albany, NY, 2004).

Gilbert, Pamela K. (ed.), *Imagined Londons* (Albany, NY, 2007).

Gilbert, Pamela K., 'The Victorian Social Body and Urban Cartography', in Pamela K. Gilbert (ed.), *Imagined Londons* (Albany, NY, 2007).

Gladwell, Malcolm, 'Annals of Medicine: The Pima Paradox', *New Yorker*, 2 February 1998.

Goodbody, Bridget L., '"The Present Opprobrium of Surgery": "The Agnew Clinic" and Nineteenth-Century Representations of Cancerous Female Breasts', *American Art*, 8 (1994), 32–51.

Gould, Stephen J., *The Mismeasure of Man* (New York and London, 1981).

Granshaw, Lindsay, '"Fame and Fortune by Means of Brick and Mortar": The Medical Profession and Specialist Hospitals in Britain, 1800–1948', in Lindsay Granshaw and Roy Porter (eds.), *The Hospital in History* (London, 1991).

Granshaw, Lindsay, and Porter, Roy (eds.), *The Hospital in History* (London, 1991).

Hacking, Ian, *The Taming of Chance* (Cambridge, UK, 1990).

Hamlin, Christopher, 'Providence and Putrefaction: Victorian Sanitarians and the Natural Theology of Health and Disease', *Victorian Studies*, 28 (1985), 381–11.

Hamlin, Christopher, *Public Health and Social Justice in the Age of Chadwick: Britain, 1800–1854* (Cambridge, UK, 2008).

Hamlin, Christopher, *Cholera: The Biography* (Oxford, 2009).

Hardy, Anne, *The Epidemic Streets: Infectious Disease and the Rise of Preventive Medicine, 1856–1900* (Oxford, 1993).

Harley, J. B., *The New Nature of Maps: Essays in the History of Cartography* (Baltimore, MD, 2002).

Hartman, M. S., and Banner, L. (eds.), *Clio's Consciousness Raised: New Perspectives on the History of Women* (New York, 1974).

Hawkins, Mike, *Social Darwinism in European and American Thought, 1860–1945* (Cambridge, UK, 1997).

Higgs, Edward, 'Registrar General's Reports for England and Wales, 1838–1858', Online Historical Population Reports, http://histpop.org/, accessed 13 October 2016.

Higgs, Edward, 'The Annual Report of the Registrar-General, 1839–1920: A Textual History', in Eileen Magnello and Anne Hardy (eds.), *The Road to Medical Statistics* (Amsterdam, 2002).

Higgs, Edward, *Life, Death and Statistics: Civil Registration, Censuses and the Work of the General Register Office, 1836–1952* (Hatfield, 2004).

Hitchcock, Tim, and Shoemaker, Robert, *London Lives: Poverty, Crime and the Making of a Modern City, 1690–1800* (Cambridge, UK, 2015).

Hodgkinson, Ruth G., 'Social Medicine and the Growth of Statistical Information', in F. N. L. Poynter (ed.), *Medicine and Science in the 1860s: Proceedings of the Sixth British Congress on the History of Medicine* (London, 1968).

Hunt, Edward, and Pam, S. J., 'Responding to Agricultural Depression, 1873–96: Managerial Success, Entrepreneurial Failure?', *Agricultural History Review*, 50 (2002), 225–52.

Innes, Joanna, 'The "Mixed Economy of Welfare" in Early Modern England: Assessments of the Options from Hale to Malthus (c.1683–1803)', in Martin J. Daunton (ed.), *Charity, Self-Interest and Welfare in the English Past* (New York, 1996).

Jacobs, Natasha X., 'From Unit to Unity: Protozoology, Cell Theory, and the New Concept of Life', *Journal of the History of Biology*, 22 (1989), 215–42.

Jacyna, L. S., 'The Romantic Programme and the Reception of Cell Theory in Britain', *Journal of the History of Biology*, 17 (1984), 13–48.

Jacyna, L. S., 'The Laboratory and the Clinic: The Impact of Pathology on Surgical Diagnosis in the Glasgow Western Infirmary, 1875–1910', *Bulletin of the History of Medicine*, 62 (1988), 384–406.

Jacyna, L. S., '"A Host of Experienced Microscopists": The Establishment of Histology in Nineteenth-Century Edinburgh', *Bulletin of the History of Medicine*, 75 (2001), 225–53.

Jacyna, L. S., 'Abernethy, John (1764–1831)', in *Oxford Dictionary of National Biography* (Oxford, 2004).

Jacyna, L. S., 'Bell, Sir Charles (1774–1842)', in *Oxford Dictionary of National Biography* (Oxford, 2004).

Jain, S. Lochlann, *Malignant: How Cancer Becomes Us* (Berkeley, CA, 2013).

Jalland, Pat, *Death in the Victorian Family* (Oxford, 1996).

Jenner, Mark S. R., 'Body, Image, Text in Early Modern Europe', *Social History of Medicine*, 12 (1999), 143–54.

Jenner, Mark S. R., 'Tasting Lichfield, Touching China: Sir John Floyer's Senses', *Historical Journal*, 53 (2010), 647–70.

Jenner, Mark S. R., and Wallis, Patrick (eds.), *Medicine and the Market in England and Its Colonies* (Basingstoke, 2007).

Jewson, Nicholas D., 'The Disappearance of the Sick-Man from Medical Cosmology, 1770–1870', *Sociology*, 10 (1976), 225–44.

Jones, John, 'Baillie, Matthew (1761–1823)', in *Oxford Dictionary of National Biography* (Oxford, 2004).

Jordanova, Ludmilla, 'Science and National Identity', in R. Chartier and P. Corsi (eds.), *Science et Langues en Europe* (Paris, 1996).

Jordanova, Ludmilla, 'Science and Nationhood: Cultures of Imagined Communities', in G. Cubitt (ed.), *Imagining Nations* (Manchester, 1998).

Joyce, Patrick, *The Rule of Freedom: Liberalism and the Modern City* (London, 2003).

Kaartinen, Marjo, *Breast Cancer in the Eighteenth Century* (London, 2013).

Kearns, G., 'The Urban Penalty and the Population History of England', in A. Brandstrom and L. G. Tedebrand (eds.), *Society and Healthy during the Demographic Transition* (Stockholm, 1988).

Kidd, Colin, *The Forging of Races. Race and Scripture in the Protestant World, 1600–2000* (Cambridge, UK, 2006).

Kline, Wendy, *Building a Better Race: Gender, Sexuality, and Eugenics from the Turn of the Century to the Baby Boom* (Berkeley, CA, 2001).

Koblenz, Lawrence, 'From Sin to Science: The Cancer Revolution of the Nineteenth Century' (Columbia University, PhD Thesis, 2013).

Koch, Tom, *Cartographies of Disease: Maps, Mapping and Medicine* (Redlands, CA, 2005).

Koch, Tom, 'Social Epidemiology as Medical Geography: Back to the Future', *GeoJournal*, 72 (2009), 99–106.

Koch, Tom, *Disease Maps: Epidemics on the Ground* (Chicago, 2011).

Krige, John, and Pestre, Dominique (eds.), *Science in the Twentieth Century* (Amsterdam, 1997).

Kümin, Beat, and Usborne, Cornelie, 'At Home and in the Workplace: A Historical Introduction to the "Spatial Turn"', *History and Theory*, 52 (2013), 305–18.

Lakoff, George, and Johnson, Mark, *Metaphors We Live By* (Chicago, 2003).

Lawrence, Christopher, '"Incommunicable Knowledge": Science, Technology and the Clinical Art in Britain 1850–1914', *Journal of Contemporary History*, 20 (1985), 503–20.

Lawrence, Christopher, 'Democratic, Divine and Heroic: The History and Historiography of Surgery', in Christopher Lawrence (ed.), *Medical Theory, Surgical Practice: Essays in the History of Surgery* (London, 1992).

Lawrence, Christopher (ed.), *Medical Theory, Surgical Practice: Essays in the History of Surgery* (London, 1992).

Lawrence, Christopher, 'Medical Minds, Surgical Bodies: Corporeality and the Doctors', in Christopher Lawrence and Steven Shapin (eds.), *Science Incarnate: Historical Embodiments of Natural Knowledge* (Chicago, 1998).

Lawrence, Christopher, and Shapin, Steven (eds.), *Science Incarnate: Historical Embodiments of Natural Knowledge* (Chicago, 1998).

Lawrence, Susan C., 'Private Enterprise and Public Interests: Medical Education and the Apothecaries' Act, 1780–1825', in R. French and A. Wear (eds.), *British Medicine in an Age of Reform* (London, 1991).

Lawrence, Susan C., 'Educating the Senses: Students, Teachers and Medical Rhetoric in Eighteenth-Century London', in W. F. Bynum and Roy Porter, *Medicine and the Five Senses* (Cambridge, UK, 2005).

Lawton, Julia, *The Dying Process: Patients' Experiences of Palliative Care* (London, 2000).

Ledger, Sally, and Luckhurst, Roger (eds.), *The Fin-de-Siècle: A Reader in Cultural History, c.1880–1900* (Oxford, 2000).

Ledger, Sally, and McCracken, Scott (eds.), *Cultural Politics at the Fin de Siècle* (Cambridge, UK, 1990).

Lenoir, Timothy, *The Strategy of Life: Teleology and Mechanics in Nineteenth-Century German Biology* (Chicago, 1989).

Lerner, Barron H., *The Breast Cancer Wars: Fear, Hope, and the Pursuit of a Cure in Twentieth-Century America* (Oxford, 2011).

Levitan, Kathrin, *A Cultural History of the British Census: Envisioning the Multitude in the Nineteenth Century* (Basingstoke, 2011).

Lilienfeld, Abraham M. (ed.), *Times, Places, and Persons* (Baltimore, MD, 1980).

Loudon, Irvine, *Medical Care and the General Practitioner 1750–1850* (Oxford, 1987).

Loudon, Irvine, 'The Vile Race of Quacks with which this Country is Infested', in W. F. Bynum and Roy Porter, *Medical Fringe and Medical Orthodoxy 1750–1850* (London, 1987).

Löwy, Ilana, 'Cancer: The Century of the Transformed Cell', in John Krige and Dominique Pestre (eds.), *Science in the Twentieth Century* (Amsterdam, 1997), 461–77.

Löwy, Ilana, *Preventive Strike: Women, Precancer, and Prophylactic Surgery* (Baltimore, MD, 2010).

Löwy, Ilana, '"Because of their Praiseworthy Modesty, They Consult Too Late": Regime of Hope and Cancer of the Womb, 1800–1910', *Bulletin of the History of Medicine*, 85 (2011), 356–83.

Mackenzie, Donald A., *Statistics in Britain 1865–1930: The Social Construction of Scientific Knowledge* (Edinburgh, 1981).

McKeown, Thomas, *The Modern Rise of Population* (London, 1976).

Magnello, Eileen, and Hardy, Anne (eds.), *The Road to Medical Statistics* (Amsterdam, 2002).

Marcus, Alan I., *Malignant Growth: Creating the Modern Cancer Research Establishment 1875–1915,* (Tuscaloosa AL, 2018).

Marks, Harry, '"Until the Sun of Science . . . the True Apollo of Medicine Has Risen": Collective Investigation in Britain and America, 1880–1910', *Medical History*, 50 (2006), 147–66.

Martel, Catherine de, Ferlay, Jacques, Franceschi, Silvia, Vignat, Jérôme, Bray, Freddie, Forman, David, and Plummer, Martyn, 'Global Burden of Cancer's Attributable to Infections in 2008: A Review and Synthetic Analysis', *The Lancet*, 13:6 (2012), 607–15.

Mazumdar, Pauline M. H., *Eugenics, Human Genetics and Human Failings: The Eugenics Society, Its Sources and Its Critics in Britain* (London, 1992).

Mediratta, S., 'Beauty and the Breast: The Poetics of Physical Absence and Narrative Presence in Frances Burney's Mastectomy Letter (1811)', *Women: A Cultural Review*, 19 (2008), 188–207.

Miller, Ian, *Reforming Food in Post-Famine Ireland: Medicine, Science, and Improvement, 1845–1922* (Manchester, 2014).

Mitchell, W. J. T. (ed.), *Landscape and Power* (Chicago, 2002).

Mitman, Gregg, and Numbers, Ronald L., 'From Miasma to Asthma: The Changing Fortunes of Medical Geography in America', *History and Philosophy of the Life Sciences*, 25 (2003), 391–412.

Mooney, Graham, 'Professionalization in Public Health and the Measurement of Sanitary Progress in Nineteenth-Century England and Wales', *Social History of Medicine*, 10 (1997), 54–78.

Mooney, Graham, 'Response: Infectious Disease and Epidemiological Transition in Victorian Britain? Definitely', *Social History of Medicine*, 20 (2007), 595–606.

Moscoso, Javier, *Pain: A Cultural History* (Basingstoke, 2012).

Moscoso, Javier, 'Exquisite and Lingering Pains: Facing Cancer in Early Modern Europe', in Rob Boddice (ed.), *Pain and Emotion in Modern History* (Basingstoke, 2014).

Moscucci, Ornella, *The Science of Woman: Gynaecology and Gender in England, 1800-1929* (Cambridge, UK, 1993).

Moscucci, Ornella, 'Denman, Thomas (1733-1815)', in *Oxford Dictionary of National Biography* (Oxford, 2004).

Moscucci, Ornella, 'Gender and Cancer in Britain, 1860-1910', *American Journal of Public Health*, 95 (2005), 1312-21.

Moscucci, Ornella, *Gender and Cancer in England, 1860-1948* (London, 2016).

Mukherjee, Siddhartha, *The Emperor of all Maladies: A Biography of Cancer* (New York, 2011).

Newton, Hannah, *Misery to Mirth: Recovery from Illness in Early Modern England* (Oxford, 2018).

Nicolson, Malcolm, 'Simpson, Sir James Young, First Baronet (1811-1870)', in *Oxford Dictionary of National Biography* (Oxford, 2004).

Nicolson, Malcolm, 'Commentary: Nicholas Jewson and the Disappearance of the Sick Man from Medical Cosmology, 1770-1870', *International Journal of Epidemiology*, 38 (2009), 639-42.

O'Connor, Erin, *Raw Material: Producing Pathology in Victorian Culture* (Durham, NC, 2000).

Omer, Zehra B., Hwang, E. Shelley, Esserman, Laura J., Howe, Rebecca, and Ozanne, Elissa M., 'Impact of Ductal Carcinoma in Situ Terminology on Patient Treatment Preferences', *JAMA Internal Medicine*, 173 (2013), 1830-1.

Omran, A., 'The Epidemiological Transition: A Theory of the Epidemiology of Population Change', *Milbank Quarterly*, 83 (1971), 731-57.

Otis, Laura, *Membranes: Metaphors of Invasion in Nineteenth-Century Literature, Science, and Politics* (Baltimore, MD, and London, 1999).

Otis, Laura, *Müller's Lab* (Oxford, 2007).

Ottoway, Susannah, 'The Elderly in the Eighteenth-Century Workhouse', in Jonathan Reinartz and Leonard Schwarz, *Medicine and the Workhouse* (Rochester, NY, 2013).

Patterson, James T., *The Dread Disease: Cancer and Modern American Culture* (Cambridge, MA, 1989).

Payne, Lynda, *With Words and Knives: Learning Medical Dispassion in Early Modern England* (London, 2007).

Pearson, Karen S., 'The Nineteenth-Century Colour Revolution: Maps in Geographical Journals', *Imago Mundi*, 32 (1980), 9–20.

Pernick, Martin S., *A Calculus of Suffering: Pain, Professionalism, and Anesthesia in Nineteenth-Century America* (New York, 1985).

Perry, Ruth, 'Colonizing the Breast: Sexuality and Maternity in Eighteenth-Century England', *Journal of the History of Sexuality*, 2 (1991), 204-34.

Pick, Daniel, *Faces of Degeneration: A European Disorder, c.1848–1918* (Cambridge, UK, 1989).

Pickstone, John V., *Ways of Knowing: A New History of Science, Technology and Medicine* (Chicago, 2001).

Pickstone, John V., 'Contested Cumulations: Configurations of Cancer Treatments through the Twentieth Century', *Bulletin of the History of Medicine*, 81 (2007), 164–96.

Pickstone, John V., 'Commentary: From History of Medicine to a General History of "Working Knowledges"', *International Journal of Epidemiology*, 38 (2009), 646–9.

Poovey, Mary, *Making a Social Body: British Cultural Formation, 1830–1864* (Chicago, 1995).

Porter, Dale H., *The Thames Embankment* (Akron, OH, 1998).

Porter, Dorothy, and Porter, Roy, *In Sickness and in Health: The English Experience 1650–1850* (London, 1988).

Porter, Roy, 'The Patient's View: Doing Medical History from Below', *Theory and Society*, 14 (1985), 175–98.

Porter, Roy, *Health for Sale: Quackery in England, 1660–1850* (Manchester, 1989).

Porter, Roy, 'Bodies of Thought: Thoughts about the Body in Eighteenth-Century England', in Joan H. Pittock and Andrew Wear (eds.), *Interpretation and Cultural History* (London, 1991).

Porter, Roy, *The Greatest Benefit to Mankind: A Medical History of Humanity from Antiquity to the Present* (London, 1999).

Porter, Roy, 'The Rise of Physical Examination', in W. F. Bynum and Roy Porter (eds.), *Medicine and the Five Senses* (Cambridge, UK, 2005).

Porter, Roy, and Rousseau, G. S., *Gout: The Patrician Malady* (New Haven, CT, 2000).

Porter, Roy, and Teich, Mikulas (eds.), *Fin de Siècle and Its Legacy* (Cambridge, UK, 1990).

Power, D'Arcy, 'Pearson, John (1758–1826)', rev. Michael Bevan, in *Oxford Dictionary of National Biography* (Oxford, 2004).

Power, D'Arcy, 'Sims, James (1741–1820)', rev. Kaye Bagshaw, in *Oxford Dictionary of National Biography* (Oxford, 2004).

Poynter, F. N. L. (ed.), *Medicine and Science in the 1860s: Proceedings of the Sixth British Congress on the History of Medicine* (London, 1968).

Rather, L. J., *The Genesis of Cancer: A Study in the History of Ideas* (Baltimore, MD, 1978).

Rather, L. J., Rather, Patricia, and Frerichs, John B., *Johannes Müller and the Nineteenth-Century Origins of the Tumor Cell Theory* (Canton, MA, 1986).

Reeves, Carol (ed.), *A Cultural History of the Body in the Age of Enlightenment* (Oxford, 2007).

Reinartz, Jonathan, and Schwarz, Leonard, *Medicine and the Workhouse* (Rochester, NY, 2013).

Reynolds, Andrew, 'Amoebae as Exemplary Cells: The Protean Nature of an Elementary Organism', *Journal of the History of Biology*, 41 (2008), 307–37.

Richmond, Marsha L., 'Protozoa as Precursors of Metazoa: German Cell Theory and Its Critics at the Turn of the Century', *Journal of the History of Biology*, 22 (1989), 243–76.

Roberts, M. J. D., 'The Politics of Professionalization: MPs, Medical Men, and the 1858 Medical Act', *Medical History*, 53 (2009), 37–56.

Roper, Lyndal, 'Beyond Discourse Theory', *Women's History Review*, 19 (2010), 307–19.

Roper, Michael, 'Slipping Out of View: Subjectivity and Emotion in Gender History', *History Workshop Journal*, 59 (2005), 57–72.

Rose, C., 'Politics and the London Royal Hospitals, 1683–92', in Lindsay Granshaw and Roy Porter (eds.), *The Hospital in History* (London, 1991).

Rosenberg, Charles E., *The Cholera Years: The United States in 1832, 1849, and 1866* (Chicago, 1962).

Rosenberg, Charles E., 'The Therapeutic Revolution: Medicine, Meaning and Social Change in Nineteenth-Century America', *Perspectives in Biology and Medicine*, 2 (1977), 485–502.

Rosenberg, Charles E., *Explaining Epidemics and Other Studies in the History of Medicine* (Cambridge, UK, 1992).

Rosenberg, Charles E., 'The Tyranny of Diagnosis: Specific Entities and Individual Experience', *Milbank Quarterly*, 80 (2002), 237–60.

Rosenberg, Charles E., and Golden, Janet Lynne (eds.), *Framing Disease: Studies in Cultural History* (New Brunswick, NJ, 1992).

Saler, Michael (ed.), *The Fin-de-Siècle World* (London, 2015).

Santosa, Aliana, Wall, Stig, Fottrell, Edward, Högberg, Ulf, and Byass, Peter, 'The Development and Experience of Epidemiological Transition Theory over Four Decades: A Systematic Review', *Global Health Action*, 23567 (2014).

Schama, Simon, *Landscape and Memory* (London, 1995).

Schlich, Thomas, 'Why Were Surgical Gloves Not Used Earlier? History of Medicine and Alternative Paths of Innovation', *The Lancet*, 386 (2015), 1234–5.

Schlich, Thomas (ed.), *The Palgrave Handbook of the History of Surgery* (Basingstoke, 2017).

Schoenberg, Bruce, 'A Program for the Conquest of Cancer: 1802', *Journal of the History of Medicine and Allied Sciences*, 30 (1975), 3–22.

Scholten, C. M., '"On the Importance of the Obstetrick Art": Changing Customs of Childbirth in America 1760–1825', *William and Mary Quarterly*, 3rd ser., 34 (1977), 426–45.

Shaw, Alexander, Moore, Charles H., De Morgan, Campbell, and Henry, Mitchell, *Report of the Surgical Staff of the Middlesex Hospital, to the Weekly Board and Governors, upon the Treatment of Cancerous Diseases in the Hospital, on the Plan Introduced by Dr. Fell* (London, 1857).

Sherwin, Susan, *The Politics of Women's Health: Exploring Agency and Autonomy* (Philadelphia, PA, 1998).

Shortt, S. E. D., 'Physicians, Science, and Status: Issues in the Professionalization of Anglo-American Medicine in the Nineteenth Century', *Medical History*, 27 (1983), 51–68.

Skuse, Alanna, 'Wombs, Worms and Wolves: Constructing Cancer in Early Modern England', *Social History of Medicine*, 27 (2014), 632–48.

Skuse, Alanna, *Constructions of Cancer in Early Modern England: Ravenous Natures* (Basingstoke, 2015).

Snow, Stephanie J., *Operations without Pain: The Practice and Science of Anaesthesia in Victorian Britain* (Basingstoke, 2006).

Sontag, Susan, *Illness as Metaphor and AIDs and Its Metaphors* (London, 2013).

Stanley, Peter, *For Fear of Pain: British Surgery, 1790–1850* (Amsterdam, 2003).

Stanley, Peter, 'How Did Civil War Surgeons Cope?', *Surgeon's Call*, 19 (2014), 3–5.

Starr, Paul, 'The Politics of Therapeutic Nihilism', *Hastings Center Report*, 6 (1976), 24–30.

Steere-Williams, Jacob, 'The Perfect Food and the Filth Disease: Milk-Borne Typhoid and Epidemiological Practice in late Victorian Britain', *Journal of the History of Medicine and Allied Sciences*, 65 (2010), 514–45.

Steere-Williams, Jacob, 'Performing State Medicine during Its "Frustrating" Years: Epidemiology and Bacteriology at the Local Government Board, 1870–1900', *Social History of Medicine*, 28 (2014), 82–107.

Steven, Connor, *The Book of Skin* (London, 2004).

Stocking, George W., *Race, Culture and Evolution: Essays in the History of Anthropology* (Chicago, 1982).

Stocking, George W., *Victorian Anthropology* (London, 1991).

Stolberg, Michael, 'Metaphors and Images of Cancer in Early Modern Europe', *Bulletin of the History of Medicine*, 88 (2014), 48–74.

Szabo, Jason, *Incurable and Intolerable: Chronic Disease and Slow Death in Nineteenth-Century France* (New Brunswick, NJ, 2009).

Szreter, Simon, 'The GRO and the Public Health Movement in Britain, 1837–1914', *Social History of Medicine*, 4 (1991), 435–63.

Szreter, Simon, 'Introduction: The GRO and the Historians', *Social History of Medicine*, 4 (1991), 404–14.

Szreter, Simon, *Fertility, Class and Gender in Britain, 1860–1940* (Cambridge, UK, 1996).

Szreter, Simon, 'The Importance of Social Intervention in Britain's Mortality Decline c. 1850–1914: A Re-Interpretation of the Role of Public Health', *Social History of Medicine*, 1 (2012), 1–38.

Szreter, Simon, and Mooney, Graham, 'Urbanization, Mortality and the Standard of Living Debate: New Estimates of the Expectation of Life at Birth in Nineteenth-Century British Cities', *Economic History Review*, 51 (1998), 84–112.

Terry, J., and Urla, J. (eds.), *Deviant Bodies* (Bloomington, IN, 1995).

Timmermann, Carsten, *A History of Lung Cancer* (Basingstoke, 2013).

Timmermann, Carsten, and Toon, Elizabeth (eds.), *Cancer Patients, Cancer Pathways: Historical and Sociological Perspectives* (Basingstoke, 2012).

Tomes, Nancy, *The Gospel of Germs: Men, Women, and the Microbe in American Life* (Cambridge, MA, 1999).

Toon, Elizabeth, '"Cancer as the General Population Knows it": Knowledge, Fear, and Lay Education in 1950s Britain', *Bulletin of the History of Medicine*, 81 (2007), 116–38.

Triolo, Victor A., 'The Institution for Investigating the Nature and Cure of Cancer: A Study of Four Excerpts', *Medical History*, 13 (1969), 11–28.

Vernon, James, 'Who's Afraid of the Linguistic Turn? The Politics of Social History and Its Discontents', *Social History*, 19 (1994), 81–97.

Waddington, Ivan, *The Medical Profession in the Industrial Revolution* (Dublin, 1984).

Waddington, Keir, 'Unsuitable Cases: The Debate over Outpatient Admission, the Medical Profession and Late-Victorian London Hospitals', *Medical History*, 42 (1998), 26–46.

Waddington, Keir, *Charity and the London Hospitals, 1850–1898* (Woodbridge, 2000).

Waddington, Keir, 'The Dangerous Sausage: Diet, Meat and Disease in Victorian and Edwardian Britain', *Cultural and Social History*, 8 (2011), 51–71.

Waddington, Keir, '"In a Country Every Way by Nature Favourable to Health": Landscape and Public Health in Victorian Rural Wales', *Canadian Bulletin of Medical History*, 32 (2014), 183–4.

Wall, Rosemary, 'Using Bacteriology in Elite Hospital Practice: London and Cambridge, 1880–1920', *Social History of Medicine*, 24 (2011), 776–95.

Warner, John Harley, 'Science in Medicine', *Osiris*, 1 (1985), 37–58.

Warner, John Harley, *The Therapeutic Perspective: Medical Practice, Knowledge, and Identity in America, 1820–1885* (Cambridge, MA, 1986).

Warner, John Harley, 'Ideals of Science and Discontents in Late Nineteenth-Century American Medicine', *Isis*, 82 (1991), 454–78.

Warner, John Harley, 'The Rise and Fall of Professional Mystery: Epistemology, Authority and the Emergence of Laboratory Medicine in Nineteenth-Century America', in A. R. Cunningham and J. P. Williams (eds.), *The Laboratory Revolution in Medicine* (Cambridge, UK, 1992).

Warren, Kenneth S., and Bowes, John Z. (eds.), *Parasitology: A Global Perspective* (New York, 1983).

Weatherall, Mark W., 'Making Medicine Scientific: Empiricism, Rationality, and Quackery in Mid-Victorian Britain', *Social History of Medicine*, 9 (1996), 175–94.

Webb, W. W., 'Warren, Pelham (1778–1835)', rev. Patrick Wallis, in *Oxford Dictionary of National Biography* (Oxford, 2004).

Weisser, Olivia, 'Boils, Pushes, and Wheals: Reading Bumps on the Body in Early Modern England', *Social History of Medicine*, 22 (2009), 321–39.

Weisz, George, 'The Emergence of Medical Specialization in the Nineteenth Century', *Bulletin for the History of Medicine*, 77 (2003), 536–75.

Weisz, George, *Divide and Conquer: A Comparative History of Medical Specialization* (Oxford, 2006).

Weisz, George, *Chronic Disease in the Twentieth Century: A History* (Baltimore, MD, 2014).

Weisz, George, and Olszynko-Gryn, Jesse, 'The Theory of Epidemiologic Transition: The Origins of a Citation Classic', *Journal of the History of Medicine and Allied Sciences*, 65 (2010), 287–326.

Welshman, John, 'The Medical Officer of Health in England and Wales, 1900–1974: Watchdog or Lapdog?' *Journal of Public Health*, 19 (1997), 443–50.

Wendell, Susan, 'Toward a Feminist Theory of Disability', *Hypatia*, 4 (1989), 104–24.

Wiltshaw, Eve, *A History of the Royal Marsden Hospital* (Edgware, 1998).

Winter, Alison, *Mesmerized: Powers of Mind in Victorian Britain* (Chicago, 1998).

Woods, R. I., 'The Effect of Population Redistribution on the Level of Mortality in Nineteenth-Century England and Wales', *Journal of Economic History*, 45 (1985), 645–51.

Woodward, John, *To Do the Sick No Harm: A Study of the British Voluntary Hospital System to 1875* (London, 1974).

Worboys, Michael, 'The Emergence and Early Development of Parasitology', in Kenneth S. Warren and John Z. Bowes (eds.), *Parasitology: A Global Perspective* (New York, 1983).

Worboys, Michael, *Spreading Germs: Disease Theories and Medical Practice in Britain, 1865–1900* (Cambridge, UK, 2000).

Online Resources

'Good Health and Well-Being', http://www.undp.org/content/undp/en/home/sustainable-development-goals/goal-3-good-health-and-well-being.html, accessed 22 May 2020.

'Is Cancer a Modern Disease?', https://scienceblog.cancerresearchuk.org/2010/10/14/claims-that-cancer-is-only-a-%E2%80%98modern-man-made-disease%E2%80%99-are-false-and-misleading/, accessed 22 May 2020.

London Lives 1690 to 1800, https://www.londonlives.org/static/Hospitals.jsp, accessed 22 May 2020.

'Malignant, adj. and n.', https://www.oed.com/view/Entry/112926?redirectedFrom=malignant, *OED Online* (Oxford, 2017), accessed 22 May 2020.

'Survival Statistics', http://www.cancerresearchuk.org/about-cancer/what-is-cancer/understanding-cancer-statistics-incidence-survival-mortality#survival, accessed 22 May 2020.

Wellcome Library, https://wellcomelibrary.org/moh/, accessed 22 May 2020.

'Why Some Cancers Come Back', http://www.cancerresearchuk.org/about-cancer/what-is-cancer/why-some-cancers-come-back, accessed 22 May 2020.

Index

Printed and bound by CPI Group (UK) Ltd, Croydon, CR0 4YY